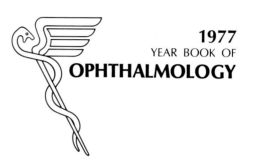

**1977**
YEAR BOOK OF
**OPHTHALMOLOGY**

# THE 1977 YEAR BOOKS

The YEAR BOOK series makes available in detailed abstract form the essence of the best of the recent international medical literature. The material is selected by distinguished editors who critically review more than 500,000 journal articles each year.

**Medicine**
Drs. Rogers, Des Prez, Cline, Braunwald, Greenberger, Bondy and Epstein.

**Surgery**
Drs. Schwartz, Najarian, Peacock, Shires, Silen and Spencer.

**Family Practice**
Dr. Rakel.

**Anesthesia**
Drs. Eckenhoff, Bruce, Brunner, Holley and Linde.

**Drug Therapy**
Dr. Azarnoff.

**Obstetrics & Gynecology**
Dr. Pitkin.

**Pediatrics**
Dr. Gellis.

**Diagnostic Radiology**
Drs. Whitehouse, Bookstein, Gabrielsen, Holt, Martel, Thornbury and Wolson.

**Ophthalmology**
Dr. Hughes.

**Otolaryngology**
Drs. Strong and Paparella.

**Neurology & Neurosurgery**
Drs. De Jong and Sugar.

**Psychiatry & Applied Mental Health**
Drs. Braceland, Freedman, Friedhoff, Kolb, Lourie and Romano.

**Dermatology**
Drs. Malkinson and Pearson.

**Urology**
Dr. Grayhack.

**Orthopedics & Traumatic Surgery**
Dr. Coventry.

**Plastic & Reconstructive Surgery**
Drs. McCoy, Dingman, Hanna, Haynes, Hoehn and Stephenson.

**Endocrinology**
Drs. Schwartz and Ryan.

**Pathology & Clinical Pathology**
Drs. Carone and Conn.

**Nuclear Medicine**
Dr. Quinn.

**Cancer**
Drs. Clark and Cumley.

**Cardiology**
Drs. Harvey, Kirkendall, Kirklin, Nadas, Paul and Sonnenblick.

**Dentistry**
Drs. Hale, Hazen, Moyers, Redig, Robinson and Silverman.

# The YEAR BOOK of
# Ophthalmology
# 1977

Edited by

## WILLIAM F. HUGHES, M.D.

*Chairman, Department of Ophthalmology,
Presbyterian-St. Luke's Hospital (Chicago);
Professor of Ophthalmology, Rush University,
and University of Illinois
Abraham Lincoln School of Medicine*

**YEAR BOOK MEDICAL PUBLISHERS, INC.**
CHICAGO • LONDON

Printed in U.S.A.

Library of Congress Catalog Card Number: 58-1522

International Standard Book Number: 0–8151–4775–9

# Table of Contents

The material covered in this volume represents literature reviewed up to January, 1977.

# Questions for Clinicians

1. What is one reason why epithelial outgrowths into the anterior chamber are not more frequent after intraocular surgery? (p. 75)
2. What are the ophthalmic findings in multiple endocrine neoplasia, type 2b? (p. 99)
3. What is the best method of removing deep rust rings in the cornea? (p. 103)
4. What is the "faden" operation? (p. 25)
5. What are the causes, methods for prevention and treatment of blinding trachoma? (p. 54)
6. Are local corticosteroids contraindicated in conjunctivitis? (p. 55)
7. What is the proper treatment of carcinoma of the conjunctiva? (pp. 59–65)
8. How would you manage a patient with ocular hypertension without visual field defects? (p. 115)
9. What method would you select for extraction of a cataract in your eye, and why? (pp. 167 and 173)
10. Of what value is infrared photography in the diagnosis of fundus tumors? (p. 192)
11. What is the proper management of small malignant melanomas of the choroid? (p. 197)
12. What are the indications for pars plana vitrectomy? (p. 199)
13. In what type of perforating injuries is pars plana vitrectomy of value? (pp. 214 and 215)
14. What are the ocular signs of thrombotic thrombocytopenic purpura and disseminated intravascular coagulopathy? (p. 237)
15. What prognostic signs for vision are revealed by fluorescein angiography after central retinal vein occlusion? (p. 242)
16. What are the earliest changes which can be demonstrated in the eyes of diabetics? (pp. 243 and 244)

7

17. What is the present status of photocoagulation of diabetic retinopathy? (pp. 246–249)
18. What are the many diverse noxious agents which can affect the pigment epithelium of the retina? (p. 254)
19. What are the differences between Stargardt's disease and fundus flavimaculatus? (p. 255)
20. What is a relatively safe dose of chloroquine, and what are the earliest signs of macular damage? (p. 259)
21. What is the probable sequence of pathologic changes leading to senile macular degeneration and disciform degeneration of the macula? (p. 260)
22. Do survivors of retinoblastoma have any tendency for development of other malignancies? (p. 265)
23. When should retinoschisis be treated? (p. 266)
24. Of what practical value is the diagnosis of opsoclonus in children? (p. 278)
25. What are the ocular signs of cytomegalovirus infection in the infant? (p. 288)
26. Of what value is the carotid compression tonography test? (p. 295)
27. What is the differential diagnosis of chalazion, and in what cases should histologic study be performed? (p. 14)
28. What diseases produce changes in the orbital bones? (p. 21)
29. What examination should be performed to determine the prognosis of occlusive therapy for amblyopia? (p. 29)
30. What is the proper management of infantile alternating esotropia? (p. 30)
31. How should a patient with thyroid ophthalmopathy be managed? (pp. 22 and 34)
32. What is the source of infection of inclusion conjunctivitis, and how can it be diagnosed and treated? (p. 45)
33. What is a new treatment of vernal conjunctivitis instead of local steroids? (pp. 56 and 58)
34. What is the etiology of recurrent erosions of the cornea and how are they treated? (p. 77)
35. What is the best method for demonstrating fungi in a corneal scraping? (p. 84)
36. What are the ocular signs of infection by amoeba? (p. 86)
37. How would you manage a Mooren's corneal ulcer? (pp. 90–92)

38. How can you differentiate epithelial disease caused by herpes simplex or herpes zoster virus? (p. 92)
39. Is thermokeratoplasty a safe procedure? (p. 103)
40. Of what value is clinical specular microscopy? (p. 105)
41. What is the basic cause of glaucomatous optic atrophy? (pp. 123–131)
42. Of what value is the water-drinking test in early detection of open-angle glaucoma? (p. 136)
43. What is the proper treatment for toxoplasmosis retinochoroiditis? (p. 177)
44. In which ocular diseases is immunosuppressive therapy effective? (p. 188)
45. What treatable lesion can be associated with opsoclonus in children? (p. 278)

# The Lids, Lacrimal Apparatus and Orbit

Introduction

In years past, the ophthalmologist was often presented with the dilemma of separating orbital mass lesions from unilateral thyroid eye disease. The thyroid suppression test was widely used as a means of making this distinction. Unfortunately, this test was not infallible and unnecessary orbital explorations were performed.

During the past 4 years, we have seen the introduction of orbital ultrasonography and computed tomography as a means of looking at the orbital structures involved. This has led to a high degree of accuracy in distinguishing between those lesions that are caused by a mass in the orbit and those abnormalities which are referred to as thyroid eye disease or inflammatory orbital disease. This heavy reliance on the newer diagnostic procedures has diverted our attention from the continuing efforts to understand the basic mechanisms of euthyroid Graves' disease.

Graves' disease is now recognized as a multisystem disease having one or more pathognomonic components: hyperthyroidism due to diffuse goiter; infiltrative dermopathy (pretibial myxedema); or infiltrative ophthalmopathy. It is widely felt that the pathogenesis of this disorder is an autoimmune disease in a genetically susceptible host. This is supported by the frequent findings of antibodies (IgG) directed against thyroid antigen. The most notable of these antibodies are long-acting thyroid stimulator (LATS) and long-acting thyroid stimulator-protector. The presence of one or both of these antibodies in the presence of nonsuppressibility of the thyroid gland is virtually diagnostic of Graves' disease. The common association of Hashimoto's thyroiditis coexisting with Graves' disease has been suggested as the reason for decreased output of thyroid hor-

mones in the face of continued stimulation by the immunoglobulins. Hence, we frequently see euthyroid Graves' disease.

When we study a group of patients with euthyroid Graves'
disease, it becomes apparent that a number have no evidence of thyroid-stimulating immunoglobulins and have
normal suppressibility of the thyroid gland. We therefore
have a subgroup of patients with clinical findings of Graves'
ophthalmopathy but absolutely no evidence of thyroid disease. It has been suggested that we are really looking at a
group of autoimmune diseases consisting of Graves' hyperthyroidism, Hashimoto's thyroiditis and Graves' ophthalmopathy. The coexistence of different autoimmune diseases
is well recognized. It seems likely then that "thyroid eye disease" has little to do with the thyroid but does share a common basis as an autoimmune disease. Further research into
this group of diseases will certainly lead to clinically available methods of distinguishing between them and hopefully
to a basic understanding of the mechanisms involved in
Graves' ophthalmopathy.

Charles F. Sydnor, M.D.
Duke University

**Lid Lesions of Childhood: Histopathologic Survey at
the Wilmer Institute (1923–74).** Marcos T. Doxanas, W.
Richard Green, Juan J. Arentsen and Frederick J. Elsas[1]
(Johns Hopkins Med. Inst.) analyzed data on 398 superficial eyelid lesions seen in a 51-year period in 385 children
seen at birth through age 15. This is the first comprehensive
clinicopathologic evaluation of eyelid lesions in children.
The findings are summarized in the table.

Chalazion was the most frequent lesion, accounting for
about 20% of the series. Dermoid cysts and papillomas followed closely, at 16.3 and 14.2%, respectively. About a quarter of the dermoid cysts were present at birth and another
10% appeared in the first 3 months of life. Papillomas occurred most frequently on the lid margins as raised cauli-
flower-like, occasionally pedunculated lesions with varying
degrees of pigmentation. Granuloma pyogenicum accounted

(1)   J. Pediatr. Ophthalmol. 13:7–39, January, 1976.

RELATIVE FREQUENCY OF LID LESIONS OF CHILDHOOD*

| | Totals | | Age: Years | | | |
|---|---|---|---|---|---|---|
| | Number | Percent | 0 | 1-5 | 6-10 | 11-15 |
| Chalazion | 82 | 20.05 | 0 | 21 | 29 | 32 |
| Dermoid cyst | 65 | 16.3 | 5 | 37 | 11 | 12 |
| Papilloma | 57 | 14.2 | 0 | 19 | 18 | 20 |
| Granuloma pyogenicum | 37 | 9.3 | 2 | 11 | 12 | 12 |
| Nevus | 36 | 9.1 | 0 | 4 | 17 | 15 |
| Hemangioma | 28 | 7.1 | 17 | 4 | 4 | 3 |
| Neurofibroma | 10 | 2.5 | 0 | 3 | 3 | 4 |
| Molluscum contagiosum | 10 | 2.5 | 0 | 4 | 3 | 3 |
| Chronic inflammation | 10 | 2.5 | 0 | 1 | 1 | 8 |
| Lymphangioma | 9 | 2.25 | 0 | 0 | 4 | 5 |
| Epithelial inclusion cyst | 7 | 1.75 | 0 | 2 | 4 | 1 |
| Foreign body | 6 | 1.5 | 0 | 2 | 3 | 1 |
| Pilomatrixoma | 5 | 1.25 | 0 | 1 | 4 | 0 |
| Pseudo-rheumatoid nodule | 4 | 1.0 | 0 | 4 | 0 | 0 |
| Apocrine hydrocystoma | 4 | 1.0 | 0 | 1 | 1 | 2 |
| Juvenile xanthogranuloma | 3 | 0.75 | 0 | 3 | 0 | 0 |
| Scar tissue | 3 | 0.75 | 0 | 0 | 2 | 1 |
| Pseudo-epitheliomatous hyperplasia | 3 | 0.75 | 0 | 2 | 0 | 1 |
| Embryonal rhabdomyosarcoma | 2 | 0.5 | 1 | 0 | 1 | 0 |
| Calcinosis cutis | 2 | 0.5 | 0 | 0 | 0 | 2 |
| Fibrous histiocytoma | 2 | 0.5 | 0 | 1 | 0 | 1 |
| Basal cell carcinoma with fibroepithelioma | 1 | 0.25 | 0 | 0 | 1 | 0 |
| Squamous cell carcinoma | 1 | 0.25 | 0 | 1 | 0 | 0 |
| Metastatic embryonal carcinoma | 1 | 0.25 | 0 | 1 | 0 | 0 |
| Fibroepithelioma | 1 | 0.25 | 0 | 0 | 1 | 0 |
| Chondroid syringoma | 1 | 0.25 | 0 | 0 | 0 | 1 |
| Syringocystadenoma papilliferum | 1 | 0.25 | 0 | 0 | 0 | 1 |
| Hair nevus | 1 | 0.25 | 0 | 1 | 0 | 0 |
| Dermatofibroma | 1 | 0.25 | 0 | 0 | 0 | 1 |
| Lipoid Proteinosis | 1 | 0.25 | 0 | 0 | 1 | 0 |
| Lid-orbital varix | 1 | 0.25 | 0 | 0 | 1 | 0 |
| Palpebral lobe of lacrimal gland | 1 | 0.25 | 1 | 0 | 0 | 0 |
| Complex choristoma | 1 | 0.25 | 0 | 1 | 0 | 0 |
| Hamartoma | 1 | 0.25 | 0 | 0 | 0 | 1 |

*From Wilmer Institute records of excised lesions during a 51-year period.

for 9.3% of these lesions, which often result from trauma with secondary bacterial invasion but were most often seen in association with chalazion. The characteristic soft, dull red appearance of the pedunculated nodule is due to its vascular framework. Nevi accounted for about 9% of the lesions in this series. There were 23 compound nevi and 10 dermal nevi, 4 and 1, respectively, having a papillary configuration. One patient each had a blue nevus, a cellular blue nevus and a spindle and epithelioid cell nevus. Hemangiomas, seen in 7.1% of patients, frequently were diffuse with involvement of deep lid structures, conjunctiva and orbit. Almost half of the lesions were of the hypercellular capillary type, all of which occurred before age 5 in a striking correlation of cell type with age.

Neurofibromas, tumors of Schwann cell origin, were found in 10 patients in this series. Of these, 5 tumors were plexiform, in which cell proliferation was confined by the nerve sheath. The other patients had tumors of a diffuse pattern or a combination of both. There were 10 patients with molluscum contagiosum, a mildly contagious disease of viral etiology. Chronic inflammation of the lid was found in 10 patients, 5 of whom had a history of surgery or trauma. Lymphangioma accounted for 9 lesions; they presented as lid swellings, but often extended deeper into the orbit and because of diffuseness were generally not accessible to excision. There were 7 epithelial inclusion cysts and 6 foreign-body granulomas in the series. Five lesions were classified as pilomatrixoma or benign calcifying epithelioma of Malherbe. There were 4 pseudorheumatoid nodules and 4 apocrine hydrocystomas. In 3 patients, scar tissue was the only pathologic diagnosis. Two patients had embryonal rhabdomyosarcoma, the most common primary orbital malignancy in children, 2 had fibrous histiocytoma and 2 had malignant epithelial tumors: a basal cell carcinoma with fibroepithelioma and squamous cell carcinoma, both of which were excised with no recurrence in a 12 and 7 year follow-up, respectively.

► [This article contains many clinical histologic illustrations. — Ed.] ◄

**Erroneous Clinical Diagnosis of Chalazion.** D. v. Domarus, E. N. Hinzpeter and G. O. H. Naumann[2] (Univ. of Hamburg). This frequently occurring ocular lesion is generally regarded as one easily diagnosed and managed. It presents as a slowly developing, roundish, firm tumor without acute inflammatory symptoms, mostly seen on the upper lid. Histologic examination reveals a zonal granulomatous inflammation, giant cells and fatty macrophages surrounding fatty vacuoles. However, other benign and even malignant tumors may well present a similar clinical picture and are erroneously diagnosed.

During 1966 – 74, 1,260 lid tumors were examined, including 138 with a clinical diagnosis of chalazion. This diagnosis

(2)  Klin. Monatsbl. Augenheilkd. 163:175 – 181, February, 1976.

was erroneous in 33 cases (25%), revealing instead another benign lesion in 23 patients and a malignant process in 10. Differential diagnosis must include systemic granulomatous inflammations such as tuberculosis, lues and various mycotic infections, and even sarcoidosis as well as foreign body and pyogenic granuloma. Most benign lesions masquerading as chalazion proved to be epithelial processes. Sebaceous gland carcinoma (4 cases) is considered the most important differential diagnosis, however, particularly because the origin of both processes is identical. In fact, the reported high mortality rate of carcinoma of the Meibomian gland (6–12%) may be based on the fact that it was likely mistaken for a chalazion until several recurrences occasioned histologic investigation.

The excised chalazion should be subjected to histologic examination in case of the presence of atypical preoperative or operative findings, recurrence on the same site, palpable regional lymph nodes, advanced age of patient or unilateral seemingly intractable "conjunctivitis."

**"Lazy-T" Correction of Ectropion of Lower Punctum** is described by Byron Smith[3] (New York Med. College). Minimal ectropion of the lower lid punctum may be tolerated in the absence of symptoms that would justify surgery. Cauterization is an uncontrolled procedure and horizontal resection of tissues inferior to the lower canaliculus has limited indications. In more severe deformities, a "lazy-T" method has been successfully used for some years. The procedure uses a vertical excision of a full-thickness "V" of the lid to remedy the horizontal relaxation and an excision of the horizontal segment of conjunctiva and tarsus to invert the lid to the proper position. Either local or general anesthesia may be used; if local anesthesia is used, a 15- or 20-minute interval should be allowed before starting surgery.

TECHNIQUE. — A lacrimal probe is placed in the lower canaliculus and a horizontal incision made 7 mm below the level of the canaliculus for about 1-1.5 cm, to section conjunctiva and tarsus. The inferior margin of the incision is undermined and 3-5 mm of tarsus and conjunctiva is excised. A vertical incision is made through all layers of the lower lid from the lid margin 3 mm lateral to the puncta down into the depth of the lower fornix. Sufficient full-thickness tissue is excised to correct horizontal laxity of the lid and bring the punctum into apposition with the globe. The horizontal wound margins are apposed and closure is carried out with interrupted 7-0 gut sutures. The vertical transmarginal incision is closed as a simple lid laceration. Two buried muscle sutures of 7-0 chromic gut are placed and tied. The rest of the skin incision is closed with 8-0 silk and a moderate nonadherent absorbent dressing is applied.

This procedure restores the lid margin to its normal relationship with the globe and the punctum is reestablished in its normal anatomic position in the proximity of the lacrimal lake. The cosmetic blemish resulting from the surgical scar is insignificant. The "lazy-T" operation is the method of choice for the correction of ectropion of the nasal third of the lower lid. Experience with the results of the operation has been gratifying.

► [This article, illustrated with line drawings, combines horizontal excision of tarsus below the punctum to invert the punctum with vertical excision of skin, orbicularis, and tarsus to correct horizontal laxity leading to ectropion. – Ed.] ◄

**Experiences with Magnet Implantation in Lagophthalmos** are reported by E. Riehm and E. N. Hinzpeter[4] (Hamburg), based on treatment of 29 patients with keratopathy due to lagophthalmos associated with facial palsy. In contrast to the frequently practiced lateral tarsorrhaphy, the present method does not alter the form or size of the palpebral fissure nor does it impede the visual field. The technique described by Mühlbauer et al. has been practiced since 1974.

The magnets are made of an alloy of platinum (77 – 78%) and cobalt to follow the bend of the eyelid, 16 – 16.5 mm in length, with a diameter of 1.0, 1.2 or 1.5 mm (Fig 1). The surgery is performed under local anesthesia on an outpatient basis. Skin incisions are carried out 6 – 8 mm parallel to the lid edge, corresponding to the length of the magnet, and the skin is dissected off of the orbicularis muscle to the lid margin. The magnet is then affixed with four 6 – 0 nylon sutures on the tarsus beneath the orbicularis (Fig 2), close to the lid edge. The polarity of the magnets must be considered. The skin is then closed with continuous silk sutures.

(4)  Klin. Monatsbl. Augenheilkd. 169:524 – 528, October, 1976.

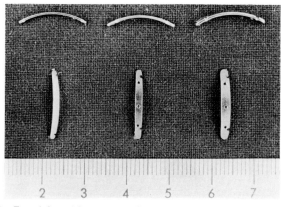

**Fig 1.** – From left to right, magnets of 1.0, 1.2 and 1.5 mm in diameter. (Courtesy of Riehm, E., and Hinzpeter, E. N.: Klin. Monatsbl. Augenheilkd. 169:524 – 528, October, 1976.)

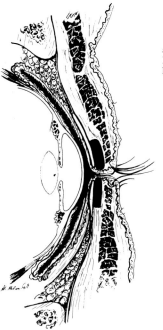

**Fig 2.** – Position of magnets in upper and lower lids. (Courtesy of Riehm, E., and Hinzpeter, E. N.: Klin. Monatsbl. Augenheilkd. 169:524 – 528, October, 1976.)

Correction of the lower lid ectropion and upper lid blepharo-
chalasia is usually carried out at the same time.

Twenty-four of the 29 patients were available for follow-
up at a postoperative interval of 1 – 11 months (average, 5.3).
In 2 patients the lower lid magnets had to be removed due
to perforation of the skin. In another patient, 5 months after
trouble-free implantation, further surgery caused considerable collateral lid swelling and subsequent perforation of
the skin by the magnets. In 23 patients a lid-closing defect of
0 – 3 mm persisted after implantation of the magnets.

The procedure should be carried out as soon as possible
after onset of palsy to prevent contracture of the palpebral
levator muscle. Although originally intended as a temporary measure, the favorable experiences to date allow consideration of this technique in patients with irreversible
nerve damage. None of the patients had subjective complaints.

► [The results in this study of implanting magnets over the tarsus near
the lid margins to aid in closing the lids appear to be satisfactory. The idea
is similar to that described for correction of ptosis (see the 1974 YEAR
BOOK, p. 7) in which extrusion occurred in 2 of the 3 cases. – Ed.] ◄

**Surgical Treatment of Lagophthalmos in Lepers.**
Lagophthalmos threatens the leper's eye with keratitis and
subsequent blindness. G. F. Maillard and A. Chamay[5]
(Univ. of Lausanne, Switzerland) report experience in treating this condition at a leper station in Iran.

Facial palsy is particularly frequent in the tuberculoid
and dimorphic forms of the disease, generally involving the
superior branch of the facial nerve; the resulting lagophthalmos leaves the cornea exposed. The cornea often
is anesthetized from concomitant involvement of the
ophthalmic division of the trigeminal nerve. Among 300
plastic procedures on the face and limbs, 61 eyelids were
operated on. Lagophthalmos may be corrected either by a
static operation to narrow the palpebral fissure and counteract the paralytic ectropion or by a dynamic procedure to
reanimate both eyelids actively. Among static procedures,
lateral tarsorrhaphy may result in a "sad" eye and medial
tarsorrhaphy may result in telecanthus.

Among dynamic operations is the temporalis transplant

(5)   Chir. Plast. 3:113 – 123, 1975.

of Gillies and Andersen (Fig 3) involving an arciform incision along the scalp, preparation of 2 aponeurotic tongues 4 mm wide extending to 5 mm above the temporal crest and isolation of a segment of periosteum above the crest. A muscular slip, at least 3 cm wide at its base, is used to ensure vascularization and innervation. An anterior triangle of temporal aponeurosis is resected for better rotation of the musculoaponeurotic strip which, after passing through a temporal subcutaneous tunnel, is exteriorized through an incision 1 cm from the external angle of the eye. Arion's needle was used in 29 temporalis transfers. The 2 tongues are passed beneath the medial canthal ligament and fixed with strong tension, making the upper lid overlap the lower by at least 3 mm.

A modification giving a direct line of action has been described to avoid distortion of the external canthus. Clodius hollows a gutter in the external orbital rim in which the strips can glide, to prevent drawing forward or "uplift" of the outer third of the lids and loss of contact with the globe. Re-education is not difficult postoperatively.

The temporalis transplant of Gillies and its recent modifications are preferred for correcting lagophthalmos in lepers.

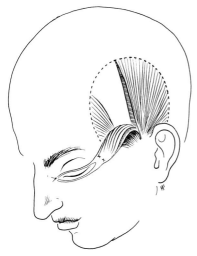

**Fig 3.** — Technique of Gillies' temporalis transfer in severe bilateral lagophthalmos. (Courtesy of Maillard, G. F., and Chamay, A.: Chir. Plast. 3:113–123, 1975.)

This procedure reanimates the eyelids and protects the eye from the risks of corneal involvement and blindness.

**Lower Eyelid Reconstruction by Tarsal Transposition.** Reconstruction of the lower eyelid can be difficult; satisfactory functional and cosmetic results often require complicated, multistage operations. Eva H. Hewes, John H. Sullivan and Crowell Beard[6] (Univ. of California, San Francisco) describe a one-stage technique in which the lower lid is reconstructed with a tarsoconjunctival flap transposed from the upper eyelid and hinged at the lateral canthal tendon. This flap makes occlusion of the eye unnecessary. The operation was performed on 13 patients with an average age of 60 years who had malignant tumors. They were observed for 10–70 months. After tumor excision with frozen-section control, the flap operation (Fig 4) was carried out. The medial extent of the tarsoconjunctival strip should be 2 or 3 mm temporal to that of the surgical defect in the lower lid. The anterior lamella of the lower lid was most often reconstructed by use of an advancement skin flap. When the lower lid lesion involved the lateral commissure, the flap was based higher in the preseptal orbicularis oculi muscle, without inclusion of the lateral canthal tendon.

Cosmetic results were excellent; no upper lid deformity was observed. In 3 eyes, rounding of the lateral canthal angle was repaired by lateral canthoplasty, with cosmetically acceptable results. The tarsoconjunctival flap was too long in 3 eyes, resulting in ectropion of the lower lid, but this was not symptomatic. Keratitis was not observed. Ectropion repair gave satisfactory results in all instances. Two patients had trichiasis from dermal hairs but required no further correction. No tumor recurrence was observed.

This technique provides the lower eyelid with a skeletal structure and a lining and permits a one-stage repair without prolonged occlusion of the eye. The lateral canthal angle is preserved. The viability of this narrow-based flap is believed to result from the abundant vascular supply to the eyelid. The functional and cosmetic results have been equal or superior to those of tarsoconjunctival advancement flaps. The technique is best suited to lesions involving the lateral

(6)   Am. J. Ophthalmol. 81:512–514, April, 1976.

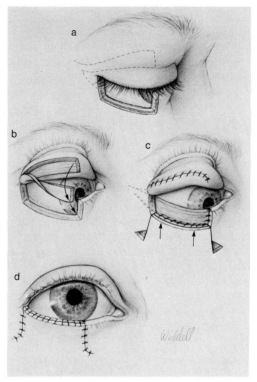

**Fig 4.** – Tarsal transposition technique. (Courtesy of Hewes, E. H., et al.: Am. J. Ophthalmol. 81:512 – 514, April, 1976.)

aspect of the lower lid, but it can be applied to lesions of the central and medial parts of the lid.

**Pathologic Changes of the Orbital Bones** are reviewed by Frederick C. Blodi[7] (Univ. of Iowa). The orbital bones may exhibit nearly all the pathologic changes seen in the skull and face. Computerized axial tomography has become valuable in diagnosing orbital lesions. The orbit may be involved in many anomalies of the cranial and facial bones, including simple carniosynostoses, Crouzon's disease, Apert's syndrome, hypertelorism, Engelmann's disease and

(7)   Trans. Am. Acad. Ophthalmol. Otolaryngol. 81:26 – 57, Jan. – Feb., 1976.

osteopetrosis. Any congenital or early acquired space-occupying lesions, such as orbital dermoids and hemangiomas, that grow slowly but steadily may enlarge the bony orbit. Large orbital defects may occur in neurofibromatosis. Orbital shrinkage may also occur if an enucleation or exenteration is performed at an early age.

Benign bone tumors that may involve the orbit include osteoma, osteoblastoma and chondroma. Tumors of indeterminate behavior, such as giant cell tumor and fibrous dysplasia, may affect the orbit. One case of orbital involvement by hemangioendothelioma of bone has been reported. Osteosarcoma may involve the orbit and may follow radiation damage. Other malignant lesions that may involve the orbit include chondrosarcoma, mesenchymal chondrosarcoma, chordoma, myeloma and Ewing's sarcoma, which carries the gravest prognosis of all primary bone tumors.

Several tumor-like lesions may involve the orbit. They include aneurysmal bone cyst, a benign, expansile lesion, and eosinophilic granuloma. In Hand-Schüller-Christian disease, an orbital infiltrate may produce exophthalmos. The bony orbit may be invaded by adjacent tumors such as meningiomas and systemic neurofibromas. Rhabdomyosarcomas have also been found to invade the orbital bones.

► [This 32d Edward Jackson Memorial Lecture was presented at the 1975 meeting of the American Academy of Ophthalmology. The article is profusely illustrated with clinical appearances, roentgenographic changes, some ultrasonic alterations and histology. — Ed.] ◄

**Indications and Results of Prednisone Treatment in Thyroid Ophthalmopathy.** Objective ocular symptoms occur in 50 – 80% of the patients with hyperthyroidism and include eyelid disturbances, edema of the intraorbital and preorbital tissues and limitation of ocular movements from eye muscle fibrosis. R. C. Apers, J. A. Oosterhuis and J. J. M. Bierlaagh[8] (Univ. of Leiden) evaluated prednisone therapy in 10 women and 3 men with thyroid ophthalmopathy. The indications for steroid therapy included cosmetic changes, bilateral asymmetrical limitation of elevation causing annoying diplopia and multiple limitations of eye movements without deviation in the primary position. The patients were fully controlled endocrinologically before

(8)   Ophthalmologica 173:163 – 167, 1976.

prednisone therapy. All had diplopia and 7 women were also treated for cosmetic reasons.

Treatment began with 60 mg prednisone daily for about 3 – 4 weeks, followed by weekly dose reductions by an average of 5 mg to a daily dose of 20 mg, and then slower reductions, usually by 2.5 mg every 2 or 4 weeks. Patients were hospitalized for the first 3 – 4 weeks of treatment.

Prednisone had to be stopped because of gastric hemorrhage in 1 patient. All patients obtained distinct cosmetic improvement due to a reduction in upper lid retraction and lid edema and regression of the exophthalmos. Exophthalmos was reduced by 2 mm or more in 6 of 12 patients. The fellow eye showed identical regression of the exophthalmos. Eye movements improved considerably in 5 patients and moderately in 2 others. In 5 patients the field of binocular single vision increased by 10 degrees or more and in 2 it increased by less than 10 degrees. Improvement in ocular motility was not more obvious in patients who had had double vision for several months than in those affected for a year or longer.

A daily dose of 60 mg prednisone appears adequate for treating nonmalignant exophthalmos in hyperthyroid patients. If no response is obtained after a month of prednisone therapy, further improvement should not be expected. The results have remained the same during follow-up for 1 – 3 years after the cessation of prednisone therapy.

# Motility

The most interesting topic at motility meetings during the past year has been Cüppers' faden operation or posterior fixation suture. This was presented at the 2d Congress of the International Strabismological Association by C. Cüppers. The procedure consists of placing a suture in a rectus muscle, 12–14 mm behind the insertion, and attaching the muscle to the sclera at that point. This limits the function of that muscle only in its field of action but has no effect on the primary position.

For the most part, muscles cause the eye to rotate in much the same way that a string (faden) attached to a pulley causes the pulley to rotate. Rotation is possible only until the string can unwind from the pulley. When the fixed portion of the string (the insertion) has reached a point where the preceding portion no longer has any arc of contact with the pulley, no further rotary action is possible. Pulling on the string will only cause the entire system to be drawn toward the direction of pull. Anchoring part of the string to the pulley posterior to the primary point of attachment reduces the length of string that can unwind, thus limiting the degrees of angular rotation possible. This is the principle of Cüppers' faden operation.

Cüppers advocated this procedure to produce what he calls artificial palsies. This will balance real palsies and will result in less deviation and better coordinated eye movements in the field of action of the palsied muscle. Consider a patient who has a congenital right lateral rectus palsy and is orthophoric in the primary position (a frequent occurrence in congenital paretic deviations). Recessing the right medial rectus and resecting the right lateral rectus might help the action of the paretic right lateral rectus but might produce an exotropia in the primary position and certainly will produce an exotropia in the left field of gaze. A faden operation on the left medial rectus would have no effect on the primary position but would minimize the deviation and uncoordination in the right field of gaze.

The faden operation can also be used in conjunction with or following conventional surgery for paretic deviations, when the purpose of the conventional surgery is to correct the deviation in the primary position. The faden operation is then used to produce coordinated movements in the field of action of the paretic muscle. This can be particularly helpful when the patient has residual diplopia in that field.

Consider a patient with a left superior oblique palsy who has had his hyperdeviation in the primary position corrected by surgery on the obliques but still demonstrates a left hyperdeviation with diplopia in the down and right field of gaze. Recessing the right inferior rectus might produce a right hyperdeviation in the primary position, while the faden operation on the right inferior rectus could limit the action of the right inferior rectus, coordinate binocular movements in the down and right field and have no effect on the primary position.

The faden operation has also been advocated for the nystagmus blockage syndrome. Patients with this syndrome demonstrate an esotropia and nystagmus. The deviation is usually present from birth. The nystagmus is eliminated in the adducted position but is present and increases with abduction. In other words, convergence of the deviating eye blocks the nystagmus of the fixing eye. In its classic form, when either eye is covered, the youngster will turn his head away from the covered eye in order to bring the uncovered eye into the adducted position where his nystagmus is eliminated and his vision improves. Some children are believed to overconverge, increasing the esotropia, and by so doing permit the fixing eye to abduct to the straight ahead position without nystagmus. This would suggest that it is convergence rather than adduction that is responsible for blocking the nystagmus. At any rate, many European ophthalmologists advocate the faden operation as well as recession of the medial rectus for this condition. That is, recess the medial and place a posterior fixation suture behind the recession. Muhlendyck believes the nystagmus blockage syndrome to be a common condition and performed the faden operation in 200 of 278 patients on whom he performed surgery for a convergent deviation. Most ophthalmologists in the United States find the syndrome much less common and suspect that many cross-fixers with functional limitation of abduction were included in this series reported by Muhlendyck at the 3d International Orthoptic Congress.

Von Noorden suggested that the faden operation might be helpful for patients with alternating hyperdeviations or dissociated vertical divergence (Orthoptic Symposium of the 1976 meeting of the American Academy of Ophthalmology and Otolaryngology). Scott and Jampolsky reported using a modification of the faden operation (Orthoptic Symposium of the 1976 meeting of the American Academy of Ophthalmology and Otolaryngology) for patients with Duane's syndrome. They believe the upshoot and downshoot of the affected eye in adduction can be eliminated by a posterior fixation suture of the lateral rectus in that eye.

Thus you can see why Cüppers' faden operation has stimulated so much interest.

Eugene R. Folk, M.D.
University of Illinois

**Use of Random-Dot Stereograms in the Clinical Assessment of Strabismic Patients** is described by J. P. Frisby, J. Mein, A. Saye and A. Stanworth[9] (Sheffield, England). Random-dot stereograms have been used recently to study anomalies in stereopsis. They provide a very pure test of stereopsis because they present disparity information in the absence of all other clues to depth and are subject to unfakeable test procedures. Patient responses to the usual type of random-dot stereogram and to a novel type containing prominent uniocularly identifiable features (Fig 5) were evaluated.

Random-dot stereograms are complex stimuli with many ambiguities concerning which element in the left field is to be fused with the element in the right. In practice, the binocular combination process produces a fusion of the fields in which relatively dense surfaces are preferred to "lace-like" patterns which have individual elements scattered in many

_____

(9)   Br. J. Ophthalmol. 59:545–552, October, 1975.

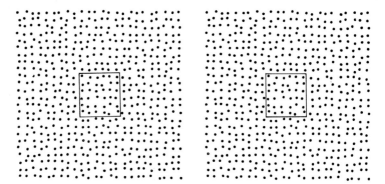

**Fig 5.** — Contoured stereogram used in the experiment. (Courtesy of Frisby, J. P., et al.: Br. J. Ophthalmol. 59:545–552, October, 1975.)

different depth planes. The Wirt test figures are relatively simple stereograms with little ambiguity; this difference may explain the asymmetry in stereoability noted between both procedures in pilot studies.

Twenty-seven strabismic patients, aged 8–18 years, were shown contoured and noncontoured stereograms, all containing a disparity of 12′. Eleven subjects obtained normal stereopsis with both types of stereogram; 10 obtained normal stereopsis with the contoured stereogram only and 6 did not obtain normal stereopsis with either type of stereogram. Subjects in the 1st group had, in general, never completely lost normal bifoveal binocular single vision, while this was true of only 1 subject in the 2d group. In the latter subjects, the prolonged presence of a constant deviation probably leads to an impairment in stereopsis or to a failure to develop it normally. In the 3d group, the diagnoses generally were more severe; 4 of the 6 subjects could obtain only gross stereopsis with the Wirt test.

The property of uniocular identifiability could make the execution of appropriate vergence movements much easier in the contoured stereogram task. Random-dot stereograms can discriminate between patient categories. The simple uncontoured stereogram is unlikely to be fused successfully by any patient who has lost bifoveal binocular single vision for any length of time but many such patients can fuse stereograms if helped by the inclusion of a contour. This fact may be very revealing in assessing the consequences for stereopsis in a patient with a history of disturbed binocular single vision.

▶ [Relatively gross stereopsis can be determined by the Wirt (or Titmus) housefly test object, a picture of two superimposed stereoscopic images polarized at right angles to each other, and giving a three-dimensional effect (the wings appearing closer than the body) when viewed through polarizing spectacles (vectograph). The commonly used Wirt stereotest consists of vectograph cards showing circles within which are four dots, one pair of which are relatively closer together and appear closer when viewed through polaroid glasses. Twelve graded steps of decreasing disparity (or increasing stereoscopic difficulty) from 0.028 to 1.939 mm (14 seconds of arc to 17 minutes of arc) test the degree of stereopsis. Reinecke and Simons (see the 1975 YEAR BOOK, p. 40) used random-dot stereograms similar to the one shown here, in one of which the letter "E" is shown in varying degrees of disparity related visual acuity (detection of the "E" at 4 minutes of disparity being normal). In the present study, a central, nonstereoscopic contour square, containing the disparate dots, helped detection of fusion in many patients who otherwise failed the noncontour stereogram. – Ed.] ◀

**Importance of Functional and Electrophysiologic Examinations in Amblyopia.** According to S. Korol and C. Fiore[1] (Geneva, Switzerland), these tests provide indispensible complementary information and permit, in most cases, detection of organic forms not apparent on clinical examination. They analyzed the results of orthoptic treatment with regard to the values obtained by functional and electrophysiologic examination in two groups of patients with a clinical diagnosis of amblyopia.

The first group consisted of 8 patients who had undergone treatment for functional amblyopia, but who actually presented changes in the retina or in the optic nerve.

Girl, 9, had had divergent strabismus of the right eye since the first months of life. At age 4 years, anisometropia with amblyopia of the right eye was diagnosed. Eyeglasses were prescribed, and the left eye was totally occluded for nearly 12 months. At age 9 years, operation was followed by esotropia, for which she was examined by the authors.

The orthoptic examination showed slight esotropia without fixation in the right eye. Contact lenses did not improve visual acuity. The electrophysiologic responses – electroretinogram (ERG) and visual evoked response (VER) – were pathologic on the right. Diagnosis was dysfunction of the photopic system, more marked on the right side.

(1)  Arch. Ophtalmol. (Paris) 36:297–312, April, 1976.

In all 8 cases, manifestations of a disease of the retina or of the optic nerve were evident. In 3 cases, there were familial patterns of tapetoretinal degeneration or malformations. The electrophysiologic examinations always showed significant changes.

The second group consisted of 29 patients with functional amblyopia. In all patients, electrophysiologic examinations revealing the abnormalities in the amblyopic eyes gave normal results in the corresponding eyes. These patients were classified into two groups according to failure or improvement by orthoptic treatment. Also, they were separated according to type of amblyopia in each group. The VER was pathologic in 15 of the 20 patients in whom the condition had not improved; the ERG was pathologic in 2 of the 5 patients examined. The ERG was pathologic and the VER normal in 1 patient (retinal dysfunction). The patients with a normal VER included an untreated man aged 40 years. In the 9 patients whose condition had improved after treatment, the VER was normal in 8 and subnormal in 1. The ERG was normal in the 5 patients examined. The ages of the amblyopic patients in the two groups ranged between 3 and 12 years, except for the man aged 40.

Once the clinical forms of amblyopia have been determined, the VER study in functional amblyopics permits a prognosis regarding the result of orthoptic treatment. Those patients in whom the VER is pathologic are not treated as there is no possibility of benefit.

▶ [This study indicates the need of ophthalmoscopy, ERG to rule out retinal pathology, and VER to avoid hopeless attempts at treatment of amblyopia. — Ed.] ◀

**Management of Infantile Esotropia.** The management of congenital esotropia is controversial, partly because of problems in definition of the entity. The usual definition as constant esotropia starting in the first 6 months of life is too broad, as it includes a heterogeneous group with different causes and prognoses. R. Scott Foster, T. Otis Paul and Arthur Jampolsky[2] (Smith-Kettlewell Inst. of Visual Sciences, San Francisco) attempted to clarify these issues by critically examining a selected group of cases of infantile esotropia,

(2)   Am. J. Ophthalmol. 82:291–299, August, 1976.

with onset of constant esotropia before age 6 months, no evidence of fusion in any gaze position and habitually equal vision, alternating esotropia. No patient had been operated on and none had received orthoptic treatment other than patching. None had neurologic dysfunction or evidence of ocular disease other than strabismus. All patients were followed for at least 1 year after the last surgery. Thirty-four patients were studied. The goal of initial surgery was full mechanical alignment in the primary position and restoration of comitancy in all gaze positions. Spectacle orthoptics were used postoperatively in many patients, and withdrawal from this treatment was gradual.

Patients were followed for an average of about 5 years after final surgery. Refractive errors at first surgery averaged +0.92 D. There was no anisometropia greater than 0.75 D, and no patient had amblyopia. Three to six muscles were operated on in each patient, and satisfactory alignment, to within several prism diopters of orthotropia, was obtained in 79.4% of patients with one operation. Seven patients required secondary procedures, 2 because of technical difficulties at surgery. Satisfactory alignment was independent of age at final surgery, although bifoveal fusion was more frequent in patients operated on before age 2 years. Preoperative A patterns greater than 10 prism D were reduced below 10 prism D in 3 of 5 patients. In 25 patients with significant V patterns, there were no residual V patterns greater than 15 prism D. Eight of 15 patients who underwent postoperative spectacle orthoptic therapy obtained bifoveal fusion. Five of 7 undercorrected patients who received spectacle prism orthoptic treatment achieved bifoveal fusion. Four of 8 overcorrected patients who were treated with minus lenses, with or without prisms, obtained conversion to bifoveal fusion.

Infantile esotropia can be cured after realignment. Surgery should be planned, with the least number of surgical sessions, between ages 12 and 18 months. Postoperative management is directed toward equal vision and motor bifoveal fusion.

► [These authors find no evidence in the literature or in their own experience that operation on alternating esotropes before the age of 1 year improves the prognosis for bifoveal fusion, although operation after 2 years does diminish the prognosis for bifoveal fusion. The authors try to straighten the eyes with one operation, usually doing three to five muscles including the obliques; the number of muscles determined by preoperative basic measurements, voluntary and forced ductions. This approach yielded 79% satisfactory realignment as compared with 42–54% good results reported in the literature after operation on fewer muscles in the first procedure. Undercorrections of less than 10 prism diopters received ''spectacle orthoptics'' consisting of full prismatic correction of either horizontal or vertical deviations, and minus lenses (or reduction in plus refractive error correction) with or without prisms for overcorrections less than 10 prism diopters. This increased the incidence of bifoveal fusion (determined by cover-uncover test rather than stereoscopic tests) from 6% after surgery alone to 53% with surgery and postoperative spectacle orthoptics. – Ed.] ◄

**Evaluation and Treatment of Superior Oblique Muscle Palsy.** David Mittleman and Eugene R. Folk[3] (Univ. of Illinois Eye and Ear Infirmary, Chicago) reviewed the records of 100 consecutive patients in whom a diagnosis was of pure superior oblique muscle palsies. All patients were referred to the University of Illinois Eye and Ear Infirmary during 1966–73. Symptoms began in the 1st year of life in 36 patients. Twenty-two cases followed severe closed-head trauma associated with loss of consciousness. No definite cause of paresis was identified in 42 cases, although many of these probably represented decompensated congenital palsies. Diabetes or vascular disease was not implicated in any case. Seven of the traumatic patients had bilateral involvement. The amount of vertical deviation varied inversely with the patient's age, being greatest in the congenital-onset group. Vertical deviation was generally greatest in upward gaze in this group, and in downward gaze in the posttraumatic cases.

Eighty-five patients underwent a 10–12 mm recession of the homolateral inferior oblique muscle or a 4–5 mm recession of the contralateral inferior rectus, or both. Complete relief of symptoms was obtained in all patients with this surgical combination. One patient underwent resection of the homolateral inferior rectus to correct a large deviation in downward gaze apparently caused by underaction of that synergistic muscle. The average reduction in deviation in the primary position after inferior oblique recession was 9Δ, and the average reduction in deviation after recession of the contralateral inferior rectus was 14Δ. In patients

(3) Trans. Am. Acad. Ophthalmol. Otolaryngol. 81:893–898, Sept.–Oct., 1976.

having both procedures, the average reduction in deviation was 31Δ.

If deviation in the primary position is 25Δ or less in unilateral superior oblique muscle palsy, recession of only the homolateral inferior oblique muscle is recommended, or contralateral inferior rectus muscle recession if the greatest vertical deviation is in downward gaze. Some of these patients may be undercorrected and may require weakening of the other muscle. Where the deviation is greater than 25Δ, simultaneous recession of both the homolateral inferior oblique and contralateral inferior rectus muscles appears to be indicated.

▶ [In this series of palsies of the superior oblique results were quite satisfactory after recession of the homolateral inferior oblique, contralateral inferior rectus, or both. This avoids a possible Brown's syndrome which can follow a tuck of the superior oblique. To avoid drooping of the lower eyelid following recession of the inferior rectus, the authors insist on careful, complete dissection of the muscle for at least a distance of 15 mm posterior to its insertion, thus severing all the muscle's connections with the lower eyelid. — Ed.] ◀

**Surgical Treatment of True Brown's Syndrome** was investigated by J. S. Crawford[4] (Toronto, Ont.). Brown described a group of patients who could not actively elevate the eye above the horizontal plane when it was rotated medially and ascribed it to shortening of the anterior part of the superior oblique tendon sheath, presumably due to a developmental anomaly after congenital complete paralysis of the inferior oblique muscle. "True" Brown's syndrome is characterized by limitation of elevation in adduction, so severe that the eye cannot be raised voluntarily above the midhorizontal plane; little or no overaction of the homolateral superior oblique muscle; widening of the palpebral fissure on adduction; and an unequivocally positive traction test on attempted elevation in adduction. Many surgeons question whether true Brown's syndrome is due to a tight sheath on the anterior part of the superior oblique tendon.

In cadaver studies, a Z tenotomy on the superior oblique tendon allowed an increase in muscle length of about 3–4 mm. A split tendon lengthening allowed an increase in length of about 5–7 mm, and a complete tenotomy allowed an 8–10-mm increase in length. None of 28 patients operat-

(4) Am. J. Ophthalmol. 81:289–295, March, 1976.

ed on for typical true Brown's syndrome during 1960–75 had a tight superior oblique tendon sheath. Forced duction testing showed that the eye elevated above the midline in adduction after a Z tenotomy; rotated well above the horizontal plane after a split tendon lengthening; and rotated normally after a complete tenotomy or a tenectomy. Nine of 16 patients having the superior oblique tendon cut just medial to the superior rectus muscle had excellent results, 1 had a good result and 3 were improved. One patient did not improve. Tenectomy produced excellent results in 2 patients.

True Brown's syndrome is not due to a tight sheath on the tendon of the superior oblique muscle. The cause is a tight tendon, and a safe and effective surgical treatment consists of cutting it just medial to the superior rectus muscle.

**Indications and Results of Eye Muscle Surgery in Thyroid Ophthalmopathy.** R. C. Apers and J. J. M. Bierlaagh[5] (Univ. of Leiden) operate on the affected muscle in patients with motility disturbances from thyroid disease, which are presumably due to fibrosis of the extraocular muscles. Indications for eye muscle surgery include singular limitation of eye movements with diplopia in the primary position and multiple limitations with a large angle of deviation in the primary position. Six months are allowed before considering surgery for the deviation to remain static. Patients should be euthyroid when operated on.

Ten patients with diplopia due to thyroid ophthalmoplegia have been operated on; in 3 only one muscle was treated. Limited elevation was treated by recession of the inferior rectus and limited abduction by recession of the medial rectus. Forced duction tests were done during surgery to evaluate limitations in the various fields of gaze. It is useful to place the sutures far enough back so that they will not detach.

The 3 patients having surgery on one muscle were improved except for residual diplopia in the extreme fields of gaze. All patients having surgery on multiple muscles had a large field of binocular single vision postoperatively, with an average diameter of 50–60 degrees.

(5) Ophthalmologica 173:171–179, 1976.

A decompression operation should be done first if necessary, but eye muscle surgery should precede eyelid surgery. The antagonist of the pseudoparalytic muscle should be recessed. Recession of the inferior rectus may be large, even 8–10 mm; recession of the medial rectus is 5 mm. The check ligaments are always cut to prevent limitation of movement of the operated muscle. The patient should be told that the lower lid will drop and that more surgery might be necessary.

# Vision, Refraction and Contact Lenses

INTRODUCTION

After a lull, the FDA has approved two more soft contact lenses; the Aqua-lens (Union Corporation) and the Natur-vue-lens (Milton Roy Corporation). Other soft lenses are close to receiving approval so that we will shortly see a more competitive race, and this is all to the good. The ophthalmologist will then have available several different types of soft lenses with different parameters which will enable him to fit more patients with these comfortable lenses.

The search continues for a long-term-wearing soft lens which would be of tremendous value for those aphakic patients who cannot master insertion and removal. Currently under investigation are the Sauflon-lens and deCarle-lens available in England, and a soft lens by Corneal Sciences in Boston. Such lenses might help neutralize the rushing avalanche of intraocular lens implantation. There also is renewed interest in the gas-permeable hard contact lens, the RX-56 lens.

It has been estimated that in 1977 from 50,000–75,000 intraocular implantations of plastic lenses after cataract extraction will be made in the United States. Although this procedure is valuable in selected cases, there is a higher surgical complication rate. During the past year, there were several incidents which must be investigated carefully. One batch of intraocular lenses sterilized by radiation caused rather severe reactions when implanted, and another batch from one laboratory resulted in approximately a dozen Pseudomonas infections postoperatively. The need for careful controls in the manufacture and sterilization of these lenses is obvious. Although the technical skill of implanting the lenses has been attained by many surgeons, determination of the proper refractive lens is still in the Dark Ages because most ophthalmologists merely guess at the power required.

A panel of ophthalmologists at the 1976 meeting of the American Academy of Ophthalmology concluded that automated refractors were essentially accurate and useful in saving time for the ophthalmologist. However, this is strictly an objective refraction, and still requires subjective testing and modification by the ophthalmologist. The art of subjective refraction and prescribing for a particular patient will prevent many of them from returning with complaints about incorrect glasses.

Jack Hartstein, M.D.
Washington University, St. Louis

**Keratoconus and Contact Lenses.** M. Massin, A. Denis-Morère and G. Ninine[6] (Paris) reviewed the data on 82 patients with keratoconus with follow-up of 1 – 12 years. Sixteen patients were not fitted with contact lenses for one or more of the following reasons: (1) better vision with spectacles; (2) advanced cases (4th degree of Amsler) where fitting is impossible; (3) unilateral keratoconus; and (4) associated diseases such as trachomatous pannus and allergic keratoconjunctivitis. Scleral lenses are used less frequently today because of the improvement in hard lenses. These have a short radius of curvature (4 – 7 mm), an overall diameter of 8 – 11 mm and an optic diameter of 5 mm. They are fitted under fluorescein and mobility must be good. Visual acuity is good and 80% of the patients could wear their lenses 10 hours or more a day. The lenses do not affect the progression of the keratoconus. Sometimes keratoconus has appeared in patients already fitted for several years to correct a myopic astigmatism but it is uncertain whether there is any etiologic relationship. If a contact lens must be worn after corneal transplantation, the daily wearing time must be halved to avoid corneal neovascularization.

**Aphakia and Contact Lenses** were studied by J.-P. Gerhard[7] (Univ. Louis Pasteur) to determine the tolerance of contact lenses in 588 unilateral and 72 bilateral aphakic

---

(6)   Klin. Monatsbl. Augenheilkd. 168:24 – 32, January, 1976.
(7)   Ibid., pp. 44 – 49.

patients. After 1 year, tolerance is excellent: 61% wear the contact lenses 10–12 hours a day, 18% wear them 6–8 hours a day and 21% lost courage. There is a parallel between binocular vision and tolerance. Dusty atmosphere decreases the tolerance which is also affected by the local state of the tissues. Fifteen years later, the situation had changed: 72% gave up the contact lenses completely and only 15% wear them 10–12 hours a day. The reasons for abandonment were diplopia, inflammation and local complications.

▶ [These tolerance figures over the long term for aphakes corrected with contact lenses are certainly poor and should provide fuel for the fire of plastic lens implanters and those working on the development of a soft contact lens which does not have to be removed by the more elderly patients. – Ed.] ◀

**Optic Correction of Aphakic Patients with Fresnel Plastic Sheets** is discussed by Antoine Aiva, Festus Sallah and Hans Jürgen Torjan[8] (Univ. of Lomé, Togo). Auguste Fresnel first used these lenses at the beginning of the 19th century. Concentric rings are pressed into a sheet of thin plastic, so that the microprisms thus formed refract the light beams toward the center like a convex lens. The light rays that touch the outer edge of the sheets are more strongly refracted than those at the center. Thus a true convex lens is formed. The optic qualities cannot always rival those offered by massive convex lenses. However, since the sheets have been promoted by a New York firm inexpensively ($12 per hundred), their mediocre optic qualities can be tolerated.

These simple sheets are available only with a refracting power of +15 diopters. For a diameter of 3.7 cm in the model available, there are 90 concentric circles, whereas the posterior side is flat. The flexibility of these sheets allows easy placement on all normal eyeglasses.

These lenses were tried on 52 aphakic eyes. Uncorrected vision was about 0.05, the same as that with a sheet fixed onto a flat glass, but if the sheet was placed on eyeglasses of –3 diopters, a visual acuity of 0.3 would be obtained.

It should be remembered that the Fresnel lenses are intended only for those who cannot finance correction in an-

(8)  Ann. Ocul. (Paris) 209:257–260, April, 1976.

other form, in underdeveloped countries, or as a temporary lens.

**Correction of Anisomyopia with Contact Lenses** is discussed by M. Dreifus, H. Tschopp and Ch. Bosshard[9] (Univ. of Zürich). Currently, it is believed that correction of anisomyopia with contact lenses is contraindicated because most are axial. However, the dioptric aniseikonia is smaller than generally believed. In childhood, it is advisable to correct an anisomyopia fully as early as possible because the distortion of room perception by spectacles seems to play a much bigger role in higher anisomyopia than the functional aniseikonia.

**Special Indications for Use of Soft Contact Lenses as Drug Release System** are discussed by G. B. Bietti, C. De Caro, J. Pecori Giraldi and E. Romani[1] (Univ. of Rome). Two criteria must first be ascertained, i.e., that impregnation with a given substance not alter the optical properties of the lens and that it be appropriate for dispensation of a given substance, because impregnation of soft lenses occurs in inverse proportion to the molecular weight of the medication and take-up may be inadequate or dispensation too rapid. However, this method may prove advantageous for a more prolonged and sustained effect compared to the usual way of administration, especially for antiglaucomatous substances, antimetabolites and mydriatics and for the possibility of reducing concentration and avoiding local discomfort or systemic side effects without loss of effectiveness. The lens (12.5 – 15 mm in diameter) may be presoaked in the liquid or drops may be regularly instilled after the lens is inserted or the two techniques may be combined.

In the present study the use of hydrophilic lenses with osmotically active substances (to obtain better and more protracted dehydration of the cornea) were examined in vitro and in vivo. The following substances were tested: 10% propyleneglycol, 10% glycerol, 10% glucose and 5% sodium chloride. Within 30 minutes the lenses had taken up enough liquid to double their weight; one exception was propyleneglycol, where the amount of liquid absorbed exceeded eightfold the original weight of the lens; it was still dispensed in

(9)  Klin. Monatsbl. Augenheilkd. 168:50 – 54, January, 1976.
(1)  Ibid., pp. 33 – 43.

demonstrable quantity after 150 minutes, twice as long as all other substances tested. These experimental data were then supplemented by a clinical study of 45 patients with edematous bullous keratopathy. Propyleneglycol was the best substance for use with soft contact lenses; for protracted administration the addition of an antibiotic (4% chloramphenicol) is suggested.

Substances designed to increase lacrimal secretion were also studied. Application of lenses presoaked in an eledoisin solution (extracted from an octopus) with subsequent 3-times daily drops of the polypeptide solution (with the lens in place) gave better results in 14 patients (23 eyes) with keratoconjunctivitis sicca than the regular method of administration; increase of lacrimal secretion was not only more pronounced, but lasted 3 times longer. With physalaemin extracted from the skin of a batrachian results were less spectacular; demonstrable amounts after 8 hours were less by twice as much as those found after 15 minutes extraction time (5 times less than with eledoisin).

Results with antiglaucomatous products showed that the concentration of propranolol could be reduced to 0.01 – 0.10%, that of clonidine to 0.06% and prostigmine to 1.5%, when the lenses were presoaked or when instillation was carried out at regular intervals after lens insertion. Another important advantage was that this method allowed the use of substances with a high molecular weight, which could not be handled by other drug release systems.

**Changing Views on Myopia** are discussed in an editorial.[2] Kepler proved that, in myopia, parallel light rays focus in front of the retina, presumably because of the length of the eyeball, and ophthalmoscopic observations in the last century showed temporal crescents at the optic disc and retinal changes at the posterior pole of the myopic eye, apparently supporting Kepler's theory. It was believed that the eyeball could be lengthened by contraction of the extraocular muscles. Inculpation of excessive accommodation led to the use of atropine and of tenotomy of the horizontal rectus muscle; others attacked the oblique muscles surgically. Some even performed iridectomy to keep the ocular tension

(2)  Br. J. Ophthalmol. 59:527 – 528, October, 1975.

low. The progress of myopia has certainly not been limited, nor its frequency reduced. Steiger pointed out in 1913 that the concept of axial myopia cannot explain all cases and postulated that corneal refraction and axial length were freely variable, genetically determined components, the chance union of which could produce any refractive error. Steiger did not appreciate that the lens is also a variable. There are far more cases of emmetropia than would be expected were refractive errors merely variables on a curve of frequency. There are also more cases of high myopia than would be expected.

If the lens is considered a unit, the refractive system of the eye consists of two components, the cornea and the lens, separated by the depth of the anterior chamber. The relation of the focal plane of this refractive system to the perceptive plane is of decisive importance. The power of the cornea and of the lens and the value of axial length show wide variation in emmetropia and the same powers and values are observed in myopia up to $-4$ D. In the emmetropic eye the different powers are coordinated with the axial length, but no such coordination exists in moderate myopia and this is the distinguishing feature of the ametropic eye. The eye becomes myopic during childhood when changes in the cornea and lens do not keep pace with axial elongation. Abnormal components, essentially abnormal axial length, appear in high refractive errors. High errors constitute not more than 5% of refractions in the general population. Questions that remain to be answered include whether the effects of contact lenses and phenylephrine seen are temporary or permanent, which types of myopia are influenced thereby and whether moderate myopia is advantageous for those living in developed societies.

**Early and Late Results of Fascia Lata Transplantation in High Myopia.** A. P. Nesterov, N. B. Libenson and A. V. Svirin[3] (Moscow) reviewed the results of strengthening the sclera with a strip of fascia lata in 184 eyes of 108 patients, aged 8–52 years, treated for progressive myopia. The mean degree of myopia was 18 diopters (D) and the range was 7–39 D. Seventy-eight eyes were astigmatic, and

(3)   Br. J. Ophthalmol. 60:271–272, April, 1976.

70 had profound degenerative changes in the choroid and retina. The myopia was definitely progressive in 128 eyes.

TECHNIQUE. — A fascial strip from the outer surface of the thigh is made into a Y-shaped transplant. Through conjunctival-tenon incisions in three quadrants of the eyeball, the lateral rectus muscle is cut off, and the graft is placed behind the globe. Its narrow arms run above and below the optic nerve and through the superonasal and inferonasal incisions, and the broad arm runs along the horizontal meridian at the temporal side. Each arm is fixed to the sclera with 2 silk sutures, and the lateral rectus is resutured to the globe.

Visual acuity had improved by a mean of 0.08 without correction in 93% of the eyes at 3 – 4 weeks postoperatively. Corrected acuity had improved by 0.25 – 0.5 in 24%. Either concentric or sectorial field narrowing was found in 177 eyes; this widened by 10 – 25 degrees in at least two directions in 160 instances. Myopia had decreased in 92% of the eyes by a mean of 3.1 D.

Long-term follow-up was for 1 – 9 years in 67 patients having 105 eyes treated. Visual acuity had improved in 72% of the eyes, the mean improvement being 0.05 without correction and 0.18 with correction. The degree of myopia had decreased in 88% of the cases by a mean of 4.2 D. The power of glasses required decreased in 91 eyes by a mean of 3.8 D.

In 29 patients having one eye operated on and followed for 1 – 7 years, myopia increased in 5 treated eyes and in 24 untreated eyes. Retinal detachment occurred in only 1 eye.

The risk of complications from this procedure is small. The beneficial effect of the operation appears to be due to support of the posterior sclera by the fascial graft, reduction in ocular tension and improvement in the blood supply to the scleral tissue.

▶ [If this was not published in the eminent British Journal of Ophthalmology, one would be skeptical of these favorable results. — Ed.] ◀

# The Conjunctiva

A recent review of oculogenital disease emphasized the resurgence of venereally acquired ocular infections, of which inclusion conjunctivitis (IC) is the most prevalent.[1] In this country IC is the most common infectious type of ophthalmia neonatorum and is a frequently encountered form of follicular conjunctivitis in the adult.[1-3] Inclusion disease probably is the major single cause of nonbacterial, "nonspecific" urethritis and cervicitis and may even be the most prevalent of all venereal diseases.[4-6]

Unfortunately, there is widespread lack of awareness and recognition of these infections, despite the fact that IC has been known as a clinical entity since the early years of this century.[2] Knowledge of the disease is sufficient now that its diagnosis and management should be within the capability of every opthalmologist.

Inclusion conjunctivitis is a chlamydial infection. *Chlamydiae* are bacteria-like microorganisms that have incomplete mechanisms for the production of metabolic energy and so are obligate intracellular parasites.

Some dispute exists with regard to the naming and classification of *chlamydiae*. There are those who believe that the agents of IC and trachoma are identical and that the agent causes a spectrum of clinical disease; those who hold this view call the organism *Chlamydia trachomatis* or refer to the organism simply as the TRIC (*TR*achoma-*I*nclusion *C*onjunctivitis) agent.[7-9] Others (including myself) believe that these diseases are caused by two distinct agents and refer to *C. trachomatis* (trachoma) and *C. oculogenitalis* (IC and genital infection).[1, 2, 10] Other chlamydial agents that affect man include *C. lymphogranulomatis* (lymphogranuloma venereum) and *C. psittaci* (psittacosis, ornithosis). *Chlamydiae* have been implicated irregularly in cases of Reiter syndrome.

Laboratory techniques have been developed for culturing chlamydial agents and for detecting and immunotyping their antigens and antibodies.[8, 11] Unfortunately, these tests are not generally available and so are of little practical value to most clinicians.

The only laboratory aid that is of any real use to the practicing ophthalmologist is the examination of Giemsa-stained or Wright-stained scrapings of the conjunctival epithelium.[12] Four findings are important: (1) inclusions, (2) polymorphonuclear leukocytes (PMNs), (3) multinucleated giant epithelial cells, and (4) absence of bacteria. Inclusions and giant cells can be found only in epithelial scrapings; smears of exudate are useful for demonstrating inflammatory cells, but no more so than scrapings.

The basophilic inclusion bodies are in the cytoplasm of conjunctival epithelial cells and are identical in appearance to the Halberstaedter-von Prowazek inclusions that are found in trachoma. When fully developed, the inclusion tends to lie against the nuclear membrane and to project into the cytoplasm in a semicircular configuration. Each inclusion consists of a packet of infectious chlamydial particles called elementary bodies. Elementary bodies are roughly round in shape, are of approximately equal sizes (300 nm), have discrete and sharp-edged cell walls, and are light purple with Giemsa or Wright stain. Individual particles of a suspected inclusion should be scrutinized for these characteristics to avoid being misled by pseudoinclusions such as pigment granules, stain granules, bacteria, and extrusions of nuclear chromatin. Initial bodies may be found. An initial body is the swollen, metabolically active particle into which the elementary body transforms after entering the host cell. Initial bodies are slightly larger ($1 \mu$) than elementary bodies and stain dark blue, often in a bipolar fashion.

Inclusions can be found readily in untreated infants with IC but may be difficult to find in adults unless the conjunctivitis is of rather recent onset.

The predominant inflammatory cell in IC is the PMN, but moderate numbers of mononuclear cells may appear in the chronic stages of the disease.

Chlamydial infections sometimes cause the production of multinucleated giant epithelial cells, although such cells are more common in herpetic infections. Giant cells consist of several tightly packed nuclei surrounded by cytoplasm and a single cell wall.

Epidemiology is as follows.[2, 13, 14] The primary reservoir of infection with *C. oculogenitalis* is in the urethra or cervix (and sometimes the rectum), and the disease is transmitted venereally. Neonatal IC (inclusion blennorrhea) is contracted during the infant's passage through the birth canal and is not prevented by silver nitrate. Ocular infection in the adult is the result of contamination of the eye by infected genital secretions. Contamination may occur directly or by way of fingers or fomites and may occur in the individual who harbors the genital infection or in other persons. Eye-to-eye transmission is rare.

Early reports of postneonatal IC incriminated swimming pools as sources of infection, and in the past the disease was called "swimming-pool conjunctivitis." Water that has been contaminated by urine or genital secretions can transmit the infection, but such cases are rare now because the organism is killed by chlorination. Present-day "swimming-pool conjunctivitis" is more likely to be caused by adenovirus.

Neonatal IC is characterized by swelling of the lids, purulent or mucopurulent exudate (PMN response), chemosis and hyperemia of the bulbar conjunctiva, and papillary hypertrophy of the tarsal conjunctiva. Conjunctival pseudomembranes of fibrin are not uncommon. There is no preauricular adenopathy or follicular response of the conjunctiva because of the immaturity of infantile lymphoid tissues, but follicles may appear if the disease persists to between age 6 weeks and 3 months. Contrary to former belief, superficial vascularization of the cornea is common; such micropannus extends usually 2 mm. or less into the peripheral cornea. Dot-like foci of epithelial keratitis, sometimes with small areas of underlying stromal haze and infiltrate, may occur anywhere in the cornea but tend to be more numerous peripherally.

The disease resolves spontaneously in several weeks to slightly more than a year, but the infant may be left with micropannus and a few tiny, subepithelial, corneal scars; mild scarring of the conjunctiva may be seen if the disease has been membranous.[15, 16]

Extraocular involvement has been recognized infrequently in infants, but vaginitis,[16] rhinitis,[16] and pneumonitis[17] (with recovery of *chlamydiae* from the sputum) have been reported.

Because of its frequency (up to 3% of all newborns in some series[18, 19]) the possibility of IC should be considered strongly in every case of ophthalmia neonatorum, but the first consideration must be to determine whether the infection is caused by the gonococcus or meningococcus. Scrapings and cultures (including chocolate agar or Thayer-Martin medium for *neisseriae*) are mandatory. These procedures help also to determine whether the infection is caused by "everyday" bacteria such as staphylococci, coliforms, streptococci, pneumococci or others.

Time of onset is of some value in differentiating the causes of neonatal conjunctivitis. IC and most of the bacterial infections do not appear clinically until the fifth day of life or later. Conjunctivitis caused by herpes simplex frequently begins after the fifth day but may be present even at the time of birth. Neisserial infections are evident usually by the third day. If the mother had premature rupture of membranes, the infant can be infected in utero; and any of these postnatal times of clinical onset can be earlier. Chemical conjunctivitis from Credé prophylaxis appears within 24 hours after instillation of the silver nitrate.

Chemical conjunctivitis is normally mild and of only a few days' duration, but high concentrations of silver nitrate can give rise to purulent exudate and even conjunctival membranes. Membranes are more suggestive, however, of IC or neisserial, streptococcal, or herpetic infections. Herpetic conjunctivitis is associated typically with vesicular blepharitis or occasionally even with disseminated infection. Herpes is the only cause of ophthalmia neonatorum that produces a nonpurulent, mononuclear, cytologic response; PMNs appear only when the conjunctivitis is membranous. Additional aids for diagnosing herpetic infection include viral cultures, examination of scrapings by the fluorescent-antibody technique, serum antibody titers, the finding of typical herpetic corneal involvement and observation of the natural course of the disease. The conjunctival inflammation of herpes simplex and of nearly all other nonchlamydial causes of ophthalmia neonatorum resolves spontaneously in 2–3 weeks, although corneal complications can persist longer.

If scrapings and cultures from the untreated patient are negative for bacteria and if there are no cutaneous or systemic signs to suggest herpetic infection, a neonatal conjunctivitis should be presumed to be IC until proved otherwise. Certain other clinical features (table) can lend additional support to the diagnosis; and the finding of inclusions, of course, settles the matter. Approached in this way the diagnosis of neonatal IC is not difficult even when sophisticated laboratory tests for chlamydial infection are not available.

Inclusion conjunctivitis in the adult begins with an acute onset of redness of the eye(s), swelling of the lids, purulent or mucopurulent discharge, conjunctival follicles and preauricular adenopathy. The follicles are most prominent inferiorly, and follicles at the limbus or on the semilunar fold or caruncle are particularly suggestive of chlamydial infection. It is interesting that the adult form of IC never has been known to be membranous or pseudomembranous, and conjunctival scarring does not occur. Micropannus and superficial focal keratitis like that of the infantile disease are common.

DIFFERENTIAL DIAGNOSIS OF INCLUSION CONJUNCTIVITIS: SELECTED FEATURES

| | DURATION > 3 WEEKS | PURULENT EXUDATE | MEMBRANES POSSIBLE | FOLLICLES |
|---|---|---|---|---|
| Neonatal inclusion | + | + | + | −* |
| Adult inclusion | + | + | − | + |
| Bacteria | −† | + | + | − |
| Silver nitrate | − | −‡ | −‡ | − |
| Adenovirus | − | −§ | + | + |
| Primary herpes | − | −§ | + | + |
| Drugs (IDU, miotics) | + | + | − | + |
| Molluscum | + | − | − | + |
| Trachoma | + | + | − | + |

*Follicles develop between 6 weeks and 3 months of age.
†Chronicity rare in infants, uncommon in adults.
‡High concentrations produce purulence and membranes.
§Mildly purulent if membranous.

The duration of the disease is the same as in infants, weeks to months. Micropannus and minute corneal scars, but not conjunctival scarring, may remain after resolution of the disease.

Most patients or their consorts have associated genital infection although it may be asymptomatic. Salpingitis and other pelvic inflammatory disease, presumably of chlamydial origin, and arthritis (Reiter syndrome?) are fairly common among parents of infants with inclusion blennorrhea.[13, 16] Otitis media appeared in 14% of volunteers with experimentally induced IC, and naturally occurring cases have been reported.[20]

Inclusion conjunctivitis should be considered in any case of follicular conjunctivitis in an adult since most of these cases in the United States are caused either by *C. oculogenitalis* or adenovirus. Adenovirus produces a watery discharge with mononuclear cytology, whereas IC produces a PMN response. Cytologic study of the exudate should be made, but often its nature can be surmised clinically. Purulent exudate may be evident by simple inspection; if not, a history of the patient's eyelids being sealed by "matter" in the mornings is evidence that PMNs are present. Pseudomembranous or membranous adenoviral infection can give rise to a PMN response and even to sealing of the lids, but membranes in an adult are inconsistent with the diagnosis of IC. One or 2 weeks after onset the keratitis of IC has a clear tendency to be peripheral, whereas adenoviral keratitis remains central and becomes nummular.[21]

Prolonged topical use of IDU or miotics can produce chronic follicular conjunctivitis with low-grade PMN response, micropannus or gross pannus, diffuse punctate keratopathy, and conjunctival scarring; but simple inquiry as to the use of these drugs may serve to eliminate them as possible etiologies. In contradistinction to the follicles of IC, which are large and succulent, drug-induced follicles are small and irregular in size.

Trachoma produces follicles and a PMN response but can be differentiated by the presence of gross pannus extending several millimeters into the superior cornea, a follicular response that is greatest on the superior tarsal conjunctiva, conjunctival scarring, and Herbert's peripheral pits. Except on Indian reservations trachoma is far less common in the United States than is IC.

Infection of the lid margin by molluscum contagiosum can produce chronic follicular conjunctivitis and most or all of the signs of IC, trachoma or drug-induced follicular conjunctivitis; but molluscum elicits a mononuclear discharge. Nevertheless, it is advisable to search for molluscum nodules before making a diagnosis of IC.

Primary herpetic conjunctivitis is follicular but is rare in adults. The discharge is mononuclear unless membranes are present, and vesicles are usually present on the lids; the keratitis evolves into dendritic, geographic, or disciform patterns.

Of the follicular conjunctivitides that have PMN exudates, only IC, trachoma and drug reactions persist more than three weeks.

The clinical lesson that emerges is that purulent or mucopurulent, nonmembranous, follicular conjunctivitis in an adult (particularly if chronic) is very likely to be IC even if inclusions cannot be demonstrated (table).

Inclusion conjunctivitis can be treated successfully with tetracycline (usually considered to be the drug of choice), erythromycin or sulfonamide. Infants should be treated with topical ointment, rather than drops, 4 – 6 times daily for 3 weeks. Adults need to be treated systemically to ensure eradication of ocular and genital disease. Tetracycline or erythromycin is given orally in a dosage of one gm per day for patients under 70 kg, or 1.5 gm per day for patients over 70 kg, in 3 – 4 divided doses daily for 3 weeks. Sulfonamides may be given as triple sulfa (Terfonyl) in a dosage of 70 mg/kg daily, in 3 – 4 divided doses. Tetracycline should be avoided during pregnancy, in nursing mothers, and in children under age 8 years because of the risks of staining of teeth and hypoplasia of enamel. Systemic sulfonamides pose some risk of erythema multiforme, among other adverse effects.

Inclusion disease clinically is resistant to neomycin, bacitracin, polymyxin, penicillin, ampicillin and gentamicin and is only slightly responsive to chloromycetin. Corticosteroids worsen the condition.

Consideration must be given to treatment of spouses, consorts, or parents, even if they are asymptomatic, to eliminate genital reservoirs of infection.

Fred M. Wilson II, M.D.
Indiana University

## REFERENCES

1. Ostler, H. B.: Oculogenital Disease, Surv. Ophthalmol. 20:233, 1976.
2. Thygeson, P.: Historical Review of Oculogenital Disease, Am. J. Ophthalmol. 71:975, 1971.
3. Armstrong, J. H., Zacarias, F., and Rein, M. F.: Ophthalmia Neonatorum: A Chart Review, Pediatrics 57:884, 1976.
4. Schachter, J., Hanna, L., Hill, E. C., Massad, S., Sheppard, C. W., Conte, J. E., Jr., Cohen, S. N., and Meyer, K. F.: Are Chlamydial Infections the Most Prevalent Venereal Disease?, J.A.M.A. 231:1252, 1975.
5. Holmes, K. K., Handsfield, H. H., Wang, S. P., Wentworth, B. B., Turck, M., Anderson, J. B., and Alexander, E. R.: Etiology of Nongonococcal Urethritis, N. Engl. J. Med. 292:1199, 1975.
6. Week, L. A., Smith, T. F., Pettersen, G. R., and Segura, J. W.: Urethritis Associated with *Chlamydia.* Clinical and Laboratory Diagnosis, Minn. Med. 59:228, 1976.
7. Collier, L. H.: On the Etiology and Relationship of Trachoma and Inclusion Blennorrhoea, Rev. Int. Trachome 37:585, 1960.
8. Grayston, J. T. and Wang, S.: New Knowledge of *Chlamydiae* and the Diseases They Cause, J. Infect. Dis. 132:87, 1975.
9. Editorial: *Chlamydia,* Trachoma, Genital Infection and Psittacosis, Br. J. Ophthalmol. 59:113, 1975.
10. Thygeson, P., Hanna, L., Dawson, C., Zichosch, J., and Jawetz, E.: Inoculation of Human Volunteer with Egg-Grown Inclusion Conjunctivitis Virus, Am. J. Ophthalmol. 53:786, 1962.
11. Jones, B. R.: Laboratory Tests for Chlamydial Infection, Br. J. Ophthalmol. 58:438, 1974.
12. Yoneda, C., Dawson, C. R., Daghfous, T., Hoshiwara, I., Jones, P., Messadi, M., and Schachter, J.: Cytology as a Guide to the Presence of Chlamydial Inclusions in Giemsa-Stained Conjunctival Smears in Severe Endemic Trachoma, Br. J. Ophthalmol. 59:116, 1975.
13. Thygeson, P. and Stone, W., Jr.: Epidemiology of Inclusion Conjunctivitis, Arch. Ophthalmol. 27:91, 1942.
14. Shachter, J.: Reply to Letter to Editor, J.A.M.A. 234:592, 1975.
15. Forster, R. K., Dawson, C. R., and Shachter, J.: Late Follow-up

of Patients with Neonatal Inclusion Conjunctivitis, Am. J. Ophthalmol. 69:467, 1970.

16. Mordhorst, C. H. and Dawson, C.: Sequelae of Inclusion Conjunctivitis and Associated Disease in Parents, Am. J. Ophthalmol. 71:861, 1971.

17. Shachter, J., Lum, L., Gooding, C. A., and Ostler, B.: Pneumonitis following Inclusion Blennorrhea, J. Pediat. 87:779, 1975.

18. Bettman, J. W., Jr., Carreno, O. B., Szuter, C. F., and Yoneda, C.: Inclusion Conjunctivitis in American Indians of the Southwest, Am. J. Ophthalmol. 70:363, 1970.

19. Hansman, D.: Inclusion Conjunctivitis, Med. J. Aust. 1:151, 1969.

20. Gow, J. A., Ostler, H. B., and Shachter, J.: Inclusive Conjunctivitis with Hearing Loss, J.A.M.A. 229:519, 1974.

21. Poirier, R. H.: Chlamydial Infections: Diagnosis and Management, Trans. Am. Acad. Ophthalmol. Otolaryngol. 79:109, 1975.

**Biochemical and Ultrastructural Study of Human Diabetic Conjunctiva.** The endothelial proliferative changes and basement membrane thickening of retinal capillaries in diabetes are associated with parallel basement membrane changes in the capillaries of several other tissues, including the conjunctiva. P. Kern, F. Regnault and L. Robert[4] (Paris) examined the incorporation of $^3$H-proline and $^{14}$C-glucosamine in the macromolecules of the intercellular matrix of human diabetic conjunctiva and in normal conjunctiva.

Conjunctival biopsy specimens were obtained from 72 patients aged 40–60, including 27 normal subjects, 21 diabetics diagnosed in the past 10 years and 24 diabetics diagnosed 10 years or more previously. Five diabetics in the first group and 14 in the second were insulin-dependent and 5 and 2, respectively, were managed by diet alone. Alterations of the conjunctival capillary basement membrane were studied by electron microscopy.

A decrease in $^{14}$C-glucosamine incorporation was found in fractions of diabetic conjunctiva. Percentages of $^3$H-proline incorporation in the polymeric collagen-containing fraction and structural glycoprotein-containing fraction were signif-

(4) Biomedicine 24:32–39, January, 1976.

icantly increased and the incorporation of $^3$H-proline in a "crude soluble collagen" fraction was reduced in parallel. Significant capillary basement membrane thickening was seen, with collagen-like fibrils present within the basement membrane in diabetic conjunctiva. Such fibrils were not seen in normal conjunctiva. The extent of basement membrane thickening appeared related to the appearance of collagen-like fibrils.

These findings suggest abnormal regulation of the relative rate of biosynthesis or excretion of extracellular matrix macromolecules, such as collagen and structural glycoproteins, as part of the metabolic disorder characterizing diabetes. The parallelism between increased proline incorporation in the polymeric collagen fraction and the appearance of collagen fibrils and thickening of the basement membrane supports this hypothesis.

**Communicable Ophthalmia: Blinding Scourge of the Middle East** is discussed by Barrie R. Jones, Sohrab Darougar (London), H. Mohsenine (Univ. of Teheran) and Robert H. Poirier[5] (Univ. of Texas, San Antonio). From a public health point of view, blinding and nonblinding forms of trachoma should be distinguished. Trachoma can be a multicyclic infection in which each cycle adds damage. The continuing pressure of reinfection in a community determines the severity of the disease and the ultimate degree of damage that occurs. Eye-seeking flies appear to provide the added dimension to transmission of infection that escalates the pressure and the duration of exposure into a life-long environmentally determined reinfection with *Chlamydia trachomatis* and the pathogenic ocular bacteria, resulting in a mass blinding scourge. Blinding hyperendemic trachoma is the central core of communicable ophthalmia. It occurs in communities with open fecal and rubbish disposal, poor personal hygiene and short interpersonal distances in climates favorable to the production of a high density of the synanthropic eye-seeking flies.

All communities with suspected blindness from communicable ophthalmia must carry out surveys of suspected rural communities. All ages must be surveyed for corneal blind-

(5) Br. J. Ophthalmol.60:492 – 498, July, 1976.

ness, potentially blinding trachomatous deformities of the lids and severe grades of upper tarsal conjunctival inflammation. Present mass control programs are based on the use of a tetracycline ointment in both eyes twice a day for 5 days monthly, for 3 or preferably, 6 months. Continuous-delivery systems in children are at least as effective as twice-daily ointment regimens. Long-acting oral tetracycline chemotherapy has potential advantages in terms of ease, certainty and continuity of delivery. Real control of communicable ophthalmia must come from fly control. Governments must take responsibility for implementing large-scale surveys and chemotherapy programs. There is an urgent need for financial support to establish academic centers in preventive ophthalmology to ensure exposure of trainees to the challenges of community ophthalmology and to encourage the recruitment of persons of high caliber into this field.

▶ [These and previous studies indicate that either trachoma or bacterial conjunctivitis alone do not produce serious corneal or visual damage. However, *Chlamydia trachomatis* from eyes or nasal mucous membrane of infected individuals is transmitted via flies bred in human feces to produce a mixed *C. Trachomatis*-bacterial infection and reinfection of eyes with resultant blinding disease. Although intermittent therapy with tetracycline ointment or oral tetracycline is effective, public health measures are even more important in these substandard communities. — Ed.] ◀

**Human Conjunctivitis: II. Treatment.** Howard M. Leibowitz, Mary V. Pratt, Inger J. Flagstad, Amado R. Berrospi and Ruth Kundsin[6] (Boston Univ.) conducted a prospective study to determine the relative effects of various topically administered medications on patients with conjunctivitis.

A total of 143 patients with acute conjunctivitis or blepharoconjunctivitis was studied. In the first study, patients received a steroid preparation only. Treatment was with 0.125% prednisolone acetate (Econopred), 0.25% prednisolone acetate (Sterofrin), 2.5% hydrocortisone acetate (Hydrocortone) and 0.1% dexamethasone (Maxidex). Two drops of medication was instilled 4 times daily at 4-hour intervals. In the second study, a mixture of dexamethasone, neomycin and polymyxin B sulfate (Maxitrol) was compared with dexamethasone; a mixture of neomycin and polymyxin B sulfate (Statrol); and hydroxypropyl methycellulose (Isopto Tears). Drug doses began at 2 drops 4 times daily.

(6)   Arch. Ophthalmol. 94:1752–1756, October, 1976.

Efficacy was assessed from symptom and sign severity and from the physician's impression of improvement. Reduction in symptoms and signs was most marked with 0.25% prednisolone acetate, followed by 2.5% hydrocortisone and 0.1% dexamethasone. Similar trends were apparent from physicians' assessments. The steroid alone and the steroid-antibiotic combination produced the best results and were about equal in efficacy. The combination was significantly more effective than the antibiotic alone. The various steroid preparations were comparably effective in *Staphylococcus aureus* conjunctivitis. Two patients exhibited allergy to Statrol. One patient reinstituted 0.25% prednisolone and acquired a contact dermatitis.

All the steroids compared in these studies were effective. Active conjunctivitis was better controlled by preparations containing a steroid, either alone or combined with an antibiotic. Antibiotic alone was relatively effective in controlling conjunctivitis but it did not control active inflammation as rapidly as did steroid-containing preparations. Evidence of clinical risk from any of the drugs was minimal, the average duration of treatment being 14 days or less. The steroid-antibiotic combination had to be discontinued least often because of worsening inflammation or adverse drug reaction.

► [This well-controlled clinical study produced some rather surprising results; that treatment of conjunctivitis of all types responded better after either local steroid or steroid-antibiotic than after local antibiotic alone, and much better than treatment with artificial tears. This must indicate that, if inflammation is diminished by the steroid, that natural immunity clears up the infection. I hope that primary physicians do not start treating all red eyes with steroids without examination of the cornea to rule out dendritic ulcers, especially, and probably also bacterial and fungal ulcers. – Ed.] ◄

**Tissue, Tear and Serum IgE Concentrations in Vernal Conjunctivitis.** Mathea R. Allansmith, Gary S. Hahn and Meredith A. Simon[7] postulated that vernal conjunctivitis might have as part of its mechanism a localized hyperplasia of IgE plasma cells in the cobblestone excrescences, and that locally produced IgE may raise the tear IgE level. Tarsal conjunctivas from 11 patients with vernal conjunc-

---

(7) Am. J. Ophthalmol. 81:506–511, April, 1976.

tivitis were stained for immunoglobulins, and IgE was measured in the tears and serum. All patients had typical cobblestone excrescences over the entire upper tarsal conjunctivas and many eosinophils in conjunctival scrapings. All had had severe itching and tearing for more than 2 seasons. Ten patients had an average age of 14 years, and 1 patient was a man aged 75 with clinically typical disease. Ten normal subjects aged 15–53 years were also studied, and tarsal tissue was sampled from 2 cadavers.

No predominance of IgE-staining cells was observed. Abundant extracellular immunoglobulin was present in both groups, thought to be extravascular serum protein also seen in normal patients, but more IgE seemed to be present in the extracellular stroma in the patients. Mean serum IgE concentrations were 1,031 ng/ml in patients and 201 ng/ml in controls, a significant difference. The respective mean tear IgE concentrations were 130 and 61 ng/ml, not a significant difference. The 2 patients with high IgE values had the most severe systemic and local disease.

The findings are consistent with a hyperplasia of IgA, IgD and IgE antibody-forming cells in the tarsal conjunctivas of some patients with vernal conjunctivitis and with tear IgE concentrations being a function of serum IgE concentrations. Evidence is strong that vernal conjunctivitis is an atopic disease, and the present findings support this concept. Although local IgE-mediated damage may occur in vernal conjunctivitis, a local hyperplasia of only the IgE system is not present.

▶ [Although vernal conjunctivitis is thought to be an allergic or atopic disease with many eosinophils found in the papillary tissue, the present studies were negative for local production of the hypersensitivity immunoglobulin IgE by the plasma cells. Although serum IgE appeared to be elevated in these patients, one control was discarded because of his unexplained high IgE. If this had not been done, there would not have been any statistical difference between patients and controls. In the following article only 3 of 7 patients had elevated serum IgE.

Because of complications from long-term use of local steroids, Easty et al. (Clin. Allergy 2:99, 1972) used topical instillations of sodium cromoglycate (also see next article), a non-steroid chemical which blocks the release of histamine from mast cells induced by interaction of antigen and antibody. Because histamine is a major cause of itching which is so distressing for patients with vernal conjunctivitis, sodium cromoglycate (SCG) provided early symptomatic relief although there was little effect on the papillae or corneal changes. However, a double-blind clinical trial of

SCG in Israel showed no beneficial effect (Hyams et al.: J. Pediatr. Ophthal. 12:116, 1975). — Ed.] ◄

**Sodium Cromoglycate (Intal) in Treatment of Vernal Keratoconjunctivitis and Allergic Conjunctivitis.** Prolonged steroid therapy for vernal conjunctivitis may cause undesirable side effects. Sodium cromoglycate (SCG) inhibits release of chemical mediators of immediate, IgE-mediated hypersensitivity. J. J. Kazdan, J. S. Crawford, H. Langer and A. L. MacDonald[8] (Univ. of Toronto) report results of a clinical trial of SCG, as 2% Intal drops, in patients with vernal keratoconjunctivitis and other forms of allergic conjunctivitis. Nineteen patients, including 2 siblings, with vernal conjunctivitis and 22 with allergic conjunctivitis of the acute seasonal or chronic atopic type were treated with Intal drops for 2 weeks to 16 months. Drops were instilled into both eyes 4 times daily. Some patients also received topical steroids and other medications.

Vernal conjunctivitis was well controlled with Intal drops alone in 13 of the 19 patients. Three of these patients had limbic lesions and 4 had superficial punctate keratitis, besides "cobblestone" conjunctival changes. Six patients with more severe keratitis or corneal ulceration received other types of treatment during relapses. Blood IgE values were elevated in 3 of 7 patients tested. Intal drops relieved itching and watering within a week in all 11 patients with seasonal conjunctivitis but were effective in only 4 of the 11 patients with mild chronic conjunctivitis. Conjunctival scrapings contained eosinophils in 3 of the more severe cases of acute inflammation. No side effects were observed, apart from occasional mild irritation in some cases.

Immunoglobulin E-mediated hypersensitivity appears to play a part in vernal conjunctivitis as well as in seasonal hay fever-type conjunctivitis. Intal may be more likely to be effective in atopic patients with vernal conjunctivitis. It was particularly useful in 2 patients with vernal conjunctivitis in whom steroids were contraindicated.

► ↓ In the following four articles, variable features and treatment of carcinomas of the conjunctiva are discussed. Although mucoepidermoid carcinomas are not uncommon in the salivary glands and less so in the respiratory tract, they are rarely found arising from the conjunctiva, al-

(8)  Can. J. Ophthalmol. 11:300–303, October, 1976.

though, as usual, the AFIP files contain 5 such cases. Histochemical staining of the mucus-secreting cells is diagnostic and important because
these tumors have a poor prognosis for recurrence and local invasion.
Accordingly, they should be resected widely and observed closely after
operation.

Squamous cell carcinomas of the conjunctiva can be highly pigmented
and resemble melanomas (see article by Jauregui and Klintworth).

Treatment of squamous cell carcinomas of the conjunctiva seems to
depend on whether the ophthalmologist is an aggressive surgeon or is
interested in radiation therapy. Carcinomas in situ show little invasive
character and can be excised or treated by beta radiation (see article by
Lommatzsch). Rose bengal staining of abnormal epithelial cells is a valuable adjunct in determining the outer limits of squamous cell carcinomas
(see article by Wilson) which must be excised more completely, preferably
with a lamellar corneoscleral excision replaced with a lamellar graft if
necessary. On the other hand, such carcinomas also respond well to beta
radiation, Lommatzsch recommending daily doses of 1,000 rads. The only
recurrence in his series followed a total dose of 8,000 rads. — Ed. ◄

# Mucoepidermoid Carcinoma of the Conjunctiva: Clinicopathologic Study of Five Cases

was made by
Narsing A. Rao and Ramon L. Font[9] (Armed Forces Inst. of
Pathology). All the patients were white men, with a mean
age of 70 years at diagnosis. The most common presentation
was with a conjunctival mass and redness and irritation of
the eye. Three patients had tumors at the limbus, 1 mass
was in the lower cul-de-sac and 1 was in the bulbar conjunctiva. In only 1 case was conjunctival carcinoma diagnosed
preoperatively. All tumors recurred within 6 months; 1 patient had two recurrences. Two patients had exenteration
after recurrence with orbital invasion, and 1 in whom persistent uveitis followed segmental corneoscleral resection
underwent enucleation. Another patient did well after lamellar corneoscleral resection. One patient had enucleation
after one recurrence and exenteration after a second.

All tumors exhibited an admixture of epidermoid and
mucus-secreting cells in varying proportions. All originated
in the conjunctival epithelium. Four tumors had predominantly epidermoid features. The 3 limbic lesions showed
extension into the peripheral cornea by epidermoid tumor
cells (Fig 6). One tumor exhibited a predominantly glandu-
lar pattern with foci of epidermoid differentiation. All recurrences showed more epidermoid elements than the orig-

(9)   Cancer 38:1699–1709, October, 1976.

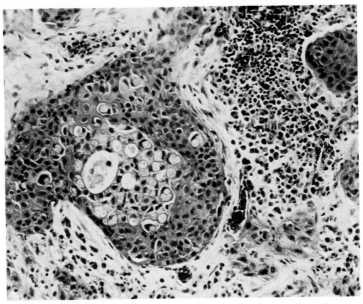

**Fig 6.**—Large epithelial lobule composed of both squamous cells and mucus-secreting cells. Note smaller infiltrating lobules surrounded by foci of lymphocytes and plasma cells. AFIP neg no. 75-9708; hematoxylin-eosin; reduced from ×210. (Courtesy of Rao, N. A., and Font, R. L.: Cancer 38:1699–1709, October, 1976.)

inal tumors. Histochemical staining for mucin was most useful in making a correct diagnosis.

Biologically these tumors appear to be locally aggressive and should be distinguished histopathologically from conventional squamous cell carcinomas of the conjunctiva, which carry a better prognosis. They should be managed by wide local excision with tumor-free margins, and frequent follow-up is necessary to detect early recurrences.

**Pigmented Squamous Cell Carcinoma of Cornea and Conjunctiva: Light Microscopic, Histochemical and Ultrastructural Study.** Hugo O. Jauregui and Gordon K. Klintworth[1] (Duke Univ.) report the first known, detailed description of a pigmented squamous cell carcinoma of the cornea and conjunctiva.

---

(1)   Cancer 38:778–788, August, 1976.

Man, 47, presented with a painful, dark swelling on the left eye. White spots had appeared 4 years before and had darkened gradually and increased in size, especially in the 6 months before hospitalization. A 15-mm tumor was present on the medial half of the cornea and conjunctiva of the left eye (Fig 7) and moderate conjunctival hyperemia was present. Visual acuity was hand movements at 2−3 ft on the left and 20/20 on the right. The tumor was excised under local anesthesia and a lamellar sclerectomy was done for residual tumor 3 weeks later. The excised tissue was replaced by a portion of preserved cornea. A large, fungating mass was present about 3 years later, covering about 80% of the cornea; the eye was enucleated.

The neoplasm predominantly consisted of pleomorphic squamous cells with large, hyperchromatic nuclei and variable amounts of brown pigment. Many squamous epithelial pearls were evident. A few atypical mitotic figures were seen in the enucleation specimen. Pigment was present in several different cell types; it manifested a marked argentaphilia and had a positive Turnbull's reaction after addition of potassium ferricyanide. Electron microscopy showed neoplastic squamous cells (Fig 8), many displaying a few mature melanosomes, cells containing rod- or racket-shaped bodies (Langerhans' cell granules), pigmented macrophages in clusters and pigmented stellate cells situated among epithelial cells.

Fig 7.−A large, pigmented tumor overlies the medial half of the cornea and conjunctiva of the left eye. (Courtesy of Jauregui, H. O., and Klintworth, G. K.: Cancer 38:778−788, August, 1976.)

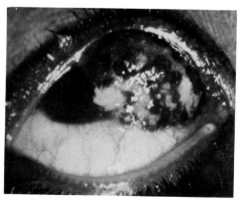

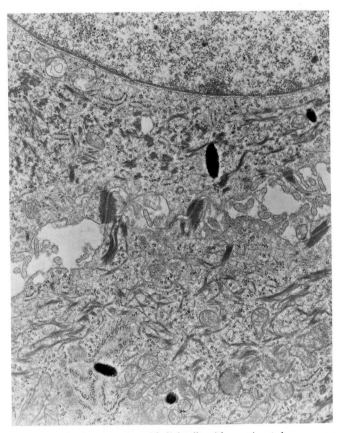

**Fig 8.**—Neoplastic squamous epithelial cells with prominent desmosomes and bundles of tonofilaments sectioned in different planes. Fully melanized melanosomes also are present; original magnification ×25,000. (Courtesy of Jauregui, H. O., and Klintworth, G. K.: Cancer 38:778–788, August, 1976.)

The pigment in this tumor had characteristic features of melanin. Desmosomes were sparse and nexuses were not seen in the neoplastic squamous cells. The melanin in the epithelial cells, macrophages and Langerhans' cells clearly originated in melanocytes. Melanin-containing cells also have been found in several tumors, including basal cell carcinomas, cutaneous squamous cell carcinomas, seborrheic keratosis, exocrine sweat gland tumors and meningiomas.

The nature of these lesions emphasizes the fact that all pigmented tumors are not melanomas.

**Rose Bengal Staining of Epibulbar Squamous Neoplasms.** Flat and inconspicuous parts of squamous neoplasms of the conjunctiva and cornea can be overlooked easily before and during operation. Fred M. Wilson II[2] (Indiana Univ.) found that vital staining of these tumors with topical 1% aqueous rose bengal solution reduces the likelihood of such oversight.

Rose bengal, an iodinated derivative of fluorescein, vitally stains degenerating and dead epithelial cells a vivid, deep red and can make areas of mild neoplasia readily apparent (Fig 9). It is impossible to state confidently that all areas of tumor involvement will stain; the staining pattern must be used only as an adjunct to careful examination. The dye will stain devitalized epithelial cells and it stains mucus intensely. Staining occurs normally along the posterior aspect of the lid margin and in a punctate manner on the nasal and inferior cornea and bulbar conjunctiva, the inferior tarsal conjunctiva and the semilunar fold and caruncle of normal eyes.

Fig 9.—**A,** unstained appearance of relatively localized epibulbar squamous neoplasm. **B,** appearance of tumor after vital staining with topical 1% rose bengal, showing that extent of epithelial abnormality is considerably greater than is evident without staining. Histopathologically, the area of diffuse conjuctival staining adjacent to the large nodule showed acanthosis, hyperkeratosis, parakeratosis, dyskeratosis and rete peg formation in various areas. (Courtesy of Wilson, F. M., II: Ophthalmic Surg. 7:21–23, Summer, 1976.)

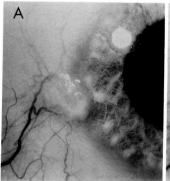 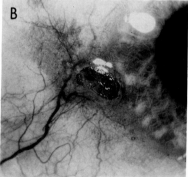

Rose bengal application often causes discomfort in the unanesthetized eye but some have found that topical anesthetics cause false positive staining. The author has found that 0.5% proparacaine and 0.5% tetracaine do not interfere with the ability of rose bengal to delineate tumor margins. The rare, spurious staining resulting from these anesthetics always has been minimal, nonconfluent and no more extensive than that seen in many normal eyes.

**Beta-Ray Treatment of Malignant Epithelial Tumors of the Conjunctiva.** Malignant epithelial tumors of the conjunctiva, though rare, require active treatment to relieve pain and prevent visual loss and metastases. P. Lommatzsch[3] (Humboldt Univ., Berlin) encountered 15 patients with malignant epithelial tumors of the conjunctiva during 1963–74 for a frequency of about 1:20,000 in the hospital population. This included 10 squamous cell carcinomas, 4 carcinoma in situ, and 1 epidermidalization. The interval between the first symptoms and referral was 1 year. Seven patients presented with a red eye and 6 with tumefaction. The nasal part of the conjunctiva was affected in 8 patients and the temporal portion in 5. Two attempts at excision before radiotherapy failed, and 2 other patients had local recurrences after surgery. A $\beta$-ray ocular applicator of either the concave mirror-like type or of a plane active surface type, filled with $^{90}Sr/^{90}Y$, was utilized. Surface doses of 10,000–18,000 rads were delivered with single daily doses of 1,000 rads. One patient was treated with 6,000 R in addition because of wide infiltration of the tarsal conjunctiva.

The 6 patients followed for over 5 years showed no recurrence or metastases after treatment. Follow-up ranged from 1 to 8 years after $\beta$-ray irradiation. Generally, the neoplasms were completely destroyed and resorbed within 1–2 months after the last $\beta$-ray application. One patient had a recurrence after treatment with 8,000 rads. No metastases to regional nodes or other organs were observed. In 3 patients in whom the tumor involved part of the cornea, a corneal scar remained after treatment. A more advanced senile cataract developed in 1 patient in the treated eye 5 years after irradiation. Another patient had a local opacity in the

(3)   Am. J. Ophthalmol. 81:198–206, February, 1976.

periphery of the lens, without any loss of visual acuity. Severe secondary glaucoma developed in 1 patient 3 years after irradiation of a limbal intraepithelial carcinoma that grew around the cornea; the treatment may have caused obstruction of Schlemm's canal. Another patient had bilateral open-angle glaucoma during follow-up which was obviously not a sequela of $\beta$-ray irradiation.

There is no uniform method of treating malignant conjunctival tumors. Beta-ray irradiation with $^{90}Sr/^{90}Y$ applicators is a successful treatment for malignant epithelial conjunctival tumors if a dose of 15,000–18,000 rads is applied to the tumor surface, and if the height of the tumor does not exceed 5 mm.

# The Cornea and Sclera

INTRODUCTION

Since the beginning of corneal transplantation, ways have been sought to prolong the storage time of donor corneas. This would allow elective scheduling of surgery, thereby providing better patient preparation, improved hospital bed utilization and a rested surgeon operating with experienced operating room personnel. In this introduction, I want to update Laibson's 1974 YEAR BOOK introduction on this subject[1] by summarizing recent experimental and clinical research on new methods of donor preservation. For a more complete discussion see the recent review by Van Horn and Schultz.[2] In addition, I will discuss some of the issues facing eye banks and speculate on future developments in this field.

An ideal storage method should fulfill a number of criteria. First, and most important, it should maintain endothelial viability, since, without it, penetrating keratoplasty is doomed to failure. A way to assess this viability during storage would be valuable. Unlimited storage duration should be possible. Sterilization of the cornea with a fail-safe indicator to detect contamination should be inherent in the method. The corneas should remain clear, thin and of normal rigidity during storage. The method should require no special equipment or material. The method should allow ease of transportability, whether it is shipped across town or across the world. No special expertise should be required so that anyone could be easily trained to perform the technical procedures involved. Finally, the method should be inexpensive. With this criteria in mind, I wish to examine the present methods of storage available to corneal surgeons today.

## 4 C Refrigeration

This is the standard storage method used successfully for the past 40 years and it is the benchmark by which all of the methods must be evaluated. It has the advantage of being technically simple, needing only a standard refrigerator as equipment and is readily transportable using insulated containers with ice. Infection following its use is rare. Because of the wide experience gained using this method, it enjoys surgeon confidence and trust. However, its major shortcoming is limited storage time. Although the limits of this time are not known, many surgeons, on an empirical basis, will not use corneas stored at 4 C beyond 24 hours.

It is assumed that endothelial death occurs in a linear fashion proportional to postmortem time at 4 C. This compels surgeons to use the tissue as soon as possible. However, Saleeby has shown an 83% success rate using 4 C stored corneas, used 50–80 hours postmortem in 148 cases followed from 3–7 years.[3] This would indicate that if cell death is proportional to postmortem time, the rate is much slower than previously assumed. It could also mean that although a large number of endothelial cells may perish at 4 C, the remaining viable cells are able to maintain graft function. In this regard, Bourne and Kaufman, utilizing clinical specular microscopy, found as few as 13% of cells remaining in some clear and thin grafts.[4] Under any circumstances, it would appear that 4 C refrigerated corneal tissue is safe to use with storage times up to 48 hours and, if necessary, this can be extended to 72 hours. Another disadvantage of this method, as well as with all other methods, is the inability to assess endothelial viability preoperatively.

### Cryopreservation

In 1965, Capella et al., reported a series of successful penetrating keratoplasties using donor corneas preserved by freezing in a special cryoprotection solution.[5] In this method, as with all other methods utilizing solutions or media, the cornea with a 2- to 3-mm scleral rim is removed from the globe and immersed in the fluid. Although there is potential for endothelial damage to occur from iris touch if the anterior chamber collapses during removal of the corneal scleral segment, it has the advantage of removing the endothelium from postmortem aqueous which may be toxic.[6] A corneal scleral segment requires posterior trephination at the time of surgery to obtain a corneal button. This has been shown to yield more endothelial cells with less damage at the cut edges than anterior trephination used in the intact globe.[7]

Cryopreservation has been recently reviewed[8] and clinical results indicate success rates equal to that of fresh 4 C stored cornea.[9] Storage duration of a year or longer is possible. However, this is a technically complicated system requiring a well trained technician, expensive equipment and can only be used for young donor tissue (under 50 years of age) with postmortem time of less than 6 hours. Thawing of the tissue is a complex and critical procedure which must be done at the time of surgery. Therefore, this tissue cannot be transported once thawed. Because of these disadvantages, its present use is limited to a few centers.

## M-K Medium

This method was developed by Bernard McCarey, Ph.D. and Herbert Kaufman, M.D., hence the abbreviation "M-K." With this method, the corneal scleral segment is immersed in TC-199 medium and stored at 4 C.[10] Dextran is added to keep the cornea thin and streptomycin-penicillin mixture is added to attempt to control infection. Laboratory studies show that animal endothelium[10, 11, 12] remains viable up to 14 days and human endothelium[11, 14] remains viable for at least 4 days when stored in M-K medium. However, some studies show no superiority over moist chamber storage.[12, 13] Clinical studies show that results with M-K stored donor corneas are as good as with 4 C refrigeration or cryopreservation when stored for up to 96 hours.[14, 15, 16, 17] McCarey et al. feel that the time from death to placement in media is critical[17] with an interval of less than 6 hours ideal.[8, 17] From all laboratory and clinical studies to date, it would appear that M-K medium at 4 C preserves human endothelial cell viability for at least 4 days, especially if time from death to placement of media is less than 6 hours. This medium is supplied for a nominal charge from Warner-Lambert Research Institute, 170 Taber Road, Morris Plains, New Jersey 07950. Surgeon acceptance of this method has been good, not only because of the longer storage duration but also because the tissue remains thin, clear and of normal texture. With this method transportability is easily accomplished using standard styrofoam eye bank containers with ice. The main disadvantage of this system is the limited storage duration. In those institutions with limited operating room time and heavy scheduling of elective cases, a storage duration of at least 7 days would be desirable. There have been disturbing reports of endophthalmitis following use of M-K medium.[18, 19, 20] This may be due to the ineffectiveness of the antibiotics in the medium at 4 C. Antibiotics are only effective against metabolizing organisms, and since metabolism is inhibited at 4 C, the presence of antibiotics in the medium is of little value. If one uses M-K medium, one must use meticulous sterile technique in preparing and handling the donor tissue.

### 37 C Organ Culture Storage

In this method, corneas are immersed in a standard tissue culture medium, minimum essential medium (Eagles) and incubated at 37 C. The medium contains serum (either calf or recipient serum) as well as an antibiotic-antimycotic combination and is changed 3 times weekly. Laboratory studies show that endothelial ultrastructure[21, 22] as well as corneal metabolism[21] are maintained for at least 5 weeks. In addition, endothelial repair of experimentally induced wounds occur during incubation.[23] Clinical studies using organ cultured corneas show that donor corneas stored for an average of 15 days (range from 2 to 35 days) have long-term success rates equal to that of cryopreserved or 4 C-refrigerated tissue or corneas stored in M-K medium.[24] The major advantage of this system is the long duration of storage it allows. This makes elective surgery possible as well as providing time to do extensive sterility checks for fungus and bacteria. Endothelial viability is maintained at room temperature with this method for at least 7 days allowing for ease of transportability without special materials or equipment for temperature control. Although antigenicity is reduced in animal models[25] clinical studies show no significant decrease in antigenicity in humans.[24] The major disadvantages of this system are its cost and complexity. It requires expensive equipment, a clean isolated room and a well-trained technician who understands tissue culture and sterile technique.

The infection potential is real. One case of fungal endophthalmitis has occurred following use of contaminated donor tissue. This contamination was either missed during the sterility checks or occurred at the time of surgery. Another disadvantage is that the organ cultured cornea is thick and cloudy. This has caused no technical difficulty at the time of surgery and in most cases the cornea clears fast enough to allow visualization of the anterior chamber detail by the end of the procedure. Further clinical studies, already under way, will determine if the cost and complexity justifies continued use of this method. If the method proves to be worthy, it would lend itself well to centralized regional eye banking.

## Eye Banking — Present and Future

As seen above, we are far from attaining the ideal storage method outlined at the beginning. Eye banking is complex and expensive. Even if one uses the standard 4 C method, costs are high in procuring this tissue, especially if technicians are involved. No longer is an unpaid volunteer working part time on donor card lists enough to constitute an Eye Bank. Just as in other tissue banks, eye banking is becoming a sophisticated endeavor. Already insurance companies are reimbursing some eye banks for a processing charge and these third-party carriers will want standards established for quality control to justify such payments. The Bureau of Biologics in the Food and Drug Administration is already involved in tissue banks utilizing blood and other organs.[26] With increasing use of media for storage, it is only a matter of time before eye banks will be under their scrutiny. In addition, product liability is forcing eye banks to examine their operations since questions have been raised regarding their liability when bad results occur.

A report at the scientific session of the Eye Bank Association of America stated that from September of 1974 to September of 1976, 18 cases of endophthalmitis occurred in a total of 13,249 transplants.[27] Since no cases of endophthalmitis following penetrating keratoplasty can be found in the literature prior to 1976[18] serious questions must be asked about the course of this apparent increase in postoperative infections. It may be that endophthalmitis previously oc-

curred and was not reported. It may be that transplant surgeons are operating on poorer-risk patients (particularly
aphakes) who are known to have increased incidence of endophthalmitis following intraocular surgery. It may be that
the use of media storage, particularly with the use of the
corneal-scleral rim, has contributed to this increase. By using the corneal-scleral rim one may convert surface contamination of the intact globe into a situation encouraging invasion of microbes into the cut scleral edges and the more vul-
nerable endothelial surface. Finally, the problem of trans-
mitting donor diseases such as those caused by slow virus
has also been of concern to eye banks.[28]

Quantity control is another problem facing eye banks.
Few eye banks have enough donor material to fill their
needs. A significant advance in this area has been the training of morticians to enucleate eyes. Thirty states now have
enabling legislation and over 1,700 morticians have been
trained since 1969.[29] This program promises to supply a
large number of donor eyes as time goes on. Another mechanism used in the state of Maryland has been legislation
that allows the cornea with a scleral rim to be removed on
all coroner cases. For this reason, the Maryland Eye Bank
processes large volumes of donor corneas for local, national
and international use and demonstrates the value of such
legislative efforts.

As to the future of eye banking, increasing standards and
regulations of eye banks is inevitable. A new allied health
category of eye bank technicians will most likely be developed. Unlimited donor material will hopefully become a
reality through legislative and public educational efforts.
Unlimited storage duration of donor material utilizing various donor methods will be possible and available to all surgeons on an elective basis. Assessment of endothelial viability will be possible. (Perhaps the clinical specular microscope will soon make this a reality.[4]) If proved to be valuable, tissue typing will be routinely performed on all donors.
Maybe antigenic modification during the storage will be
possible. Under any circumstances eye banking will become
more technically sophisticated and expensive and probably
will be limited to regional centers that can readily supply

the needs of all surgeons in that region with high-quality sterile donor corneas.

Donald J. Doughman, M.D.
University of Minnesota

## REFERENCES

1. Laibson, P. R.: Introduction – The Cornea, in Hughes, W. F. (ed.): *Year Book of Ophthalmology* (Chicago, Ill.: Year Book Medical Publishers, 1974).
2. Van Horn, D. L., and Schultz, R. O.: Corneal Preservation: Recent Advances, Surv. Ophthalmol. 21:301 – 312, 1977.
3. Saleeby, S. S.: Keratoplasty: Results Using Donor Tissue Beyond 48 Hours, Arch. Ophthalmol. 87:538 – 539, 1972.
4. Bourne, W. M., and Kaufman, H. E.: The Endothelium of Clear Corneal Transplant, Arch. Ophthalmol. 94:1730 – 1732, 1976.
5. Capella, J. A., Kaufman, H. E., and Robbins, J. E.: Preservation of Viable Corneal Tissue, Arch. Ophthalmol. 74:669 – 673, 1965.
6. Bito, L. Z., and Salvador, E. V.: Intraocular Fluid Dynamics 2. Post-mortem Changes in Solute Concentration, Exp. Eye Res. 10:273 – 287, 1970.
7. Brightbill, F. S., Pollack, F. M., and Slappey, T.: A Comparison of Two Methods of Cutting Donor Corneal Buttons, Am. J. Ophthalmol. 75:500 – 506, 1973.
8. Slappey, T. E.: Corneal Preservation, Transplant. Proc. 8, Suppl. 1, 223 – 227, 1976.
9. Kaufman, H. E.: Corneal Cryopreservation and its Clinical Application, Transplant. Proc. 8, Suppl. 1, 149 – 152, 1976.
10. McCarey, B. E., and Kaufman, H. E.: Improved Corneal Storage, Invest. Ophthalmol. 13:165 – 173, 1974.
11. Van Horn, D. L., Schultz, R. O., and DeBruin, J.: Endothelial Survival in Corneal Tissue Stored in M-K Medium, Am. J. Ophthalmol. 80:642 – 647, 1975.
12. Breslin, C. W., Sherrard, E. S., Marshall, J., and Rice, N. S. C.: Evaluation of the McCarey-Kaufman Technique of Corneal Storage, Arch. Ophthalmol. 94:1545 – 1551, 1976.
13. Friedland, B. R., and Forster, R. K.: Comparison of Corneal Storage in McCarey-Kaufman Medium, Moist Chamber or Standard Eye Bank Conditions, Invest. Ophthalmol. 15: 143 – 147, 1976.

14. Aguavella, J. V., Van Horn, D. L., and Haggerty, C. J.: Corneal Preservation Using M-K Media, Am. J. Ophthalmol. 80: 791–799, 1975.

15. Bigar, F., Kaufman, H. E., McCarey, B. E., and Binder, P. S.: Improved Corneal Storage for Penetrating Keratoplasties in Man, Am. J. Ophthalmol. 79:115–120, 1975.

16. Stark, W. J., Maumanee, A. E., and Kenyon, K. R.: Intermediate-Term Corneal Storage for Penetrating Keratoplasty, Am. J. Ophthalmol. 79:795–802, 1975.

17. McCarey, B. E., Meyer, R. F., and Kaufman, H. E.: Improved Corneal Storage For Penetrating Keratoplasties in Humans, Ann. Ophthalmol. 8:1488–1495, 1976.

18. LeFrancois, M., and Baum, J. L.: Flavobacterium Endophthalmitis Following Keratoplasty, Arch. Ophthalmol. 94:1907–1909, 1976.

19. Lemp, M. A.: Pseudomonas Endophthalmitis Following Penetrating Keratoplasty With Corneal Tissue Preserved in M-K Medium. Presented at the scientific session, Eye Bank Association of America, Oct. 5, 1976, Las Vegas.

20. Jones, D. B.: Personal Communication.

21. Lindstrom, R. L., Doughman, D. J., Van Horn, D. L., Dancil, D., and Harris, J. E.: A Metabolic and Electron Microscopic Study of Human Organ-Cultured Cornea, Am. J. Ophthalmol. 82:72–82, 1976.

22. Doughman, D. J., Van Horn, D. L., Harris, J. E., Miller, G. E., Lindstrom, R. L., and Good, R. A.: The Ultrastructure of Human Organ-Cultured Cornea, Arch. Ophthalmol. 92:516–523, 1974.

23. Doughman, D. J., Van Horn, D. L., Rodman, W. P., Byrnes, P., and Lindstrom, R. L.: Human Corneal Endothelial Layer Repair During Organ Culture, Arch. Ophthalmol. 94:1791–1796, 1976.

24. Doughman, D. J., Harris, J. E., and Schmitt, M. K.: Penetrating Keratoplasty Using 37° C Organ-Cultured Cornea, Trans. Am. Acad. Ophthalmol. Otolaryngol. 81:778–793, 1976.

25. Doughman, D. J., Miller, G. E., Mindrup, E. A., Harris, J. E. and Good, R. A.: The Fate of Experimental Organ-Cultured Corneal Xenografts, Transplantation 22:132–137, 1976.

26. Meyer, H. M.: Standards For Tissue Banks and Transplantation, Transplant. Proc. 8, Suppl. 1, 253–255, 1976.

27. McTigue, J. W., Magovern, M., and Beauchamp, G.: A Survey of Eye Banks Reporting Bacterial Infection Following Keratoplasty, Presented at the Scientific Session, Eye Bank Association of America Meeting, Oct. 5, 1976, Las Vegas, Nevada.

28. DeVoe, A. G.: Complications of Keratoplasty, Am. J. Ophthalmol. 79:907–912, 1975.
29. Fisher, Ruth: Personal Communication, Iowa Eye Bank.

**In Vitro Biology of Corneal Epithelium and Endothelium.** Myron Yanoff[4] (Univ. of Pennsylvania) studied cellular contact inhibition as it pertains to the corneal epithelium and endothelium. Primary corneal epithelial explants were prepared from adult Dutch female rabbits or adult albino rabbits. Primary corneal endothelial explants were prepared from stripped Descemet's membrane from adult rabbits. Endothelial explants were also prepared from 6-month-old pigs, and epithelial-endothelial collision studies were done using tissues from rabbits. Full-thickness corneal organ cultures were prepared from the excised corneas of adult rabbits, dogs, pigs and human beings. Autoradiographic studies were done with use of tritiated thymidine.

Modified Eagle's minimal essential medium (MEM) with-

Fig 10.—Full-thickness cornea organ culture at 48 hours. Note relatively acellular stromal zone near cut edge. *En*, endothelium; *Ep*, epithelium; culture from dog cornea. Hematoxylin-eosin; reduced from ×40. (Courtesy of Yanoff, M.: Trans. Am. Ophthalmol. Soc. 73:571–620, 1975.)

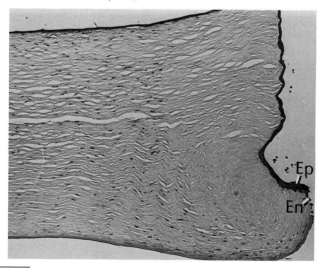

out serum proved to be the optimal method for growth of
corneal epithelium. Epithelial outgrowths and the epithelium and endothelium of corneal organ cultures migrated and
proliferated in MEM without added serum. Corneal epithelium grew rapidly in culture as a multilayered, cohesive
outgrowth with a smooth advancing edge; its growth was
limited to a period of about 2 weeks. Endothelium grew as a
monolayered cohesive outgrowth with a serrated advancing
edge. Migration was delayed up to 48 hours but then had a
steady growth pattern which was continuous and limited
only by the size of the culture dish. Epithelium and endothelium were easily differentiated in collision tissue culture
studies in which epithelial growth migrated over nearly half
of the corneal stroma until its contact with endothelium, at
which point it showed no further advance (Fig 10). In cor-

**Fig 11.** – Epithelial downgrowth in eye of patient. Note how epithelium has grown
over only posterior aspect of superior cornea, ending in a horizontally linear line
*(arrow).* (Courtesy of Yanoff, M.: Trans. Am. Ophthalmol. Soc. 73:571–620, 1975;
from Yanoff, M., and Fine, B. S.: *Ocular Pathology: A Text and Atlas* [Hagerstown:
Harper & Row, 1975, p. 133.])

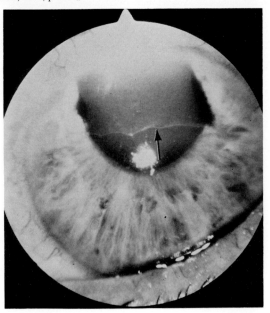

neal organ cultures, epithelium and endothelium had a mutually inhibiting effect on contact, no further migration of either tissue taking place. Clinically, epithelial downgrowth involves two thirds of the cornea surface after cataract extraction, and is inhibited on contact with healthy endothelium (Fig 11). In whole corneal organ culture, the endothelium showed some release from contact inhibition in time, the normally monolayered tissue becoming multilayered in areas. If serum was not added to MEM, the corneal epithelium became keratinized after about 4 days in culture, producing a model for the study of corneal epithelial keratinization.

The findings suggest that, if the corneal endothelium is healthy in vivo, it can inhibit epithelial growth. The inhibition observed would explain the sparing of the inferior cornea by epithelial downgrowth. If the endothelium is not healthy or is covered, the epithelium probably will not be inhibited and will grow into the eye after surgery.

► [It has been puzzling why epithelial downgrowth after corneal transplantation rarely occurs. Yanoff's thesis provides a sound experimental explanation; that is, that healthy corneal endothelium inhibits growth of corneal epithelium. Experimental epithelial downgrowths have been notoriously difficult to produce, perhaps because of intact endothelium. One cannot help but wonder if any method of cataract extraction which abuses the endothelium might increase the incidence of this dreaded complication. No doubt limbal-based conjunctival flaps and better suturing of the wound help prevent epithelial downgrowth although the endothelium has been compromised. — Ed.] ◄

**Recurrent Erosion of the Cornea.** Nicholas Brown and Anthony Bron[5] (London) studied patients presenting with suspected recurrent corneal erosion who had a history of trauma or abrasion, followed by recurrent pain with healing and then a clinical recurrence or at least two attacks suggestive of recurrent erosion without a history of trauma but associated with clinical signs of recurrent erosion at some time. The 80 patients studied were aged 24–73. The control group included 200 patients aged 20–85 without corneal symptoms or a history of corneal disease. Initial treatment was with chloramphenicol drops or chloramphenicol ointment with 0.5% hyoscine drops and padding for the eye. Large bags of loose epithelium were debrided under slit-

(5) Br. J. Ophthalmol. 60:84–96, February, 1976.

lamp control. When healing did not occur, debridement was repeated and followed by carbolization with 100% phenol. Patients then applied 5% NaCl ointment before going to bed. Treatment was continued for 3 – 18 months or longer when relapses occurred.

Macroform erosions occurred in 10% of patients, microform erosions in 56% and both types in 31%. The macroform type was more often related to trauma but 40% of cases were spontaneous in origin. The most common cause of initial trauma was a fingernail. Recurrences occurred at about the time of waking. Eye rubbing was admitted by 10% of patients. Superficial corneal dystrophies of the fingerprint lines, bleb and Bietti's lacunar (maplike) types were found in the healed state in 59% of patients. Epithelial microcysts were found in 59% of patients; they were sometimes of the Cogan type. Only 11% of patients had no corneal signs in the healed state. Control subjects had a very low incidence of dystrophies and cysts. Debridement was done initially in 12 eyes and later in 4; it assisted healing, but did not prevent recurrences. Carbolization was used to treat 7 eyes and appeared to reduce the recurrence rate. The recurrence rate increased when NaCl ointment prophylaxis was withdrawn.

Anomalous production of basement membrane material and other connective tissue sheets probably occurs in these patients. The defect is commonly present in the cornea before the initial trauma. Fluid collecting in or beneath the epithelium at night and adherence of the epithelium to the tarsal conjunctiva are possible factors leading to recurrences.

▶ [The usual keen observations of these clinicians point out that recurrent erosions of the corneal epithelium usually occur after macerating injuries or in predisposed corneas with underlying superficial disturbance of basement and Bowman's membranes (e.g., lattice dystrophy), and that residual abnormalities can often be observed between attacks which break down later. The pathogenesis may also lie in abnormal epithelium which heals poorly (see the next article), especially associated with inflammation and hyposensitivity. The corneal epithelium has amazing powers of rapid regeneration; e.g., over a corneal graft completely denuded of epithelium, when given a smooth Bowman's surface over which to glide and if the advancing edge of epithelium is composed of normal cells. Proteolytic enzymes such as collagenase in macerated or abnormal epithelium or inflammatory cells might well prevent a firm adhesion of the basement membrane to Bowman's membrane. I am a believer in clean removal of abnormal epithelium in such cases by gently scraping it off with a round-ed No. 15 Bard Parker blade, leaving a clean sharp edge, but the rationale of applying a cauterizing agent such as phenol or iodine to the denuded cornea eludes me. – Ed.] ◄

**Pathogenesis and Treatment of Persistent Epithelial Defects.** Retention of a smooth, transparent corneal surface is of major importance in maintaining normal vision, but the integrity of this surface is frequently challenged by injury or disease. H. Dwight Cavanagh, Donovan Pihlaja, Richard A. Thoft and Claes H. Dohlman[6] (Boston) followed 155 patients from 1973 to 1975 with persistent epithelial defects. Herpetic corneal disease was the cause in 74 cases. In 68 cases of simplex infection, the mean duration of disease before formation of a persistent defect was 10.2 years. Seventeen persistent defects followed chemical burns. Delayed postsurgical epithelial healing was present in 19 cases, recurrent corneal erosion in 14 and dry-eye syndromes in 10. Eight patients had anterior segment necrosis, 7 had bacterial corneal infection, 4 had neuroparalytic keratitis and 2 had fungal corneal infection.

Persistent epithelial defects usually occurred in severely damaged corneas and often were associated with reduced or absent corneal sensation. The defects had a distinct predilection for the central visual part of the cornea, and half were over 20 mm$^2$ in size. Ultrastructural study showed an irregular epithelial surface with absent microvilli and loss of the normal stratified architecture of the layer of cells near the defect edge. Cell degeneration and death were frequent in all cell layers. Cytoplasmic projections were associated with disintegration of adjacent anterior stromal collagen. Even the constant use of all types of bandage lenses failed to result in prompt healing. Only one of the 29 patients whose corneas perforated had never received topical steroids.

Early and continuous use of a soft-bandage contact lens is recommended if patching is unsuccessful, and frequent wetting with normal saline or tear substitutes is necessary. An appropriate antibiotic should be instilled twice daily. Topical steroids are used only very cautiously. A collagenase inhibitor may be useful in treating stromal melting. A conjunctival flap with subsequent penetrating keratoplasty is considered early if the potential for corneal recovery with

(6)   Trans. Am. Acad. Ophthalmol. Otolaryngol. 81:754–769, Sept.–Oct., 1976.

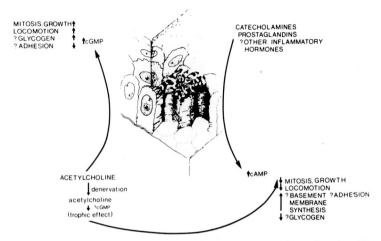

MITOSIS. GROWTH ↑
LOCOMOTION ↑
? GLYCOGEN ↑    ↑cGMP
? ADHESION ↓

CATECHOLAMINES
PROSTAGLANDINS
? OTHER INFLAMMATORY
HORMONES

ACETYLCHOLINE

↓ denervation

acetylcholine
↓ ?cGMP
(trophic effect)

↑cAMP

MITOSIS. GROWTH ↓
LOCOMOTION ↓
? BASEMENT ? ADHESION
MEMBRANE
SYNTHESIS
? GLYCOGEN ↓

**Fig 12.** — Proposed mechanism for biochemical regulation of growth and proliferation of corneal epithelium. (Courtesy of Cavanagh, H. D., et al.: Trans. Am. Acad. Ophthalmol. Otolaryngol. 81:754–769, Sept.–Oct., 1976.)

good vision is poor, especially if stromal melting is proceeding rapidly.

A proposed mechanism for corneal epithelial growth is shown in Figure 12. One would predict that the worst inhibition of epithelial wound healing would occur when inflammatory factors that increase cellular cyclic AMP levels are coupled with depression of cholinergic levels in neurotropic eyes. This combination was observed to some degree in all patients in whom persistent epithelial defects developed.

**Effects of Ophthalmic Drugs, Vehicles and Preservatives on Corneal Epithelium: Scanning Electron Microscope Study.** Scanning electron microscopy (SEM) has shown loss of microvilli, interruption of cell membranes and clumping of tonofilaments after the application of tetracycline and several other ophthalmic preparations to the corneal surface. Roswell R. Pfister and Neal Burstein[7] (Univ. of Colorado) attempted to evaluate the component effect of some commonly used topical drugs, vehicles and preservatives on the surface corneal epithelium by SEM. The preparations were tested in vivo in their clinical concentrations

(7) Invest. Ophthalmol. 15:246–259, April, 1976.

and volumes. Drug components in 0.9% saline were instilled in the eyes of albino rabbits and specimens were taken for SEM at varying intervals afterwards. Benzalkonium chloride (BAK) was evaluated after scraping off the corneal epithelium of 5 anesthetized rabbits; 2 corneal buttons were obtained for evaluation from patients with keratoconus 1 hour after application of 2% pilocarpine alone or 2% pilocarpine with 0.01% BAK.

The results are summarized in the table. Pure forms of the topical anesthetics 0.5% tetracaine and 0.5% proparacaine had no plasma membrane effects, though 0.3% gentamicin caused erection of central cellular microvilli. Significant plasma membrane injury and cell death were caused by

DRUGS, VEHICLES AND PRESERVATIVES USED IN RABBITS WITH RESPECTIVE SEM CORNEAL EFFECTS*

| Topical preparation | | SEM surface effect |
|---|---|---|
| *Preparations causing no plasma membrane effects:* | | |
| Drugs: | Atropine 1% | |
| | Chloromycetin 0.5% | Surface epithelial microvilli normal in |
| | Epinephryl borate 1% | size, shape, and distribution. |
| | Gentamicin 0.3% | |
| | Proparacaine 0.5% | |
| | Tetracaine 0.5% | No denuded cells. |
| Vehicles: | Boric acid 5% in petrolatum mineral oil | Cell junctions intact. |
| | Methylcellulose 0.5% | Plasma membranes not wrinkled. |
| | Polyvinyl alcohol 1.6% | |
| | Saline 0.9% | |
| Preservatives: | Chlorbutanol 0.5% | Usual number of epithelial "holes." |
| | Disodium edatate 0.1% | |
| | Thimerosal 0.01% | |
| *Preparations causing moderate plasma membrane effects:* | | |
| Drugs: | Phospholine iodide 0.25% | Most cells normal. |
| | Pilocarpine 2% | |
| | Fluorescein 2% | Some cells show loss of microvilli and |
| | Fluor-I-Strip (wet with one drop 0.9% saline) | wrinkling of plasma membranes. |
| | | A small number of cells showed disruption of plasma membrane with premature cellular desquamation. |
| *Preparations causing significant plasma membrane injury and cell death:* | | |
| Drugs: | Cocaine 4% | Complete loss of microvilli. |
| | Neopolycin (No BAK) | Wrinkling of plasma membranes. |
| | | Premature desquamation of top layer of cells. |
| | | Severe epithelial microvillous loss. |
| Preservatives: | Benzalkonium chloride 0.01% | Severe membrane disruption. |
| Drug + Preserva-tive: | Pilocarpine 2% or | Death and desquamation of 2 superficial |
| | Gentamicin 0.3% + Benzalkonium chloride 0.01% | layers of cells over 3-hour period. |

*Each preparation was tested in 4–6 rabbit eyes.

BAK. Loss of microvilli and premature desquamation were noted after topical 4% cocaine or neopolycin without BAK. Severe plasma membrane disruption and destruction were seen in the human corneal specimens after the application of 2% pilocarpine with 0.01% BAK. Loss of microvilli and plasma membrane destruction were seen in the surface cells after the application of 2% pilocarpine alone.

The cytotoxicity of topical ocular preparations can be tested in an in vivo model and evaluated by SEM. The extensive use of BAK in ophthalmic preparations must be reviewed critically and, if indicated, its use should be curtailed.

► [In this and the following article, the artistically abstract pictures of scanning electron microscopy of the corneal epithelium leave no doubt of the deleterious effects of the cationic surfactants, benzalkonium chloride (Zephiran) and cetylpyridinium chloride, which are used in drug solutions to preserve penetration of the drugs through the epithelium. The clinician can occasionally relieve recalcitrant healing of the epithelium by avoiding those drug preparations containing these substances. — Ed.] ◄

**Electrophysiologic and Anatomical Effects of Cetyl-pyridinium Chloride on the Rabbit Cornea.** Both benzalkonium chloride (BA) and cetylpyridinium chloride (CPC), which are cationic surfactants, have been shown to markedly increase corneal permeability to fluorescein in conjunction with lysis of the outermost cell membranes. Keith Green[8] (Med. College of Georgia) studied the effects of CPC on the cornea in electrophysiologic and anatomical studies done on in vivo and in vitro rabbit corneas. Ringer's solution containing 0.21, 0.56 and 2 mM CPC was used in the in vitro physiologic studies, whereas 0.56 mM or 2 mM CPC was used in the in vivo studies. All three concentrations of CPC were used in the anatomic studies.

Cetylpyridinium chloride caused hyperpolarization of the potential difference at all concentrations and exposure times. Longer exposure times caused greater subsequent falls in potential difference (PD). The recovery rate of the PD to normal pretreatment levels was also exposure time and concentration dependent. Patterns of PD change were similar in the in vitro and in vivo studies. Loss of microplicae from the cells was observed at 0.56 mM CPC. At 2 mM CPC the underlying cells were exposed. More extensive ap-

(8)   Acta Ophthalmol. (Kbh.) 54:145–159, April, 1976.

plication of these solutions led to surface pitting and apparent holes in the cell membrane.

In many respects the effects of CPC on the electrophysiology and anatomy of the rabbit cornea parallel those of BA. Surfactants alter the electric characteristics of the cornea and may affect fixed surface and tissue charges, but their major effect is to enhance the penetration of drugs, especially in ionic form, across the relatively impermeable epithelium. Cetylpyridinium chloride eliminates the physiologic and anatomic barrier to fluid movement in the corneal epithelium by destroying the cell membranes and causing lysis of the cells. Sanction of the use of CPC in ophthalmic preparations as a protein-drug unbinding agent appears to be premature. Long-term testing is needed to assure the safety of incorporating this surfactant in ophthalmic preparations.

**Effects of Artificial Intraocular Pressure Elevation on the Corneal Endothelium in the Vervet Monkey** *(Cercopithecus ethiops).* High intraocular pressure may lead to decompensation of the corneal endothelium that permits excess fluid to enter the corneal stroma from the anterior chamber, but it is not clear whether this is due to the high pressure itself or to secondary damage to the endothelial cells. Björn Svedbergh[9] (Univ. of Uppsala) studied the effects of a moderate rise in intraocular pressure, lasting some hours, on the ultrastructure of the corneal endothelium in 10 adult vervet monkeys. The intraocular pressure was raised by perfusion to 33 – 44 mm Hg in one eye and by a few mm Hg above the spontaneous level (12 – 15 mm Hg) in the other. Equal flow through both anterior chambers was obtained with use of infusion pumps; mock aqueous humor was used for perfusion fluid. The animals were killed after 3 – 7 hours. Autoradiography was performed with tritiated thymidine.

A patchy haze appeared in the anterior stroma of the eyes subjected to high pressures after about 2 hours, followed by epithelial bedewing. The peripheral part of the cornea was more susceptible to damage than the central part. The cells were often flattened and unevenness of the cell surface was increased toward the anterior chamber. Vacuolation oc-

(9)   Acta Ophthalmol. (Kbh.) 53:839 – 855, December, 1975.

curred both within and between cells and mitochondrial swelling was observed. The perinuclear space was slightly distended. More severe changes included a progressive loss of intracellular organization, loss of cilia and disruption of the apical cell junction. Balloon-like protrusions or blebs budded off or burst, leaving gaping craters behind. Even whole cells were lost. Repair was quite efficient; neither stromal patchy opacities nor epithelial bedewing were noted after 3 and 10 days.

Elevated intraocular pressure presumably leads to increased leakage through the intercellular spaces that is counteracted by the fluid pump up to a certain intraocular pressure level. Increased cell compression and distention of the whole bulb also occur, the latter leading to lateral stretching of the endothelial cells. Eventually the structural barriers to fluid passage are broken down and aqueous accumulates near Descemet's membrane. Similar morphologic changes have been observed in glaucoma. Probably rapid, marked endothelial cell damage occurs in acute glaucoma, whereas in chronic glaucoma the damage is more gradual, making continuous healing possible. Corneal damage may underlay the development of corneal aqueous veins in long-standing glaucoma.

► [These experiments in monkeys indicate that the degree and duration of elevated intraocular pressure is directly related to damage of the corneal endothelium. Most clinicians are aware that a later cataract extraction after a previous attack of acute angle closure glaucoma carries a high risk of development of bullous keratopathy, but perhaps are less cognizant that the same applies to a lesser extent in open-angle glaucoma. – Ed.] ◄

**Methenamine Silver-Stained Corneal Scrapings in Keratomycosis** were investigated by Richard K. Forster, Mary G. Wirta, Manuel Solis and Gerbert Rebell[1] (Univ. of Miami). Treatment of most cases of mycotic keratitis can be successful if topical antimycotic therapy is started early. Usually an immediate diagnosis is possible by examination of corneal scrapings microscopically, but the Gram and Giemsa stains and potassium hydroxide wet mount have not been entirely satisfactory. It may be difficult to detect fungi by these methods, especially in early ulcers where little

(1)   Am. J. Ophthalmol. 82:261–265, August, 1976.

fungus may be present. More satisfactory results have been obtained by staining corneal scrapings by Grocott's methenamine-silver technique. The procedure was modified to reduce the time from 2 hours to 1.

TECHNIQUE. — A drop of warm 1% gelatin solution is placed on a slide and a film is spread with another slide. Corneal scrapings from the ulcer are spread on coated slides and fixed in methenamine for 5 minutes before being stained by either the standard or the shortened methenamine-silver procedure. In the shortened method, oxidation of the slide in 5% chromic acid is limited to 30 minutes, and the slide is placed in methenamine-silver solution heated to 58–60 C. Processing by the standard Grocott procedure follows. Staining with light green is for 40 seconds.

Gram- and Giemsa-stained smears can be passed through the methenamine-silver procedure with good results. Fungous hyphae appear black against a pale green tissue background, and the septa should be clearly visible. It is often advisable to run a control histologic section containing known fungi through the staining procedure to monitor the optimal time for removal of the scrapings from the methenamine-silver solution.

Good fungus-positive slides have been obtained with this method. The authors no longer use potassium hydroxide preparations. Results were positive with methenamine-silver staining in 89% of 9 culture-positive cases, compared with 60% with the Giesma method, 54% with the Gram stain and 25% with potassium hydroxide wet mounts. The total time required is no longer than with the Giemsa method.

► [Doctor John Ayer, Professor of Pathology at Rush Medical College, states that the Grocott methenamine-silver stain is one of the best stains for general detection of fungi. – Ed.] ◄

**Treatment of External Ocular *Candida* Infections with 5-Fluorocytosine.** A. Romano, E. Segal, E. Eylan and R. Stein[2] (Tel Aviv Univ.) studied the efficacy of 5-fluorocytosine, an antimycotic agent effective in treating various clinical *Candida* infections, in the management of external ocular mycotic infections. Fifteen patients with chronic ocular *Candida* infections who had not responded to Mycostatin or amphotericin B were evaluated. They were among 77 pa-

(2) Ophthalmologica 172:282–286, 1976.

tients treated for *Candida* infections of the eye during a 3-year period.

Thirteen patients had chronic blepharoconjunctivitis and 6 of these also had canaliculitis. One patient had bilateral superficial and subepithelial keratitis and 1 a corneal ulcer. All patients with blepharoconjunctivitis were over age 40; both the other patients were young. Ten patients were women and *Candida* infection of the genital tract was present in 2 of them. A 1% solution of 5-fluorocytosine was given topically in a dose of 2-3 drops, 6 times daily. Two patients also received 5-fluorocytosine tablets in a dosage of 100–120 mg/kg daily.

Half the patients had previously received antibiotics and steroids topically for a prolonged period and Mycostatin had been used for at least 3 months. Twelve patients had not responded, 2 had recurrences and 1 had an allergic reaction to Mycostatin. In 10 patients, yeasts had persisted despite the treatment. All patients responded favorably to 5-fluorocytosine but treatment for at least 3–6 months was necessary. No resistance to treatment was observed. Topical treatment was inadequate only in the patient with bilateral recurrent keratitis but satisfactory results were obtained when oral 5-fluorocytosine was added. No side effects were noted in any patient.

It seems apparent that 5-fluorocytosine is effective in the treatment of external *Candida* ocular infections but its efficacy in intraocular infections remains to be determined. No side effects were noted in the present study and no resistance to the drug developed.

► [This halogenated pyrimidine has a relatively low spectrum of activity except against *C. albicans* and *Cryptococcus neoformans,* but resistant strains of *C. albicans* have been reported. However, this drug penetrates the eye well, and is almost nontoxic both locally and orally. – Ed.] ◄

**Amoebic Infection of the Eye: Pathologic Report.** Norman Ashton and William Stamm[3] (London) review the histologic findings in a previously reported case of acanthamebic keratitis and the findings in 756 other cases of keratitis and ulcerative keratitis with respect to this diagnosis. An initial biopsy specimen of the cornea showed only nonspecific inflammation, but later specimens yielded troph-

(3)  Trans. Ophthalmol. Soc. U.K. 95(Pt. 2):214–220, 1975.

ozoites and cysts of *Acanthamoeba (Hartmannella)* on special staining and immunofluorescence study with Ryan and A-1 antiserums (Fig 13). Electron microscopic study showed a typical trophozoite of *Acanthamoeba* and a phagocytosed polygonal cyst. *Acanthamoeba* organisms were readily isolated on nonnutrient agar plates seeded with *Escherichia coli* or *Aerobacter aerogenes.* The eye itself exhibited almost total absence of the cornea, dense stromal polymorphonuclear infiltration with abscess formation in the deep cornea and partial detachment of Descemet's membrane. The lens showed very early cortical cataractous changes anteriorly and a light inflammatory infiltrate was present in the retina, optic nerve and choroid. The sclera was normal.

To identify amoebae in tissue sections stained by routine histologic methods is extremely difficult. Special staining methods are of value in demonstrating cysts, but are of little value in identifying trophozoites. The gelatinous capsules of cysts stain intensely with Heidenhain's hematoxylin, Gomori's chromium hematoxylin, periodic acid-Schiff, Bauer chromic acid-Schiff and silver techniques. Indirect immunofluorescence staining can be used to identify trophozoites if suitable antiserums are available.

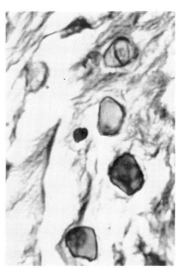

**Fig 13.** —Section of corneal disc showing several thick-walled cysts selectively stained with silver methenamine. Grocott-Gomori stain; reduced from ×750. (Courtesy of Ashton, N., and Stamm, W.: Trans Ophthalmol. Soc. U. K. 95(Pt. 2):214–220, 1975.)

Of the 756 cases of keratitis or corneal ulceration reviewed, 106 were selected for silver methenamine staining because of large cells resembling trophozoites or cysts and 20 were examined by immunofluorescence staining. No case of amoebic infection in the cornea or anterior segment was found, which suggests that the condition may be a very new entity or extremely rare, although the organisms are difficult to find in sections.

► [These are the histologic findings in the case reported by Nagington et al. (see the 1975 YEAR BOOK, p. 90). As the authors state, a review of 106 cases of keratitis with special silver methenamine staining did not reveal amoebae, although the organisms are difficult to identify in tissue.

However, in the next article, there are 2 additional cases of amoebic disciform and ring abscess type of keratitis and 1 case of amoebic uveitis. As the authors state in their discussion, amoebae are present in air, soil and water, and may infect the cornea especially after trauma and if associated with bacterial infection. Under unfavorable circumstances for the organism, it may become encysted and be resistant to treatment. Reversion to trophozoites is accompanied by greater clinical activity. Although treatment is unsatisfactory, the authors have tried paromomycin 1%, flucytosine 1%, and amphotericin B 0.1% solutions combined with antibacterial therapy. Amoebic uveitis may result from inoculation via the nasopharynx (e.g., in mice), thence transmitted to the eye via the blood stream. Thus, in a chronic ulcerative keratitis, we must suspect not only fungi but amoeba. — Ed.] ◄

### *Acanthamoeba polyphaga* Keratitis and *Acanthamoeba* Uveitis Associated with Fatal Meningoencephalitis.

*Acanthamoeba polyphaga* keratitis was identified in a South Texas rancher after corneal trauma and a second case of *A. polyphaga* corneal infection complicating herpes simplex keratitis was confirmed in a Houston nurse the following year. *Acanthamoeba* was confirmed as the cause of uveitis and fatal meningoencephalitis in a Texas youth in retrospective studies. *Acanthamoeba* has now been confirmed as a new, diverse ocular pathogen. D. B. Jones, G. S. Visvesvara and N. M. Robinson[4] reviewed the previously reported cases of ocular *Acanthamoeba* infection.

The trophozoites of *A. polyphaga* are generally uninucleate and the cysts are double walled. All strains have grown well on standard media without the addition of bacteria. Both inoculation into monkey kidney cell cultures and intranasal inoculation of trophozoites into young mice have

---

(4) Trans. Ophthalmol. Soc. U.K. 95(Pt.2):221–232, 1975.

produced positive results. Pathologic studies in the case of uveitis revealed severe necrosis, chronic inflammatory exudate and multiple amoebic trophozoites. Brain sections showed diffuse edema, multiple cortical abscesses and periventricular necrosis. Amoebic trophozoites were abundant in the cerebral grey matter, cerebellum and medulla. Cysts were not demonstrated. Postmortem cultures of cerebrospinal fluid and brain tissue were negative. Autopsy study of the eye showed acute and chronic inflammation of the iris, ciliary body and vitreous and hemorrhage and necrosis of the ciliary body. The retina exhibited chronic perivascular inflammation and the optic disc was edematous. The patient had waded in drainage ditches and might have been immersed in a cattle trough.

Amoebic keratitis, characterized by disciform disease with epithelial ulceration and dense suppuration along segments of the perimeter, can be diagnosed with the use of standard microbiologic stains and media. The confirmation of *Acanthamoeba* as a cause of human uveitis merits further investigation.

► ↓ In the following three articles, Brown and his associates make a case for the presence of collagenase and proteoglycanases in the conjunctiva adjacent to Mooren's corneal ulcer. This tissue contains large numbers of plasma cells, suggesting an immune mechanism. In the immunofluorescent study of limbal conjunctiva in 3 cases of Mooren's ulcer, the second of the three articles, IgG, IgM and C3 complement were found, but in the first article, Brown stated that "repeated attempts to identify immune globulins in the conjunctiva via fluorescent antibody staining were negative."

Ophthalmologists are painfully aware that treatment of a typical Mooren's ulcer has been unsatisfactory. Many treatments have been tried without notable success; e.g., antibiotics, corticosteroids, subconjunctival heparin, anticollagenase inhibitors such as cysteine, acetylcysteine and sodium ethylenediamine tetra-acetic acid, cryotherapy, conjunctival flaps, delimiting keratotomy, excision of superficial corneal tissue in front of the ulcer or lamellar grafts which usually melt. In view of the evidence that the adjacent conjunctiva contains proteolytic enzymes, Brown, in the third article, found excision of 4 mm or more of conjunctiva adjacent to the Mooren's ulcer to be curative in 8 of 10 cases. Doctors Wilson, II, Grayson and Ellis (Br. J. Ophthalmol. 60:713, 1976) reported good results in 7 cases and 1 failure after "limbal conjunctivectomy" in diverse conditions with marginal ulceration such as Mooren's ulcer, gonococcal keratoconjunctivitis, rheumatoid arthritis with marginal ulcer, keratoconjunctivitis sicca, rosacea keratitis and thermal burn. There is a spectrum of etiology and severity of marginal degenerations, some of which like Terrien's gutter dystrophy respond well to lamellar corneal transplantation, but in others like a classic Mooren's ulcer which progresses "relentlessly" to the center of the cornea, a resection of limbal conjunctiva might be tried in view of the above evidence. — Ed. ◄

**Mooren's Ulcer: Histopathology and Proteolytic Enzymes of Adjacent Conjunctiva.** The conjunctiva adjacent to Mooren's ulcers has been reported to exhibit collagenolytic activity. Stuart I. Brown[5] (Univ. of Pittsburgh) examined excised limbal conjunctiva adjacent to Mooren's ulcers by light and electron microscopy. Collagenolytic activity was assayed in tissue cultures of normal human conjunctiva and collagenase was assayed with use of radioactive collagen prepared from guinea pig skin with $^{14}$C-glycine.

Excised, ulcerated corneal tissue exhibited many lymphocytes and polymorphonuclear leukocytes. The conjunctival epithelium was intact in most sections, whereas the subepithelial tissues were packed with plasma cells. Similar findings were recorded in 4 specimens of conjunctiva. Fewer cells were seen in specimens from an eye having multiple excisions of conjunctiva. Growth of excised conjunctiva on collagen gels resulted in total gel lysis within 48 hours; lesser lysis was seen with conjunctiva from normal eyes. Cysteine, sodium ethylenediamine tetra-acetic acid and serum did not prevent gel lysis by conjunctiva from eyes with Mooren's ulcer. Harvest media completely lysed radioactive collagen gels and reduced the specific viscosity of a solution of collagen. Viscosity of corneal proteoglycan was degraded by the harvest media. Heat inactivated the enzymatic activity of the media. Polyacrylamide gel electrophoresis of the reaction mixture showed collagen breakdown products typical of mammalian collagenase.

Excised corneal epithelium and limbal conjunctiva from cases of Mooren's ulcer contain a true collagenase. Collagen gel breakdown by the conjunctiva was at least 10 times greater than that caused by a similar quantity of diseased corneal tissues previously examined. The conjunctiva adjacent to Mooren's ulcers contains large numbers of plasma cells and produces a collagenolytic enzyme and probably a proteoglycanolytic enzyme. The ulcers heal after excision of

(5)  Br. J. Ophthalmol. 59:670–674, November, 1975.

this tissue, indicating that the conjunctiva is intimately involved in the pathogenesis of Mooren's ulcers.

**Autoimmune Phenomenon in Mooren's Ulcer.** Mooren's ulcer is a chronic, painful ulceration of unknown etiology, starting in the corneal periphery and progressing relentlessly, at last centrally, to involve the entire cornea. Recent studies have shown that metabolic products from tissue culture of the adjacent conjunctiva can degrade collagen and corneal proteoglycan, and study of the excised conjunctiva has shown it to be heavily infiltrated with plasma cells and lymphocytes. Stuart I. Brown, Bartly J. Mondino and Bruce S. Rabin[6] (Univ. of Pittsburgh) documented autoimmune phenomena directed to the conjunctiva in 3 cases of Mooren's ulcer. Direct immunofluorescence studies were done on conjunctival tissue taken from adjacent to the corneal ulcers in 2 cases and adjacent to a healed corneal ulcer in the third. Indirect immunofluorescence studies used normal human conjunctiva and cornea as controls.

The 2 patients with active disease had IgG, IgM and C3 in the intercellular spaces of the surface epithelium and, in some parts of the biopsy specimens, within the epithelial cell cytoplasm. One patient also had IgM along the conjunctival basement membrane and both IgG and IgM within the connective tissue of the conjunctiva. The patient with inactive disease had IgG within epithelial cells but no complement. Fibrinogen was absent in all cases. All 3 patients had circulating antibodies binding to the epithelial cell cytoplasm of normal human cornea and conjunctiva. In 2 cases the titer was higher to conjunctiva than to cornea. Two patients had low titers of antibody to parietal cells. All 3 patients had the HL-A 2 antigen. Two had polyclonal elevations of serum IgA. The 2 studied had normal levels of C3 and C4.

Immunoglobulins localized to the conjunctival epithelium were demonstrated in these 3 cases of Mooren's ulcer, and complement was also present in the 2 active cases. All 3 patients had circulating antibodies to conjunctival and corneal epithelium. Other significant immune alterations were not demonstrated in these patients.

---

(6)   Am. J. Ophthalmol. 82:835–840, December, 1976.

**Mooren's Ulcer: Treatment by Conjunctival Excision.** Mooren's ulcer is a chronic, painful ulceration of unknown cause, starting in the corneal periphery and progressing relentlessly, first circumferentially and then centrally to involve the entire cornea. Consistent healing has not been obtained with any form of treatment. Stuart I. Brown[7] (Univ. of Pittsburgh) reports the results of excision of limbal conjunctiva in eyes with progressive Mooren's ulcers in 7 patients.

Ten eyes with progressing Mooren's or similar ulcers were treated by excising a 3 to 4 mm ring of limbal conjunctiva adjacent to the ulcer. Eight eyes healed within 3 weeks and 7 have remained healed, whereas 1 eye has had repeated ulcers that healed when re-treated by conjunctival excision. In the latter case, repeated conjunctival excisions limited the progress of ulceration to the periphery until a secondary infection caused a dense central corneal opacity. In the 2 eyes that did not heal, repeated conjunctival excision has reduced the severe pain and the size of the ulcers. Complete healing after conjunctival excision has occurred in 5 days to 3 weeks. Patching the lids closed until healing was complete, followed by hypertonic salt solutions, seemed to aid and maintain healing. When conjunctival excision had to be repeated, sharp dissection with a curved Vannas scissors facilitated excision of the conjunctiva that was tightly bound to the sclera.

Excision of conjunctiva may remove a source of antibodies and cornea-destroying enzymes if the ulcerations are an autoimmune phenomenon. There may be a relatively benign form of Mooren's ulcer that heals after a lamellar graft or conjunctival flap procedure and a severe form for which no treatment is successful. The present findings may explain reports of successful treatment of Mooren's ulcers by peritomy and freezing of the conjunctiva. Freezing of conjunctiva was tried for recurrences in 2 of the present patients; progress of the ulcers was stopped temporarily, but they did not heal until the conjunctiva was excised.

**Herpetic Corneal Epithelial Disease.** The ocular epithelial diseases caused by herpes simplex and herpes zoster may appear similar biomicroscopically. Ronald J. Marsh,

(7)  Br. J. Ophthalmol. 59:675–682, November, 1975.

DIFFERENCES BETWEEN HERPES SIMPLEX AND ZOSTER EPITHELIAL KERATITIS

| Disease | Epithelium | Stroma | Tear Film | Staining Characteristic | Mechanical Debridement | Steroid Response | Cutaneous Manifestations | Cytology |
|---|---|---|---|---|---|---|---|---|
| Herpes simplex | Fine, lacy dendrites with or without terminal end bulbs | Variable involvement | Usually normal | Edges stain with rose bengal; denuded ulcer base stains with fluorescein | Can only be removed with epithelium | May cause enlargement | Current or past history of cold sores | Ballooned epithelial cells, syncytial multinucleated giant cells, occasional epithelial cells with intranuclear eosinophilic inclusions; mononuclear leukocytes may be present |
| Herpes zoster acute | Smaller lesions, often stellate; simple raised contour; usually peripheral | None | Mucoid discharge | Stains sparingly with rose bengal and fluorescein | Can only be removed with epithelium | No apparent effect | Typical zoster rash and lid vesicles | Ballooned epithelial cells, multinucleated giant cells, margination of chromatin and glassy basophil, intranuclear inclusion bodies |
| Delayed (corneal mucus plaques) | Coarse, elevated gray-white plaques | Diffuse haze | Unstable with rapid drying time | Brilliant staining of whole lesion with rose bengal, moderate with alcian blue, and sparingly with fluorescein | Can be removed with minimal damage to underlying epithelium | No apparent effect | Typical zoster scarring on same side | Mucus adherent to ballooned epithelial cells with occasional multinucleated giant cells |

Frederick T. Fraunfelder and James I. McGill[8] (Moorfields Eye Hosp., London) reviewed methods of differentiating the dendritic pattern of herpes zoster from that of herpes simplex (table). About 1,100 new cases of ocular herpes simplex and 283 cases of herpes zoster with ocular involvement were seen during 1972 – 74.

Zoster epithelial lesions include acute epithelial dendritic keratitis and delayed corneal mucous plaques. The keratitic lesion was seen in 13% of the patients with ophthalmic zoster and the plaques in 7%. Acute epithelial keratitis is characterized by small, fine, multiple dendritic or stellate lesions which are only intraepithelial on biomicroscopy and are generally located in the peripheral cornea. The typical lesion of mucous plaque keratitis is a whitish gray plaque with sharp margins, lying on the epithelial surface; it is linear or branching in shape. The plaques are usually multiple and may appear anywhere on the cornea. Most are seen 3 – 4 months after onset of the cutaneous lesions.

The dendritic ulcers of herpes simplex have a characteristic arborescent pattern with irregular but sharply defined borders. Terminal end bulbs are present and the epithelial borders of the ulcer are elevated. Alcian blue generally does not stain the lesion appreciably but it does stain corneal mucous plaques. Rose bengal strongly stains the corneal mucous plaque and the margins of herpes simplex ulcers but it stains the small acute dendritic zoster lesions only moderately.

The dendritic lesions of both herpes simplex and zoster can be removed only if the corneal epithelium is removed but corneal mucous plaques are easily removed by gentle scraping. Topical steroids often increase the width of branches of the dendritic lesions caused by herpes simplex. Cytologic studies may be useful and herpes simplex virus can be readily isolated from the edges of its ulcers.

Topical steroids are contraindicated in epithelial herpes simplex but are of value in treating corneal mucous plaque keratitis of zoster. Idoxuridine is of use in herpes simplex keratitis but adversely affects the compromised corneal epithelium in delayed zoster lesions.

(8)   Arch. Ophthalmol. 94:1899 – 1902, November, 1976.

**Herpes Simplex Virus in Human Cornea, Retrocorneal Fibrous Membrane and Vitreous.** Herpes simplex keratouveitis is one of the major treatment problems facing the ophthalmologist. H. Barry Collin and Mark B. Abelson[9] (Massachusetts Eye and Ear Infirm.) studied a case which extends the range of tissues involved by herpes simplex to include the retrocorneal membrane and the vitreous.

Studies were done in a man, aged 60, with an 8-year history of recurrent herpetic keratouveitis. A corneal perforation was treated with a soft lens and patching and a penetrating keratoplasty and cataract extraction were done 6 months later. An opaque edematous graft resulted from violent uveitis despite intensive steroid therapy. A penetrating keratoplasty was performed 10 months after the graft. Dexamethasone and idoxuridine were used but endophthalmitis and wound melting were noted 3 months later and a repeat penetrating keratoplasty was done. A postoperative wound leak was treated with histoacrylate glue. The anterior chamber reformed but an opaque graft resulted.

The cornea removed at the first regraft exhibited a nonvascular retrocorneal membrane (RCM) extending over the posterior corneal surface, almost completely replacing the endothelium. The main cell type in the RCM resembled the fibroblast; a few inflammatory cells were present. Virus-like particles were seen within or just outside the cytoplasm of about 10% of the corneal stromal cells. About half the cells in the RCM contained virus particles and were in various stages of disintegration. Large collections of naked virus particles or "viral crystals" were seen in the nuclei of several cells. The cornea removed at the second regraft had a large proportion of disintegrated fibroblast-like cells containing viral particles. The affected cells were mainly in the center of the cornea. Several cells also showed large "crystal" accumulations of naked virus particles.

A clinical impression of a quiescent inactive cornea before keratoplasty may be deceptive. The unusually violent clinical course in the present patient seems related to the presence of active virus. The identification of cases in which the cytopathologic effect is largely due to viral proliferation and

(9)   Arch. Ophthalmol. 94:1726–1729, October, 1976.

destruction may permit greater selectivity in the use of steroids.

► [This sad story of repeated graft failures in a case of recurrent herpes simplex keratouveitis re-emphasizes the fact described by Dawson et al. (Arch. Ophthalmol. 79:740, 1968) that live "naked" virus particles (DNA cores or "crystals" without capsids and envelopes) which can be cultured may exist in otherwise quiet eyes that have had stromal keratitis. This brings up the practical decision in such cases of whether to use steroids to combat any hypersensitivity factor and reduce the increased likelihood of a graft rejection (see the next article), knowing that the steroid might encourage proliferation and spread of the virus. Perhaps the soluble derivative of vidarabine (adenine arabinoside, Vira-A), viz., Ara AMP (see article by Pavan-Langston et al.) might be used intravenously or subconjunctivally or without steroids. — Ed.] ◄

**Immune Host Response to Corneal Grafts Sensitized to Herpes Simplex Virus.** Stromal herpetic disease is of particular interest in view of its varied clinical picture and its tendency to reactivation. Herpes simplex virus (HSV) has been demonstrated in the stroma of corneas with chronic or acute herpetic disease and also in the stroma and keratocytes of experimental corneas. It has been proposed that stromal keratitis is related to a hypersensitivity mechanism, the viral infection modifying the host cells so that they are considered foreign by the host.

F. Polack, C. Siverio, F. Bigar and Y. Centifanto[1] (Univ. of Florida) studied the fate of corneas sensitized by intrastromal (convalescent) or subcutaneous injections of HSV after transplantation to HSV-sensitized hosts. Studies were done using the McKrae strain of HSV grown in human embryonic lung tissue. Adult albino rabbits received 12 injections of 0.1 ml HSV undiluted stock subcutaneously twice a week. Seventy-six penetrating keratoplasties were done.

The results are shown in Figure 14. Presumably, viral antigens stimulated an immune reaction in the sensitized host. Study of the limbal area in 2 host animals that were systemically sensitized before transplantation showed that the area was free of cellular infiltration. The interval for delayed immune response in a sensitized host was 7 – 10 days. All the grafts opacified within 10 days after transplantation, while only 2 of 16 control grafts opacified, both of

(1)   Invest. Ophthalmol. 15:188 – 195, March, 1976.

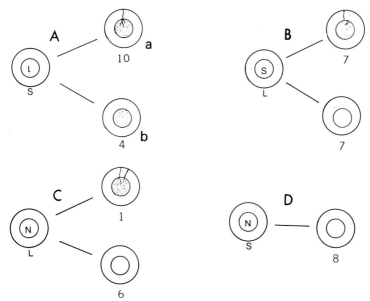

**Fig 14.**—Schema representing results in 4 groups. **A,** locally sensitized grafts in systemically sensitized hosts (14 grafts). All grafts opacified. Cloudiness and vascularization predominated in 10 grafts *(a)* and edema predominated in 4 of them *(b)*. **B,** systemically sensitized grafts in locally sensitized hosts (14 grafts). Seven of the 14 transplants opacified. **C,** normal grafts in locally sensitized hosts (7 grafts). One of 7 grafts opacified. **D,** no graft opacification occurred in this group. *L,* locally sensitized; *S,* systemically sensitized. (Courtesy of Polack, F., et al.: Invest. Ophthalmol. 15:188–195, March, 1976.)

them 3 weeks after keratoplasty. Half the grafts from systemically sensitized rabbits placed in previously infected eyes were opacified, suggesting that viral antigens reached the cornea of the donor animal. Normal corneal grafts in systemically sensitized rabbits were clear for 2 months of follow-up. Cultures of the opacified corneal grafts showed no HSV growth.

Nonspecific eye inflammation may cause cloudiness of a corneal graft but this may be transient and unrelated to an immune response unless the inflammation is by an exaggerated host response and by the introduction of antigens which may be shared by the graft cells, antigens not belonging to but present in the graft. In clinical transplantation, both donor and recipient may be sensitized to HSV since many persons have been exposed to the virus.

**Intraocular Penetration of the Soluble Antiviral, Ara AMP.** Vidarabine is superior to idoxuridine for treating ocular viral infections but little or no parent compound enters the aqueous when given topically or subconjunctivally. Low levels of the metabolite hypoxanthine arabinoside are recoverable. More recent studies have centered on the 5′ monophosphate or nucleotide form of vidarabine, Ara AMP, which appears to be equipotent with vidarabine in the treatment of acute herpetic keratitis in rabbits. Deborah Pavan-Langston, Richard D. North, Jr., Patricia A. Geary and Arlyn Kinkel[2] (Massachusetts Eye and Ear Infirm.) determined the intraocular penetration of Ara AMP after topical, subconjunctival and intravenous administration in male albino rabbits.

The animals received 0.05 ml of 3% Ara AMP solution in one eye 4 times at 15-minute intervals, 25 mg of Ara AMP subconjunctivally, 50 mg subconjunctivally or 100 mg/kg intravenously. Aqueous humor and serum samples were assayed by high-pressure liquid chromatography.

No vidarabine or Ara AMP was detected in the aqueous after topical administration or the subconjunctival application of 25 or 50 mg of Ara AMP. Trace levels of vidarabine and Ara AMP were present 1 and 2 hours after the intravenous dose of 100 mg/kg. Levels of hypoxanthine arabinoside (Ara Hx) were $1.1 - 2.4$ $\mu$g/ml in treated eyes after the instillation of drops. Higher levels, up to 9.6 $\mu$g/ml, were found after subconjunctival administration. Levels of Ara Hx in the aqueous after intravenous injection were an order of magnitude higher than those found after the subconjunctival administration of 50 mg. Serum vidarabine and Ara AMP were undetectable. Concentrations of Ara Hx in the aqueous were in the same rank order as dose.

Intravenous and possibly subconjunctival administration of Ara AMP may produce effective levels of intraocular antiviral drug, effective in the treatment of deep herpetic disease.

**Treatment of Vaccinial Keratitis with Vidarabine.** Vaccinia virus occasionally produces severe keratitis in

(2)   Arch. Ophthalmol. 94:1585–1588, September, 1976.

human beings. It may be a complication of vaccination or, rarely, the result of direct ocular contamination with cowpox virus. No previous treatment has proved wholly satisfactory. Vidarabine (adenine arabinoside) benefits systemic vaccinial infections in animals and herpetic keratitis in man. Robert A. Hyndiuk (Med. College of Wisconsin), Mas Okumoto (Univ. of California), Richard A. Damiano (Med. College of Wisconsin), Mario Valenton (Univ. of the Philippines) and Gilbert Smolin[3] (Univ. of California) determined the efficacy of vidarabine in experimental vaccinial keratitis and compared its effects on the disease in rabbits with those of idoxuridine.

Both eyes of 21 rabbits were infected with vaccinia virus, Connaught strain, by twice instilling virus suspension onto the abraded cornea. Fourteen eyes were treated 36 hours later with polyethylene glycol, 12 with 0.1% idoxuridine in water, and 14 with a 5% suspension of vidarabine in polyethylene glycol 4000. The animals were killed 1 day after treatment. Vidarabine was also instilled into the eyes of 8 normal uninfected rabbits.

Keratitis was almost completely eliminated after 5 days of treatment in the animals given vidarabine for 5 days. Significant improvement occurred with idoxuridine but it was less than in the vidarabine-treated animals. Virus titers in the idoxuridine-treated group were 1 or 2 log units lower than in control animals and the titers of vidarabine-treated animals were at least 3 log units lower. No signs of ocular toxicity appeared in the uninfected animals treated with vidarabine.

Vidarabine had a significantly greater therapeutic effect on vaccinial keratitis than did idoxuridine in rabbits in this study. Nearly complete clearing of the corneal lesions was obtained, with no signs of toxicity from the drug.

**Thickened Corneal Nerves as a Manifestation of Multiple Endocrine Neoplasia** are discussed by Dennis M. Robertson, Glen W. Sizemore and Hymie Gordon[4] (Mayo Clinic and Found). The multiple endocrine neoplasia (MEN) 2b syndrome is characterized by the association of medullary thyroid carcinoma (MTC), pheochromocytoma

(3)  Arch. Ophthalmol. 94:1363–1364, August, 1976.
(4)  Trans. Am. Acad. Ophthalmol. Otolaryngol. 79:772–787, Nov.–Dec., 1975.

and multiple mucosal tumors in patients who usually have a marfanoid habitus and other developmental anomalies. The ophthalmic findings include conjunctival and lid neuromas, keratoconjunctivitis sicca and thickened corneal nerves. In MEN 2a, mucosal neuromas and eye lesions are absent and hyperparathyroidism often occurs. The MEN type 2 syndromes may be inherited in an autosomal-dominant manner. Review was made of 29 patients with MEN type 2 syndromes; 15 had MEN 2b and 14 had MEN 2a. Ophthalmic examination was made of 15 patients with MEN 2b. Nine patients were from 2 families.

All affected members of 1 family had greatly thickened corneal nerves forming an irregular lace pattern across the entire cornea. Enlarged nerves also were common in the subconjunctival region and could be seen in bundles as flat, poorly circumscribed neuromas, generally associated with dilated perilimbal conjunctival blood vessels. Two patients in the other family had thickened lids, conjunctival neuromas and thickened corneal nerves. Some patients, who apparently represented new mutations with MEN 2b, had abnormally thickened nerves in the trabecular meshwork on gonioscopic examination. Thickened fibers were seen coursing through the iris stroma in several of these patients; funduscopy indicated increased prominence of the long ciliary nerves in some cases. Only 2 of 14 patients with MEN 2a had thickened corneal nerves. Members of 2 other families with MTC, pheochromocytomas and parathyroid hyper-

| FEATURES OF MULTIPLE ENDOCRINE NEOPLASIA, TYPE 2b | |
|---|---|
| Thyroid: | Medullary carcinoma |
| Parathyroid: | Usually normal |
| Adrenal: | Pheochromocytoma(s) |
| Eyes: | Thickened corneal nerves, keratoconjunctivitis sicca |
| Stomach, colon: | Dilated |
| Mucous membranes: | Multiple neuromas, including those of conjunctivas and lids |
| Trunk and limbs: | "Marfanoid" with relatively long limbs and increased joint laxity |
| Skin: | Attenuated flare response to intradermal histamine |

plasia did not have somatic anomalies, mucosal neuromas or thickened corneal nerves. Features of MEN 2b are listed in the table. The ophthalmologist may be the first to see these patients. When thickened corneal nerves are recognized, study for MTC is mandatory. Both MEN type 2 syndromes can be considered neuroectodermal disorders. Thickened corneal nerves may be found in both syndromes.

**Schnyder's Corneal Dystrophy and Hyperlipidemia** are discussed by R. Kaden and G. Feurle[5] (Univ. of Heidelberg). This pathologic entity is characterized by: bilateral oval, disc- or ring-shaped crystalline deposits in the central cornea, most frequently in the anterior third of the stroma immediately below Bowman's membrane; a white limbus belt (type I, Vogt) nasally and temporally in the lid area; no inflammatory phenomena, pain or sensation of dryness; onset in early youth; and autosomal dominant heredity. Other observations include an occasional pronounced arcus lipoides or xanthelasma and absence of the white limbus belt. Corneal sensibility is rarely affected; opacities progress extremely slowly, so visual acuity is relatively well preserved.

In the present study hyperlipoproteinemia was present in 5 of 8 patients examined in a kinship in which 10 members had this dystrophy. In 1 patient lipid levels were in the normal range, whereas in another (a child) hyperlipidemia was present without corneal abnormalities. All 3 members of the 2d generation had hyperlipoproteinemia, type IV in 2 and type III in 1, just as in 2 more members of the 3d generation. Five members of the kinship had manifest or subclinical diabetes mellitus; this is explained by the frequent association of type IV hyperlipoproteinemia and diabetes mellitus.

The pathogenetic relationship between disturbance of lipid metabolism and corneal degeneration remains obscure; a coincidental association is unlikely, given the frequency of observation. It is equally unlikely that the corneal cholesterol accumulation can be regarded as lipid deposits connected to the hyperlipoproteinemia. The possibility that both Schnyder's corneal dystrophy and hyperlipoproteinemia

(5) Albrecht von Graefes Arch. Klin. Ophthalmol. 198:129–138, 1976.

are expressions of a basic disturbance of lipid metabolism cannot be ruled out. Another possibility is that hyperlipoproteinemia will lead to corneal cholesterol deposits, given the presence in the cornea of additional local and hereditary disturbances of lipid metabolism.

Each ophthalmologic diagnosis of Schnyder's corneal dystrophy should require analysis of lipid metabolism in the patient and his family, with corresponding dietetic advice on cholesterol and the associated high risk of coronary heart disease.

**Ascorbic Acid Prevents Corneal Ulceration and Perforation Following Experimental Alkali Burns.** Persistent corneal epithelial defects, corneal ulceration and perforation after alkali burns of the eye have been attributed to a nutritional deficiency in the aqueous caused by damage to the ciliary body. Richard A. Levinson, Christopher A. Paterson and Roswell R. Pfister[6] (Univ. of Colorado) studied clinical changes in the corneal relation to aqueous levels of glucose and ascorbate after 6- and 12-mm alkali burns in rabbits and the influence of systemic ascorbic acid administration on the sequelae of 12-mm alkali burns.

Burns were produced with 1N NaOH in albino rabbits and aqueous was aspirated at specified times after injury. Daily subcutaneous injections of 1.5 gm ascorbic acid were administered to 10 animals given 12-mm burns of both eyes. This treatment produced maximum elevation of aqueous ascorbic acid levels 24 hours after each daily injection.

Glucose levels returned to normal by 14 days after a 6-mm burn and ascorbate levels returned to 80% of normal within 7 days. The corneas showed persistent epithelial defects and occasional peripheral vascularization. Glucose levels changed similarly after a 12-mm burn but ascorbate levels remained well below control values even at 28 days. All these corneas showed acute inflammation, persistent epithelial defects and corneal vascularization. Ulceration, descemetocele formation and perforation were frequently observed in animals maintained longer than 14 days. Eleven of 18 corneas in control animals progressed to perforation after a 12-mm burn, whereas only 3 of 18 eyes in ascorbate-treated animals showed some ulceration and this completely

---

(6)  Invest. Ophthalmol. 15:986–993, December, 1976.

reversed with continued treatment. Aqueous and plasma ascorbate levels were much higher in the ascorbate-treated animals. Little influence of elevated ascorbate levels on epithelial migration was evident.

Exogenous maintenance of adequate aqueous levels of ascorbic acid appears to overcome the relatively scorbutic state of the anterior segment induced by a 12-mm alkali burn in the rabbit eye, and reduces the likelihood of corneal ulceration and perforation.

**Corneal Rust Removal by Electric Drill: Clinical Trial by Comparison with Manual Removal.** Rust from a ferrous corneal foreign body has a toxic effect on the corneal stroma and if left in place, the stained tissue undergoes necrosis and sloughs. Desferrioxamine therapy has not been found to be superior to surgical treatment. Nicholas Brown, Richard Clemett and Rodney Grey[7] (London) compared rust removal by electric drill with manual removal. A new slim electric drill that can be held in the hand like a pencil is used. It has a spring friction chuck to hold dental burs and is operated by light finger pressure from any side on a ring. The straight drill is advanced obliquely to the eye. Patients with significant corneal rust were treated after removal of the foreign body. Electric drill treatment was given to 64 patients and manual treatment to 57.

The smaller rust rings were easily removed by either treatment method, but large, deeply infiltrated rust rings were difficult to remove completely by manual rotation of the dental bur. There was no difficulty in removing the complete rust ring with the electric drill under slit-lamp control. A smooth crater was left, in contrast with the irregular crater left after manual rust removal. No unintentional corneal excavation occurred with the electric drill method. Five patients treated manually required a second treatment. The mean duration of attendance was less for patients treated with the electric drill and pain lasted for a shorter time in this group. This treatment took less than half as long as did manual treatment. Epithelial healing time was comparable in the two groups.

**Alterations in Corneal Morphology Following Thermokeratoplasty.** Thermokeratoplasty (TKP) has been

(7)  Br. J. Ophthalmol. 59:586–589, October, 1975.

advocated as a relatively safe nonsurgical alternative to keratoplasty in cases of keratoconus but recurrent epithelial breakdown may follow the procedure, and in many patients a sufficient improvement in visual acuity has not been obtained. James V. Aquavella, Richard S. Smith and Edward L. Shaw[8] (Albany Med. College) conducted retrospective histologic studies of corneal buttons removed at penetrating keratoplasty in patients who had previously undergone TKP.

Data on 15 patients who had grafts because of healing difficulties or inadequate visual acuity, or both reasons, were evaluated. The mean patient age was 40; there were 8 men and 7 women. The average time between TKP and penetrating keratoplasty was 6 months and the average follow-up period after keratoplasty has been 12.5 months.

The 8 patients with poor and protracted epithelial healing and a relatively long interval between TKP and penetrating keratoplasty showed the most severe histologic changes, including bullous keratopathy with anterior membrane changes, severe central stromal melting with impending perforation and fibrinous iritis with hypopyon. Inadequate visual results in 7 patients with normal epithelial healing were due to either central stromal scarring or a persistent central stromal inflammatory infiltrate. In patients with retarded healing, the corneal epithelium was thin and compressed and the basal epithelial cells were often frankly edematous and exhibited bullous separation from the underlying cornea. The epithelial basement membrane was thickened, and Bowman's membrane was absent in some cases. Severe corneal melting usually began 4–11 months after TKP.

Complications of penetrating keratoplasty included 3 graft rejections, 2 of which were completely reversed. In 2 patients, the grafts ultimately opacified; in both, penetrating keratoplasty had been done on an urgent basis. Ultimate visual acuity was 20/25 to 20/20 in 3 patients and 20/40 in 8. Two patients with opaque grafts have light perception and are candidates for regrafting. One patient with Down's syndrome is not evaluable and 1 patient has been lost to follow-up.

(8)　Arch. Ophthalmol. 94:2082–2085, December, 1976.

Small variations in TKP technique can significantly affect the outcome. Although TKP may eliminate the need for penetrating keratoplasty in certain patients, the surgical option should be readily available. In addition to reduced probe temperature, other modifications are currently being studied for improving the results of TKP, including variation in the use of topical steroids and a limited number of probe applications.

▶ [The delayed healing of the corneal epithelium and the stromal melting following thermokeratoplasty for keratoconus in these 15 cases requiring penetrating corneal transplantation, plus the histopathologic changes certainly do not create much enthusiasm for this procedure. The comments made by this editor still appear valid (see 1975 YEAR BOOK, p. 113). In spite of the undesirable clinical and histologic changes produced in some cases by this procedure, the authors are still trying to modify their technique to avoid complications; e.g., a probe temperature of no more than 95 C with pulsed contact time of 1 second or less, variation in use of topical steroids, limited number of applications and increased caliber of the cannula providing constant saline irrigation. In my mind, there must be exceptional contraindications to the highly successful penetrating corneal transplantation, in cases of keratoconus which cannot be satisfactorily corrected by contact lenses, in order to warrant thermokeratoplasty with significant morbidity and impermanent results. Why subject a cornea with basic loss of tissue to further abuse? — Ed.] ◀

**Clinical Specular Microscopy.** William M. Bourne, Bernard E. McCarey and Herbert E. Kaufman[9] have modified the specular microscope to obtain an instrument that can be used easily in routine clinical examination and in photography of the corneal endothelium at high magnification ($\times 200$). The instrument has been proved reliable and durable, having taken over 7,000 endothelial photographs during clinical examinations in 1975. Light passes through a slit into a system of mirrors that directs the light through the objective lens and its attached dipping cone into the cornea. The dipping cone lens is a flat-surfaced extension on the $\times 20$ water immersion objective which applanates the cornea. The focusing knob adjusts the excursion of the dipping cone to focus the image for corneas of varying thickness. Light is reflected back through the objective lens and eyepiece lens into the single lens reflex camera. A xenon flash tube permits clear photographs to be made despite continuous small eye movements. A drop of topical anesthetic is

(9)   Trans. Am. Acad. Ophthalmol. Otolaryngol. 81:743–753, Sept.–Oct., 1976.

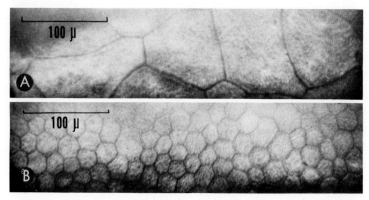

Fig 15.—A, mammoth endothelial cells in clear corneal transplant (371 cells per mm²). B, normal endothelial cells of older individual are shown for comparison (1,944 cells per mm²). (Courtesy of Bourne, W. M., et al.: Trans. Am. Acad. Ophthalmol. Otolaryngol. 81:743–753, Setp.–Oct., 1976.)

applied to the cornea before the examination. Multiple photographs may be taken rapidly with an automatic film advance attached to the camera. The most convenient final central magnification has been ×400. The examination usually lasts only a few minutes.

The results of old endothelial injury may be detected by this method when such injury is not obvious on slit-lamp examination. The earliest signs of corneal homograft rejection, such as mild anterior chamber reaction and fine keratitic precipitates, are observed. The status of an endothelial dystrophy may be documented and followed by clinical specular microscopy. One of the most valuable uses of the method is in evaluating the effects of different ocular surgical procedures on the endothelium. The technique may also be useful in intraocular lens insertion. It is useful at all stages of keratoplasty evaluation (Fig 15). The effects of different techniques of keratoplasty on the endothelium may be compared directly by postoperative specular microscopy.

Clinical specular microscopy holds great promise in improving the diagnosis, as well as the treatment, of corneal diseases.

▶ [This simple technique, with excellent pictures of the all-important corneal endothelium, certainly aids the clinician in detecting minimal amounts of endothelial degeneration preoperatively which might affect his decision to operate or choice of technique. As the authors state, the clinical specular microscope will be highly useful to evaluate the results of operations, such as different types of cataract extraction, phakoemulsification, plastic lens implantation and corneal transplantation. In addition, Bigar, Schimmelpfennig and Gieseler (Albrecht von Graefes Arch. Klin. Ophthalmol. 200:195, 1976) found that specular microscopy showed endothelial changes in 27% of 226 donor corneas, making them undesirable for penetrating corneal transplantation, although examination with a slit lamp in these cases showed no abnormality. — Ed.] ◄

**Penetrating Keratoplasty Using 37 C Organ Cultured Cornea.** Standard eye bank storage at 4 C is associated with endothelial cell death that increases with time, and the endothelial cell population is reduced by 72 – 96 hours of storage in M-K medium. Cryopreservation is technically complicated and expensive. Donald J. Doughman, John E. Harris and Mary Kay Schmitt[1] (Univ. of Minnesota) report the clinical results obtained with corneas stored by organ culture (OC) incubation at 37 C. During 1974 – 75, penetrating keratoplasties were done in 63 patients with OC-incubated corneas; 41 of these patients were followed for $5^{1}2$ months or longer. Procedures were done with sterile technique in a laminar flow hood. The globes were stored at 4 C before processing for OC. Eagle's minimum essential medium (MEM) was used with calf serum, L-glutamine and an antibiotic-antimycotic mixture added. Corneas were kept at 37 C in 95% air-5% $CO_2$, and the MEM was changed three times weekly. Anterior vitrectomy or vitreous aspiration was performed in most aphakic and some combined cataract-penetrating keratoplasty procedures.

Donor corneas were stored by OC incubation for an average of 13 days, with a range of 2 – 35 days. No bacterial or fungal infections occurred. Fourteen of the 41 transplants that were followed have failed. Two of the 22 followed for less than $5^{1}/_{2}$ months have failed. All failed grafts but one were clear at least 4 weeks before failing. Donor age, postmortem times and duration of OC storage did not influence the results. All graft failures were caused by factors unrelated to OC storage at 37 C. Twelve of the 27 long-term successes represented poor-prognosis cases.

(1) Trans. Am. Acad. Ophthalmol. Otolaryngol. 81:778– 793, Sept. – Oct., 1976.

Organ culture of human donor corneas at 37 C maintains endothelial viability for up to 35 days. The major disadvantage of this storage method at present is its cost; however, this is a first-generation method, and further research should result in simplification of the method and a reduction in its cost. The preliminary results are most encouraging.

▶ [See the Introduction to this chapter by Doughman who evaluates the various methods of preserving donor corneas, and the problems and future of eye banking. — Ed.]

▶ ↓ The following four articles pin down some of the generally accepted features of corneal graft rejection. Repeated grafts on one or both eyes increase the likelihood of graft rejection (see the first article). I have one patient in which operation on the second eye produced a graft reaction in the first eye but not in the second eye! Cytotoxic lymphocytes in the recipient's peripheral blood were demonstrated by the direct cell mediated lympholysis technique in 8 of 25 patients receiving penetrating grafts, 6 of whom developed graft rejections (see article by Grunnet et al.). Soluble mediators of inflammation and cellular immunity include the lymphokines which are "the product of the specific interaction between a sensitized lymphocyte and its sensitizing antigen," one of which is the macrophage migration inhibition factor (MIF). Sher et al. demonstrated MIF in the aqueous of rabbits coincident with allograft and xenograft reactions. No significant increased MIF activity was found in nonimmunologic inflammations but activity increased in other types of immunologic inflammations. To avoid the undesirable reactions and toxicity of heterologous antilymphocytic serum, Chandler prepared homologous rabbit antiserum by injection of thymus cells. He soaked donor rabbit cornea allographs in this serum, and found that although the time of onset of allograft rejection was delayed, the incidence of rejection was not reduced compared with controls. — Ed. ◀

**Repeated Keratoplasties and Graft Rejection.** Y. Pouliquen and C. Rocher[2] (Paris) studied 68 patients who had had one or more penetrating corneal transplants, with graft rejection reactions occurring 84 times in 118 keratoplasties.

An analysis of the results indicates that grafts performed as a primary procedure on one or both eyes develop a graft rejection of the endothelial type, which appears between the 1st and 3d month; the prognosis is good in 53–66% of the cases treated with steroids. If grafts were performed on both eyes, there was a risk of development of a graft rejection in the eye with the first graft simultaneously if one developed in the second eye.

Repeated grafts on the same eye caused development of

(2) Arch. Ophtalmol. (Paris) 35:847, November, 1975.

graft rejections of varying types; endothelial, stromal and mixed, with a much earlier appearance. The prognosis was worse: 6% cure, 33% semifailure and 60% failure.

Repeated grafts on severe leukomas (burns, leukoma adhaerens, inflammatory keratopathies with active neovascularization, etc.) practically all end in failure due either to immunologic reactions or inflammatory or cicatricial changes.

**Occurrence of Lymphocytotoxic Lymphocytes and Antibodies after Corneal Transplantation.** Opinion still differs as regards the significance of tissue compatibility for the outcome of corneal grafting. Lymphocytotoxic antibodies have been described in patients whose grafts failed from allograft rejection. Niels Grunnet, Tom Kristensen, Flemming Kissmeyer-Nielsen and Niels Ehlers[3] (Univ. of Århus, Denmark) investigated cellular and humoral sensitization in a series of 25 patients given one or several 7-mm penetrating corneal grafts. Cellular cytotoxicity was analyzed with use of the direct cell mediated lympholysis (CML) technique. Defibrinated blood lymphocytes from patients were mixed with $^{51}$Cr-labeled PHA lymphoblasts from 4 normal target subjects that possessed 14 different HLA-A and B antigens. Tubes were incubated for 6 hours under culture conditions. Patient serums were analyzed for lymphocytotoxic antibodies using the trypan blue-exclusion test.

Eight patients were positive in direct CML tests. Of these 6 had clinical signs of corneal graft rejection, making the association a significant one; another patient has been pregnant several times, and 1 was transplanted 3 weeks before study. The only patient with lymphocytotoxic antibodies with an uncomplicated course had been pregnant twice and was cornea transplanted once before the actual transplantation. There was no striking influence of the number of HLA-A and B incompatibilities on the results of direct CML tests. Only 2 of 8 positive test results were explained by mismatching of HLA antigens, but the target cells used did not possess all known HLA-A and B antigens.

These findings imply that the immune system of a corneal graft recipient may be stimulated to produce or recall cyto-

(3) Acta Ophthalmol. (Kbh.) 54:167–173, April, 1976.

toxic lymphocytes. They argue for the immunologic recognition of the allograft. Patients must be followed for long periods after corneal grafting to detect clinical rejections. In future tests target cells from the specific corneal donor will be used, and the recipients of the same donor tissue will be tested several times in the posttransplantation period to determine the predictive value of the direct CML test for clinical rejection.

**Macrophage Migration Inhibition Factor Activity in Aqueous Humor during Experimental Corneal Xenograft and Allograft Rejection.** Immunologic rejection mediated by cellular immune components is an important cause of corneal graft failure. In rabbits the resultant graft damage is mediated by mononuclear cells, mainly small lymphocytes. The stimulus for the recruitment and activation of the effector cells is unclear, but soluble mediators of inflammation such as lymphokines are a possibility. Neal A. Sher, Donald J. Doughman, Elizabeth Mindrup, Lloyd A. Minaai (Univ. of Minnesota) and Kenneth A. Foon[4] (Natl. Inst. of Health) found that significant macrophage migration inhibition factor (MIF) is demonstrable in the aqueous humor of rejecting xenografts and allografts. Penetrating corneal xenografts were performed in adult female New Zealand rabbits and interlamellar allografts in female Dutch belted pigmented rabbits.

Increased MIF activity was demonstrated in the aqueous after penetrating xenograft placement in chickens and rabbits. Activity of MIF increased markedly after interlamellar xenografting. After interlamellar allografting, marked individual variation in the course of rejection and in MIF activity was observed. No significant MIF activity was found in various types of nonimmunologic inflammation, but titers of MIF activity were increased in immunogenic uveitis. Nonimmunologic inflammation was induced by multiple paracenteses, corneal alkali burns, clove oil and mechanical debridement of the corneal endothelium.

The findings implicate an immunologic mechanism in the elaboration of MIF in the aqueous and suggest that the assay for MIF in the aqueous may provide further diagnostic

(4) Am. J. Ophthalmol. 82:858–865, December, 1976.

information as to the presence of a true immunologic rejection of a corneal graft. Study of the various immunologic mediators in accessible ocular fluids may provide better understanding of the pathophysiology of ocular inflammation and graft rejection.

**Immunologic Protection of Rabbit Corneal Allografts: Prolonged Survival of Allografts Pretreated with Homologous Antibody Against Transplantation Antigens.** Burde et al. reported that rabbit corneal allografts pretreated with heterologous antilymphocyte serum (ALS) had prolonged survival times compared with unsoaked grafts or those pretreated with normal serum. John W. Chandler[5] (Univ. of Washington) details the preparation and testing of homologous antibody against transplantation antigens for the pretreatment of rabbit corneal allografts. Homologous antibody was prepared by immunizing Dutch pigmented rabbits with New Zealand white (NZW) rabbit lymphocytes. Serums were collected and pooled 2 weeks after the intraperitoneal injection of $10^8$ thymus cells emulsified in complete adjuvant. Standard techniques were used for corneal transplantation. There were 22 recipients of unsoaked and 22 of antibody-soaked allografts; 25 rabbits received grafts soaked in normal rabbit serum. The 3 Dutch pigmented rabbits that were immunized with NZW antigens received allografts soaked in their antibody-containing serum.

The antibody was much less cytotoxic than similarly prepared heterologous guinea pig antilymphocyte serum. The homologous antibody preparation significantly prolonged corneal allograft survival. A low titer of homologous cytotoxic antibody against transplantation antigens was detected 5 weeks after initial immunization. Allografts soaked in homologous serum containing antibody against transplant antigens had a mean survival of 40.8 days compared with 26.2 days for unsoaked grafts and 30.6 days for grafts soaked in normal serum. Graft rejection was less frequent for grafts soaked in antibody-containing serum, but the difference from the incidence in the control groups was not significant.

(5) Invest. Ophthalmol. 15:213–216, March, 1976.

Homologous antibody against transplantation antigens is successful in prolonging rabbit corneal allograft survival. It appears that similar pretreatment of human corneal allografts might succeed in prolonging graft survival and even perhaps in reducing the incidence of allograft rejection.

**Aphakic Bullous Keratopathy Treated with Prosthokeratoplasty: Analysis of 34 Consecutive Cases.** Anthony Donn[6] (Columbia Univ.) reviewed the results of implantation of the Cardona keratoprosthesis as a primary procedure in 34 consecutive patients with severe aphakic bullous keratopathy. Corneal swelling was advanced in all and acuity was no better than counting fingers. Thirty patients were aphakic at the time of the keratoprosthesis and 4 had a cataract extraction done at the same time. Two thirds of the patients were over age 70. Nine had operations on both eyes. The follow-up period ranged from 6 to 72 months.

Three extrusions occurred, 2 with necrosis and infection, all within a year after surgery. None of these eyes retained useful vision, but there were no enucleations. In 2 other patients, the condition worsened, with apparently permanent late vitreous hemorrhages occurring, although the keratoprostheses remained in good position. Another patient was unimproved because of preexisting retinal disease. Twenty-eight of the 34 eyes were greatly improved during follow-up; 16 have been followed for over 2 years and 7 of these for 4 years or longer. All but 2 of these patients can read ordinary print. Four of the successfully treated patients had temporary late vitreous hemorrhages, diagnosed ultrasonographically. Final vision was worsened slightly by this occurrence in 2 of the patients. These patients have been followed for years after the vitreous hemorrhage without further loss of vision occurring.

The great advantage of the keratoprosthesis lies in the speed and ease with which useful vision can return. These are important advantages for elderly patients, who are the major sufferers from aphakic bullous keratopathy. The keratoprosthesis procedure is simpler than penetrating keratoplasty and provides a return of useful vision more quickly.

(6)   Arch. Ophthalmol. 94:270–273, February, 1976.

However, the visual field is restricted to 30 degrees and the risks of extrusion and infection must be weighed against the complications of penetrating keratoplasty in aphakic eyes.

▶ [This article summarizes the good results obtained in complete aphakic bullous keratopathy by the primary insertion of a Cardona "nut and bolt" prosthesis. The results are comparable with those using a penetrating corneal transplant in this type of case. The convalescence time is shorter, which is especially valuable in older patients. The author says the technique is easier than penetrating keratoplasty. The two major difficulties are obtaining the prosthesis made by Cardona's laboratory at Columbia University, and the restriction of the visual field to at least 30 degrees. I recently saw a patient for the first time who had had a Cardona prosthokeratoplasty performed by this group, and 10 years postoperatively the vision was 20/25 and the prosthesis was in good position. However, the other eye had two previously unsuccessful penetrating grafts for Fuchs' dystrophy, but after the third successful graft, with reported 20/200 vision, she was visually happy. Unfortunately, after a cataract extraction, the cornea decompensated to a complete bullous keratopathy. This made her completely unhappy with the Cardona implant, 20/25 vision and a restricted visual field.

In cases of heavily vascularized leucomas and chemical burns with previously unsuccessful penetrating grafts, the Columbia University group recommends an acrylic implant with intralamellar fenestrated teflon flange reinforced by overlying autogenous periosteum, the cornea or sclera covered by a conjunctival flap. This reduces the rate of extrusion, due to necrosis of the anterior layers of the cornea, to below 10%. — Ed.]

**Scleritis and Episcleritis.** Peter G. Watson (London) and Sohan Singh Hayreh[7] (Iowa City, Ia.) analyzed the data from 207 patients with episcleritis in 301 eyes and 159 with scleritis in 217 eyes seen at Moorfields Eye Hospital in the past 10 years. Follow-up for 1–8 years was possible in 91% of the cases.

Simple episcleritis was present in 170 eyes and nodular episcleritis in 47. Diffuse anterior scleritis was present in 119 eyes, nodular anterior scleritis in 134 eyes, necrotizing scleritis in 42 eyes and posterior scleritis in 6 eyes. Thirteen eyes with necrotizing scleritis were regarded as scleromalacia perforans.

The findings showed that episcleritis is a benign recurring condition, mild keratitis being the only occasional complication. It does not progress to scleritis except in cases of herpes zoster. Scleritis is always accompanied by episcleral inflammation. It is a much more severe disease than the latter,

(7)  Br. J. Ophthalmol. 60:163–191, March, 1976.

leading to loss of visual acuity from corneal changes, uveitis, cataract or retinal detachment if not treated. Connective tissue disease is the most common associated general condition; 21% of the patients with this condition and necrotizing scleritis died during follow-up. Nearly half of the patients with scleritis had a known associated systemic condition.

Biopsy is contraindicated in scleral disease because the sclera does not heal easily. Diagnosis is based on an exact clinical examination.

Apart from the few patients with a specific bacterial or viral cause, treatment consisted of suppression of the inflammation. Treatment must be continued until the disease has followed its natural course. Only 3 eyes in this series (0.6%) were lost, 1 in a patient who could not tolerate treatment.

In cases of episcleritis, oxyphenbutazone and betamethasone ointments appeared to hasten recovery by about 1 day.

Patients with scleritis received oxyphenbutazone systemically, 600 mg daily for 4 days, followed by 400 mg daily until suppression occurred and then for 1 week. An alternative treatment is systemic indomethacin, 100 mg daily, reduced to 75 mg daily when a response occurs and then continued until the condition has been quiescent for 1 week. Usually local steroids can also be used. Subconjunctival steroids are not recommended in scleritis. Systemic steroids are given in heavy suppressive doses if scleritis is very severe and fails to respond within a week, or if any avascular areas appear in the episclera. A dose of 80 mg prednisolone daily is usually sufficient initially. Surgery is very rarely necessary in scleral disease. Four patients have required corneal grafting.

► [This is a long and well-illustrated article of the clinical manifestations, differential diagnosis, associated systemic disease, and treatment of episcleritis and scleritis. — Ed.] ◄

# Glaucoma

INTRODUCTION

The search for an ideal operation for chronic glaucoma continues as it has for almost a century. Trabeculectomy, first described by Cairns in 1967, has become the most popular microsurgical procedure for glaucoma in this country.[1] Although its popularity may be well deserved, it is difficult to justify statistically. Spaeth, in a review of patients from the Wills Eye Hospital, reached the conclusion that for most persons with chronic glaucoma, a scleral cautery procedure of the Scheie type lowers pressure to a lower level for a longer duration than does trabeculectomy.[2] Data from our own service indicate that while the degree of control to be expected with trabeculectomy may be slightly better than we previously experienced with sclerectomy and Scheie procedures, the postoperative complications of flat anterior chamber, flat filtering bleb, and late cataract formation were no less frequent than with the older procedures.[3] The one area in which trabeculectomy may represent an improvement and which has not yet been documented in time or statistics is a low incidence of postoperative endophthalmitis. This may be due to a filtering bleb which is thick and unlikely to become infected during the course of conjunctivitis.

The surgical techniques described by various authors vary so widely that one could conclude that different procedures are being done. Cairns' original procedure placed the scleral incision at the limbus. Watson's later modification placed this at the other end.[4] Hetherington used a triangular scleral flap.[5] Richardson described an intentional cyclodialysis of the ciliary body at 12 o'clock as a part of his procedure, while others described incisions directed through trabecular fibers.[6, 7]

The mode of action of trabeculectomy remains unclear. Although Cairns originally proposed that the procedure worked by opening the cut ends of Schlemm's canal to direct contact with aqueous humor, Rich in our laboratories and Spencer in histologic specimens from human eyes, demonstrated that the cut ends of Schlemm's canal soon fibrosed off and direct access of aqueous humor to Schlemm's canal does not exist for long.[8, 9] In our own experience, the regurgitation of blood from Schlemm's canal into anterior chamber which can be produced by jugular compression does not appear to last for longer than a few months after successful trabeculectomy. Shields produced evidence with India ink studies that trabeculectomy acts purely as a filtering procedure with the seepage of aqueous humor along the cut edges of the scleral flap.[10] Purnell found that the sclera may exercise a blotter effect when its inner layers are excised, exposing the outer layers of the sclera to direct contact with aqueous humor.[11] The current feeling is that, although all of these may be parts of the whole, the operation functions basically as a filtering procedure for glaucoma and does not represent any new means of outflow for aqueous humor.

There does appear to be correlation between the appearance of the histologic specimen and postoperative control of intraocular pressure. In our laboratories, those specimens submitted from eyes in which only trabecular meshwork and Schlemm's canal were excised, showed a higher incidence of success than those in which either Descemet's membrane or ciliary body were included with excised trabecular meshwork.

Trabeculectomy, then, appears not to have quite lived up to its advance billing as a greatly improved operation for glaucoma, but may offer some refinements over classical filtering procedures.

Samuel D. McPherson, Jr., M.D.
Duke University School of Medicine

## REFERENCES

1. Cairns, J. E.: Trabeculectomy. Am. J. Ophthalmol. 66:673, 1968.
2. Spaeth, G. L., Joseph, N. H., and Fernand, E.: Trabeculectomy: Reevaluation after Three Years and a Comparison with Scheie's procedure. Trans. Am. Acad. Ophthalmol. Otolaryngol. 79:349, 1975.

3. McPherson, S. D., Jr., Cline, J. W., and McCurdy, D.: Recent Advances in Glaucoma Surgery, Trabeculotomy and Trabeculectomy. Ann. Ophthalmol. 9:91, 1977.

4. Watson, P.: Trabeculectomy, a Modified *Ab Externo* Technique. Ann. Ophthalmol. 2:199–205, 1970.

5. Kolker, A. E., and Hetherington, J., Jr.: *Becker-Shaffer's Diagnosis and Therapy of the Glaucomas* (4th ed.; St. Louis: C. V. Mosby Company, 1976).

6. Richardson, K.: Trabeculectomy, Presented before Advice and Dissent in Glaucoma, University of California, San Francisco, Dec. 6, 1974.

7. Schwartz, A. L., and Anderson, D. R.: Trabecular Surgery. Arch. Ophthalmol. 92:134, 1974.

8. Rich, A., and McPherson, S. D., Jr.: Trabeculectomy in the Owl Monkey. Ann. Ophthalmol. 5:1082, 1973.

9. Spencer, W. H.: Histologic Evaluation of Microsurgical Glaucoma. Trans. Am. Acad. Ophthalmol. Otolaryngol. 76:389, 1972.

10. Shields, M. B.: Personal Communication, 1977.

11. Purnell, W. D.: Scleral Permeability. Proceedings of the Annual Staff Meeting, Department of Ophthalmology, University of North Carolina School of Medicine, 1974.

# OCULAR HYPERTENSION

ROBERT A. MOSES, M.D.
*Washington University, St. Louis*

It has been recognized for many years that eyes with elevated intraocular pressure sometimes lose visual field. It is this tendency of high-pressure eyes to suffer field loss that has caused many ophthalmologists to equate elevated intraocular pressure with glaucoma. During the past several years it has been more common to classify increased intraocular pressure without visual field loss as ocular hypertension, whereas the term glaucoma is reserved for a particular type of field loss, usually, but not necessarily, associated with elevated intraocular pressure and cupped optic disc. (This mixed classification inspires me to hope that one day we will speak of things we can define and measure — intra-

(This work was supported in part by NEI Grant EY 00256 from National Institutes of Health, Bethesda, Maryland.)

ocular pressure, disc cupping, visual field – and relegate the term glaucoma to ancient history.) Ocular hypertension, the long tail of the ocular pressure distribution curve skewing out to the right, may be defined as each individual author desires, but often is considered to be pressure greater than 20 or 21 mm Hg, or perhaps 24 mm Hg or greater.

Surprisingly, in the long history of the study of glaucomatous visual field loss, relatively few controlled studies have been done. We all treat eyes which show glaucomatous field loss. Many of us also treat the fellow eye when only one eye shows glaucomatous field loss. The relationships between the level of intraocular pressure and visual field loss were studied retrospectively by Kass, Kolker and Becker in the second eye of patients with unilateral glaucomatous field loss.[1] Of their 31 patients, 9 patients developed field loss in the eye in which no loss was found at the first examination. These 9 eyes were characterized by a high initial pressure (mean 33.1 vs. 24.8 mm Hg in the nonloss group) and a tendency for the pressure to remain over 24 mm Hg and to increase with time even though all 9 eyes were treated. The authors remark: "This supports the commonly held belief that elevated intraocular pressure and glaucomatous visual field loss are directly related. From the practical point of view, treatment of the fellow eye does not protect it from the development of visual field loss unless the intraocular pressure is reduced to 24 mm Hg or less on more than 50% of the measurements." However, even mean pressure less than 24 mm HG is not absolute protection, as 10% of the eyes in the less than 24 mm Hg group lost field. Thus, second eyes of patients with unilateral glaucomatous field loss should generally be considered glaucomatous and treated, even in the absence of field loss.

The above report dealt with the prognosis of visual field loss in the second eye of asymmetric cases of primary openangle glaucoma. Of the much larger group of ocular hypertensives, can any prognostic statements be made? This group is very troublesome. Six to 10% of the population over age 40 years have increased intraocular pressure but few of these lose field. Up to this time, the ophthalmologist, when confronted with an ocular hypertensive, had two choices: (1)

to treat, or (2) to temporize and watch for the first signs of field loss before treating. The first course has a tremendous rate of apparent success because many of those treated would not have lost field even if untreated, but is undesirable because there is no anti-glaucoma treatment that is without unpleasant and sometimes dangerous side effects. The second course is hazardous since the patients may lose field but not return when told and because it may be that once field loss has begun it is more difficult to arrest. When they do return, the visits are expensive to the patients and time consuming to the ophthalmologist who will find that most of the ocular hypertensive patients have not lost field. A third possibility of management also exists—this is the treatment of selected ocular hypertensives who appear to have an increased likelihood of developing field loss without therapy. This involves evaluation of various "risk factors."

A step forward in the characterization of the open-angle glaucoma patient is that such patients are particularly likely (88%) to possess HLA-B7 or HLA-B12 antigens on their white blood cells.[2] Thus an untreated ocular hypertensive who responds to a standard course of topical dexamethasone with an intraocular pressure of more than 31 mm Hg (GG response) and who has either HLA-B7 or HLA-B12 antigen stands about a 41% chance of losing visual field in 5–10 years, about 8 times the risk when the antigens are absent.

More exciting, because it is easier and cheaper to perform, is the demonstration that ocular pressure response to 1% or 2% epinephrine twice daily may be a predictor of likelihood of visual field loss of the untreated ocular hypertensive.[3] Eighty patients with ocular hypertension and GG response to a standard course of topical dexamethasone were treated for pressure response to topical epinephrine. Thirty-four of the 80 patients had their intraocular pressure reduced by more than 5 mm Hg by epinephrine treatment. One eye was untreated (in some cases both eyes) for 5 to 10 years. During this time, 20 patients lost visual field in their untreated eye. Seventeen of these 20 (85%) had responded to epinephrine. The other 17 epinephrine responders belonged to the larger group (60 patients) who did not lose visual field. Thus, in this select group of 80 ocular hypertensive patients, a pressure response of more than 5 mm Hg predicted a 50% chance of losing visual field if untreated.

In the study of HLA antigens, there were 2 patients who lost field among the ocular hypertensive, dexamethasone responsive subjects with neither HLA-B7 nor HLA-B12. Both were diabetic. In the epinephrine response study there were three nonresponders to epinephrine who lost field. Two of these 3 were diabetic. The diabetic glaucoma population is somewhat different from the nondiabetic population, a subject explored in another paper by Becker and his group.[4]

The major importance of the above two studies is that, if confirmed, one may be able to predict future field loss in patients with ocular hypertension with an accuracy of almost 50% instead of the 5 – 7% accuracy in unselected ocular hypertensives. Therapy to a patient who has a 1 in 2 chance of developing change certainly is easier to recommend and emphasize than when the odds are 19 in 20 that the patient will do as well whether he is treated or not. The importance of documenting and confirming these reports is obvious.

Several risk factors for field loss now seem to be well established; among these are a family history of glaucoma, the degree of elevated intraocular pressure, cupping of the optic disc more extensive than usual and diabetes mellitus. The presence of diabetes tends to split the group at risk; for the nondiabetic group, the presence of HLA-B7 or HLA-B12 antigen and good pressure response to topical epinephrine may be added as risk factors. In the diabetic group, a family history of glaucoma is no longer a strong risk factor nor is presence of HLA-B7 or HLA-B12 antigen,[4] and nonresponse to epinephrine does not offer the same degree of security against field loss.

The perfect predictor of field loss in ocular hypertensives has not yet been developed and so it cannot yet be stated which ocular hypertensives must be treated to prevent field loss. But if I had neither diabetes nor a positive glucose tolerance test, yet had ocular hypertension, a family history of glaucoma, somewhat larger than average optic disc cups and a pressure fall of more than 5 mm Hg on topical epinephrine, I would most certainly want to be on antiglaucoma therapy, and I would also want my intraocular pressures maintained nice and low, certainly below 24 mm Hg.

REFERENCES

1. Kass, M. A., Kolker, A. E., and Becker, B.: Prognostic Factors in Glaucomatous Visual Field Loss. Arch. Ophthalmol. 94:1274, 1976.
2. Shin, D. H., and Becker, B.: The Prognostic Value of HLA-B12 and HLA-B7 Antigens in Patients with Increased Intraocular Pressure. Am. J. Ophthalmol. 82:871, 1976.
3. Becker, B., and Shin, D. H.: Response to Topical Epinephrine: A Practical Prognostic Test in Patients with Ocular Hypertension. Arch. Ophthalmol. 94:2057, 1976.
4. Becker, B., Shin, D. H., and Cooper, D.: Primary Open-Angle Glaucoma and Diabetes Mellitus — Histocompatibility Antigens and Parental History. Invest. Ophthalmol. 15:954, 1976.

**Optic Disc in Glaucoma: Pathogenetic Correlation of Five Patterns of Cupping in Chronic Open-Angle Glaucoma** is presented by George L. Spaeth, Roger A. Hitchings and Eliyathamby Sivalingam[8] (Jefferson Med. College). This study was supported by NIH grant no. E400677-04. Cupping is the classic sign of optic nerve damage in chronic open-angle glaucoma. Tissue loss can be responsible for this change but cupping can occur without tissue loss, with elevated intraocular pressure directly pushing the disc posteriorly. Most diseases of the optic nerve head do not result in cupping, which feature strongly suggests elevated intraocular pressure. If glaucoma is defined so as to include low-tension glaucoma and inappropriately high, though normal intraocular pressure, glaucoma is almost always responsible for acquired cupping of the optic nerve head. Optic neuritis of inflammatory origin is rarely associated with cupping.

Several distinctive types of cupping are distinguishable. Focal saucerization is a relatively shallow, sloping cup, usually located inferotemporally and associated with focal ischemia and a dense paracentral scotoma. Overpass cupping connotes tissue loss within the optic nerve head without posterior displacement of the disc surface or vessels, detectable by stereoscopic examination. In temporal unfolding, the cup enlarges in concentric circles, usually in an inferotemporal or superotemporal direction, which may be undetected unless compared with the other disk or if it shows progressive

(8) Trans. Am. Acad. Ophthalmol. Otolaryngol. 81:217–223, Mar.–Apr., 1976.

enlargement on repeated field tests. In polar notching, the extension of the cup is toward the poles. This is characterized by localized tissue loss and a dense, irreversible arcuate scotoma (Fig 16). In a fifth type of cupping, bean-pot cupping, there is extreme posterior displacement of the lamina and undermining of the neural rim.

The shallow focal saucer appears to be a sign of an ischemic type of low-tension glaucoma. Overpass cupping suggests that elevated pressure is causing tissue damage which, when detected promptly, may be reversible. This is also the case with temporal unfolding, which may be due to direct glial damage by the elevated pressure itself. Marked functional loss is usually present with even slight polar notching. In bean-pot cupping, pressure elevation and field loss are variable.

Visible alteration of the optic nerve head is a hallmark of glaucoma, but visual field examination is essential because field loss can occur with apparently normal discs. However, different patterns of cupping may help establish not only

**Fig 16.** —Superior arcuate scotoma in Bjerrum area confirmed diseased appearance of the disc. Polar notching need not be marked to be pathologic. (Courtesy of Spaeth, G. L., et al.: Trans Am. Acad. Ophthalmol. Otolaryngol. 81:217–223, Mar.–Apr., 1976.)

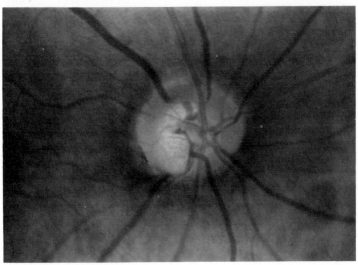

whether glaucoma is present and how it is progressing, but it may even suggest what type of disease is the underlying factor, whether mechanical or vascular.

► ↓ Each of the next five articles zeroes in on a local ischemic cause of glaucomatous optic atrophy in the region of the cribriform plate. These elaborate investigations include injection studies to determine the arterial supply to this region; measurement of perfusion pressure (the difference between pressure in the ophthalmic artery·and intraocular pressure); fluorescein angiography of the disc and surrounding choroid with experimentally raised intraocular pressure and in glaucoma, oxygen tensions and autoregulation; the enlargement of the blind spot and Bjerrum scotomas relative to intraocular pressure; and histologic changes in glaucoma. Vascular insufficiency in the region of the optic nerve head appears to be more of a primary cause of visual field defects in glaucoma than obstruction to axoplasmic flow. The literature is well reviewed in the article by Ernest.—Ed. ◄

**Pathogenesis of Glaucomatous Optic Nerve Disease** was investigated by J. Terry Ernest[9] (Univ. of Chicago).

Pressure on a nerve always presents the possibility of interference with circulation to the nerve. Block of the normal movement of axoplasm to the axon terminals may be involved in glaucomatous optic nerve disease. The vasculature of the optic disc was examined in 50 autopsied eyes from adults aged 43–87 years. Optic disc oxygen tension was measured in Rhesus monkeys. Autoregulation was examined in the monkey and also in normal man. Autoregulation was defined as a local optic disc process operating to maintain the tissue-available oxygen at a constant level despite variation in perfusion pressure. Autoregulation is a kind of local homeostasis in which the autonomic nervous system is not involved; the adjustments are made without disturbing the general circulation.

Injection studies of cadaver eyes showed that the short posterior ciliary arteries provide branches to the optic nerve near the lamina cribrosa through the incomplete circle of Haller and Zinn and through choroidal arteries. Monkey studies showed that the central retinal artery "leaks" oxygen. By autoregulation, the optic disc oxygen tension compensated for changes in perfusion pressure. In man, the visual threshold in the Bjerrum area was elevated with an increase in intraocular pressure but the eye compensated

(9)  Trans. Am. Ophthalmol. Soc. 73:366–388, 1975.

with a reduction in threshold toward normal, given ample time.

Glaucomatous optic nerve disease apparently results from failure of local homeostatic circulatory mechanisms to compensate for sustained intraocular pressure elevation. The superior and inferior temporal nerve fibers, those in highest concentration relative to the optic disc blood supply, are affected first. The first fibers affected are those midway between the disc circumference and the central retinal artery, this being the area of relatively lowest oxygen tension. Through understanding of autoregulation in the eye, it will be possible to know when to begin treatment and at what level the intraocular pressure must be maintained to prevent optic nerve damage and visual loss.

**Pathogenesis of Optic Nerve Lesions in Glaucoma** is discussed by Sohan Singh Hayreh[1] (Univ. of Iowa). The pathogenesis of visual field defects and optic nerve changes in glaucoma remains an enigma. Some views of the pathogenesis of optic disc changes and visual field defects relate to a vasogenic origin in the lesions and others to mechanical factors. The blood supply to the anterior optic nerve, except that of the surface nerve fiber layer of the disc, is essentially from the posterior ciliary arteries directly or via the peripapillary choroid. The retinal circulation appears to have efficient autoregulation, but the choroid and the prelaminar region of the optic nerve head lack such autoregulation. Available evidence indicates that the optic disc changes and field defects in glaucoma and low-tension glaucoma are vasogenic in origin, not mechanical. The vascular disturbance primarily involves not only the prelaminar vessels, but also those in the peripapillary choroid and its area of distribution, i.e., the retrolaminar part of the optic nerve. The disorder results from a fall in perfusion pressure in involved vessels, due either to raised intraocular pressure or reduced mean blood pressure in the vessels, or a combination of these factors. There is no evidence that obstruction of axoplasmic flow in the optic nerve fibers at the level of the lamina cribrosa plays any role in the optic disc changes and visual field defects in glaucoma.

(1) Trans. Am. Acad. Ophthalmol. Otolaryngol. 81:197–213, Mar.–Apr., 1976.

Since a fall in perfusion pressure in the ocular vascular bed appears to be the essential factor in the production of vascular disorders in the optic disc and of the consequent visual field defects, glaucoma and low-tension glaucoma represent two aspects of the same disorder.

**Fluorescein Angiography: Its Contributions toward Understanding the Mechanisms of Visual Loss in Glaucoma.** George L. Spaeth[2] (Thomas Jefferson Univ.) documented the fluorescein angiographic characteristics of glaucoma in a prospective study of 247 subjects. Significant differences were found in blood flow to the optic nerve and retina between normal subjects and those with chronic open-angle glaucoma. Elevated intraocular pressure causes retardation of flow in the retina, optic nerve and possibly the choroid. Optic nerve perfusion is affected in some cases by elevated pressure to a greater degree than is flow to the retina or choroid. Selective sensitivity of the choroid was not noted and observations on the peripapillary capillaries were too few to permit firm conclusions.

Persisting hypoperfusion of the optic disc was highly characteristic of glaucoma, especially in patients with low-tension glaucoma, in whom lasting hypoperfusion of the inferotemporal area of the disc was almost always present. Persistent hypoperfusion was significantly correlated with visual field loss, but transient hypoperfusion of the disc was not correlated with disease or with visual field loss. Improved disc perfusion with decreasing intraocular pressure was documented in about a third of the glaucoma patients. Localized persistent hypoperfusion of the disc was noted in 2 patients before the development of corresponding field loss. Progression of disease in the absence of demonstrated ischemia was noted in 2 patients. Intraocular pressures above 35 mm Hg without apparent ischemia were observed in 12% of patients. Angiographic findings in some of the patients are shown in Figures 17, 18, 19 and 20. The optic nerve was stained by fluorescein in 30% of glaucoma patients without apparent relation to the intraocular pressure. Staining was rare in normal subjects.

A tentative classification of glaucoma includes primary

---

(2)   Trans. Am. Ophthalmol. Soc. 73:491–553, 1975.

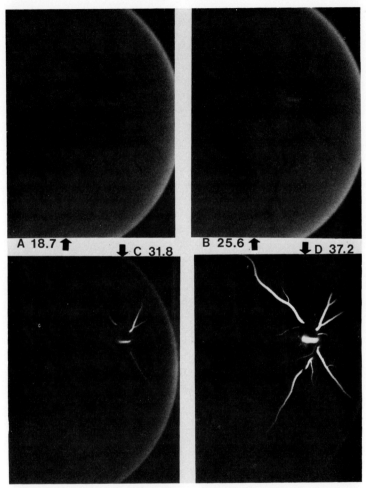

**Fig 17.** — Angiogram when the intraocular pressure was 42 mm Hg. (Courtesy of Spaeth, G. L. Photograph by L. William Bell: Trans. Am. Ophthalmol. Soc. 73:491 – 553, 1975.)

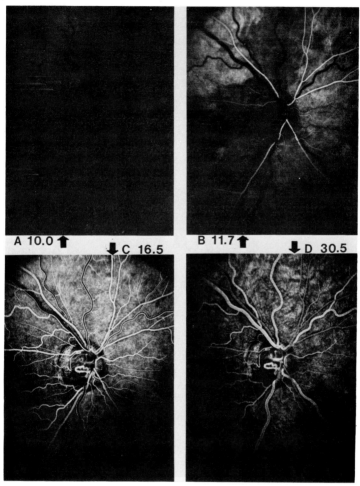

**Fig 18.** — Angiogram taken 2 months after that in preceding figure with intraocular pressure of 15 mm Hg. (Courtesy of Spaeth, G. L. Photograph by L. William Bell: Trans. Am. Ophthalmol. Soc. 73:491–553, 1975.)

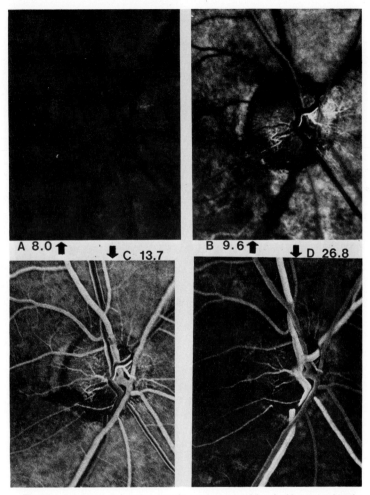

**Fig 19.** — Angiogram taken 3 years after a superonasal loss had been noted in the right eye. (Courtesy of Spaeth, G. L. Photograph by L. William Bell: Trans. Am. Ophthalmol. Soc. 73:491–553, 1975.)

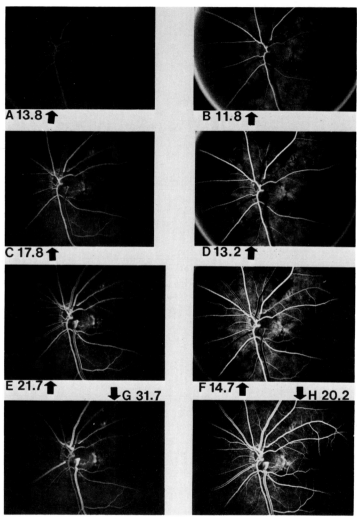

**Fig 20.** – Angiogram taken preoperatively (**A, C, E, G**) when intraocular pressure was 19 mm Hg and postoperatively (**B, D, F, H**) when intraocular pressure was 6 mm Hg. Disc filling occurs more rapidly and completely at the lower intraocular pressure (compare times in right column with those in the left). (Courtesy of Spaeth, G. L. Photograph by L. William Bell: Trans. Am. Ophthalmol. Soc. 73:491–553, 1975.)

hyperbaric cases with neuronal damage from elevated intraocular pressure, primary ischemic changes without elevated intraocular pressure and secondary ischemic changes which result from elevated pressure. Undoubtedly more than one mechanism is involved in many cases. Fluorescein angiography is of use in defining the pathogenesis of visual loss in glaucoma. It may identify the ocular hypertensive who will acquire visual field loss and help in determining the intraocular pressure level that a particular eye can tolerate.

**New Techniques for the Examination of the Optic Disc and Their Clinical Application** are discussed by Bernard Schwartz[3] (Tufts Univ.). Optic disc cupping may be measured by projecting slit beams of light on the disc, or by photogrammetric measurement. Photogrammetry, used mainly to create contour maps of terrain, is based on the use of two stereophotographs of an object that remains stationary. Several problems must be resolved before photogrammetric techniques can be confidently applied to clinical studies. Optic cup measurements may be expressed in absolute numbers, by use of a standard internal reference or by the volume-distribution curve method, in which cross-sectional areas of the cup are plotted against depth of cup from surface to bottom of cup.

Pallor can be measured by the amount of color contrast, but such measurements depend on subjective evaluation of the boundaries of the area of pallor. A more objective method involves the use of microdensitometry, measurement of the diffuse optical density of black-and-white photographic negatives of the optic disc. Variables in exposure and in film development complicate this technique. Presently an attempt is being made to obtain standard frequency distribution curves for normal populations. Eventually this method will be useful for screening and also for following glaucomatous patients to determine impending field loss by changes in disc pallor.

The area of disc pallor may not entirely represent avascular tissue but an area of glial tissue within which are vascular structures. Fluorescein angiography has been modified to obtain high-contrast, high-resolution angiograms of the

---

(3) Trans. Am. Acad. Ophthalmol. Otolaryngol. 81:227–237, Mar.–Apr., 1976.

optic disc to study the vascular structure of the area of disc pallor. Only half the angiograms have been adequate for interpretation, because of inadvertent ocular movements, reactions to fluorescein and interference by opacities in the ocular media.

These techniques will eventually prove useful in providing information that can predict which ocular hypertensive patients will go on to acquire field loss.

**Glaucomatous Cupping of the Human Optic Disc: Neurohistologic Study.** František Vrabec[4] (Prague) studied 20 cases of various primary and secondary glaucomas at enucleation or autopsy. The optic nerves and discs were cut sagitally or, in 3 cases, transversally, and sections were stained by Jabonero's silver carbonate method. Most subjects were aged 60–70. There were 6 cases of primary absolute glaucoma and 14 of secondary glaucoma of varying causes in the series. An optic disc from a control subject aged 75 without eye disease was examined as a control.

Study of a case of moderately advanced glaucoma showed a loss of retinal axons corresponding with arcuate scotomas in two areas (Fig 21) and a diffuse outgrowth of collaterals from the remaining axons adjacent to the gaps caused by degeneration of fascicles, mostly at the level of the posterior lamina cribrosa. Except for hydrophthalmic eyes the pattern of change was identical in the primary and secondary glaucomas. The retina and its axons were quite well preserved despite great functional failure in 4 of 16 patients, whereas in 4 others the retina consisted of glial tissue with all its axons lost. The lamina cribrosa was variably altered in all but 3 of 17 cases. Changes were most marked at the level of the connective part of the lamina and just behind it (Fig 22). Fiber loss in the retrolaminar-intraorbital part of the optic nerve was variable. The vessels of the lamina cribrosa and the retrolaminar part of the optic nerve showed diverse pictures. In two hydrophthalmic eyes, many enlarged arterioles invaded the optic nerve from the leptomeningeal circulation. The ciliary nerves were intact in all but 1 of the 20 eyes examined.

These findings confine the breaking point of retinal axons

(4)   Albrecht von Graefes Arch. Klin. Ophthalmol. 198:223–234, 1976.

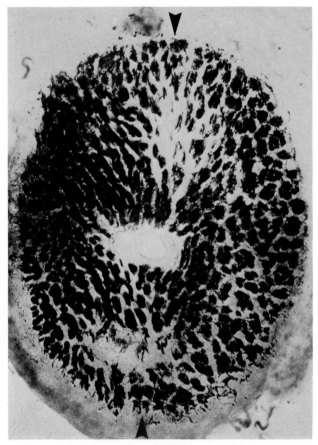

**Fig 21.** — Cross section of optic disc behind the lamina cribrosa, in a case of moderately advanced glaucoma. Above and below the central retinal vessels are areas with rarefied or entirely lacking fascicles of axons. *Arrows,* vertical meridian; optic disc is slightly elongated vertically. Jabonero's method; reduced from ×72. (Courtesy of Vrabec, F.: Albrecht von Graefes Arch. Klin. Ophthalmol. 198:223–234, 1976; Berlin-Heidelberg-New York: Springer.)

in glaucomatous atrophy of the optic nerve to the lamina cribrosa. Axonal degeneration follows the same course in primary and secondary glaucomas. The starting point is at the vertical meridian of the disc, where the great accumulation of axons corresponds to arcuate scotomas. Axons are

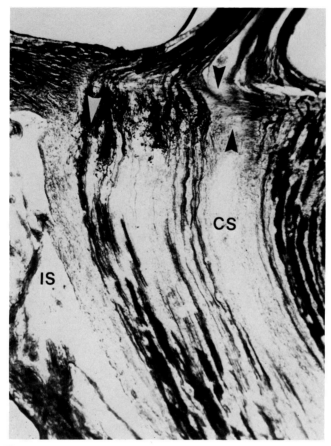

**Fig 22.** — General view of glaucomatous optic nerve head with anterior and posterior limits of the lamina cribrosa marked by *arrows*. Numerous axons of artificially detached retina at level of lamina cribrosa display countless retraction balls and cones of growth *(white arrow)* indicating level of interruption of axons. *CS,* central connective tissue strand; *IS,* intervaginal space. Jabonero's method; × 90. (Courtesy of Vrabec, F.: Albrecht von Graefes Arch. Klin. Ophthalmol. 198:223– 234, 1976; Berlin-Heidelberg-New York: Springer.)

relatively normal once they pass the danger zone within the hinder portion of the lamina cribrosa and just behind it. The area implicated is located just in front of the origin of myelin sheaths of the optic nerve.

**Low-Tension Glaucoma.** Lee C. Chumbley and Richard F. Brubaker[5] (Mayo Clinic and Found.) reviewed 45 cases of low-tension glaucoma seen in 1953–73 to determine the factors affecting the ocular course. Patients with applanation tonometric pressures exceeding 22 mm Hg in either eye at any time were excluded from the series. No patient had used topical or systemic steroids, and none had evidence of an intracranial neoplasm. Low-tension glaucoma affected 77 of the 90 eyes, with a Bjerrum-type scotoma or disc changes suggestive of glaucoma in at least one eye. The 30 women and 15 men had an average age of 66 years at diagnosis. Only 1 patient had a family history of glaucoma. Seventeen patients had follow-up visual field examinations an average of 6.4 years after presentation.

There was no significant difference in ocular prognosis between patients with a Po/C of 100 or higher and those with lower values. The presence of splinter hemorrhages at the optic disc (10% of affected eyes) or of systemic arterial hypertension with a diastolic pressure over 100 mm Hg was associated with progress of visual field defects. Patients with sudden visual loss or associated hemodynamic events, comprising 33% of the series, had a more favorable prognosis regarding stability of field defects than those without such events. Extension of visual field defects across the macula was seen in 25% of affected eyes. There was no firm evidence that treatment of low-tension glaucoma improved the ocular prognosis.

The occurrence of optic nerve head cupping and atrophy in the chronic glaucomas and in low-tension glaucoma but not in ischemic optic neuropathy may be related to a preexistent large cup, as a congenital or familial feature, or to the vascular insufficiency, which produces infarction and atrophy. The rare occurrence of extension of field defects across the macula in chronic simple glaucoma suggests that the mechanisms of low-tension glaucoma and chronic simple glaucoma differ. The results of treatment of low-tension glaucoma have been disappointing, but the data are insufficient for specific conclusions to be drawn. Presently patients who

---

(5) Am. J. Ophthalmol. 81:761–767, June, 1976.

have no history of acute or permanent visual loss but who have abnormal C values on tonography or progress of visual field loss are treated. Surgery is not helpful in preventing further deterioration of visual function in low-tension glaucoma.

▶ [The term "low tension glaucoma," indicating patients with disc and field changes suggestive of glaucoma and intraocular pressures 22 mm or less, might well be abandoned in view of this and other work which suggest that anemia and cardiovascular disorders (see the 1974 YEAR BOOK, p. 138) might be a more important cause of these field defects. – Ed.] ◀

**Comparative Tonometry with Position-Independent Manual Applanation Tonometers** was carried out by G. K. Krieglstein, V. Brethfeld and E. V. Collani[6] (Univ. of Würzburg). The development of such devices by Perkins and Draeger in accordance with Goldmann's guidelines has made possible the application of this recognized principle of intraocular pressure measurement with patients sitting or supine.

One hundred patients were examined by 2 investigators using both devices in a blind study. The statistical evaluation of data revealed an average increase of intraocular pressure of 2.5-3 mm Hg when the patient changed from a sitting to supine position. This postural response was fully reversible, a statistically significant "overshoot phenomenon" being noted; the intraocular pressure clearly decreased below the level of initial values. No relationship could be demonstrated between this postural effect, the intraocular pressure value and patient age.

The physiologic variability of intraocular pressure makes quantitative representation of short-term alterations a delicate methodologic problem due to external influences. The decrease of intraocular pressure with repeated applanation remains the crux of any comparative tonometry but the mechanism of this complex phenomenon is not yet clarified. It is doubtful that the values gained after repeated applanation may be regarded as the "resting pressure of the eye," as proposed by Kindler-Loosli and Schmidt. Several factors indicate variable ocular hemodynamics in the sitting and supine positions, which in turn will have effects on the ho-

(6) Albrecht von Graefes Arch. Klin. Ophthalmol. 199:101–113, 1976.

meostasis of intraocular pressure in the individual patient. Alterations of arterial pressure with postural change possibly have a role.

**Intraocular Pressure Registration through Soft Contact Lenses** was attempted by G. K. Krieglstein, W. K. Waller, H. Reimers (Univ. of Würzburg) and M. E. Langham[7] (Johns Hopkins Univ.). In the presence of chronic corneal disease a tonometric examination is extremely difficult, if not impossible, yet a secondary or primary glaucoma, if unrecognized and untreated, will impede the treatment of the corneal condition. The present study investigated the possibility of intraocular pressure pneumotonometric registration through soft contact lenses and involved patients with various chronic corneal diseases. Comparative measurements were carried out on the soft contact lenses as well as the diseased cornea.

Areas of scarred cornea gave incorrect values, whereas in corneal edema the values corresponded to those gained through the soft lenses and reflected accurate and reliable pressure readings. Comparative registrations in normal eyes confirmed that the presence of a soft lens did not modify the accuracy of pressure measurements. Only if the refraction of the lens exceeded 8 D did such registration result in false high values.

Although pneumotonometric registration can be reliable even on a diseased corneal surface, the use of soft contact lenses has decided advantages. Local anesthesia (always associated with an unfavorable effect on regenerating tissue) can be avoided as can the possibility of activating a chronic inflammatory process, such as a metaherpetic corneal ulcer, by the tonometric manipulations. However, this type of tonometry must be regarded as an "orientational" examination and should not lead to diagnosis of glaucoma through contact lens.

**Diagnostic Value of the Water-Drinking Test in Early Detection of Glaucoma** was tested by Knud Erik Rasmussen and Hans Alrø Jørgensen[8] (Copenhagen) in 119 eyes of 64 patients by comparing the results of the test with

(7)   Albrecht von Graefes Arch. Klin. Ophthalmol. 199:223–229, 1976.
(8)   Acta Ophthalmol. (Kbh.) 54:160–166, April, 1976.

the development of glaucoma 10 or more years later. Field defects developed in 29% of 31 eyes with initially positive tests and in 24% of 88 eyes with negative tests. Accordingly, little value can be attached to the water provocative test as either a diagnostic or prognostic aid in cases of ocular hypertension or open-angle glaucoma. Lowering or raising the value of 8 mm Hg rise after drinking 1 liter of water as being negative or positive, respectively, would not improve the value of this test. There was no correlation between the initial tension and the development of visual field defects and both positive and negative reactors with or without treatment developed later field defects in a significant number of cases.

► ↓ The following two articles are concerned with the detection of ocular hypertensives which are likely to develop glaucoma with visual field defects (see the Introduction to this chapter by Moses). Ocular hypertensives have abnormally high blue-green and yellow thresholds indicating central retinal dysfunction, but this has not been related as yet to later field changes (see next article). In a series of steroid-responders and ocular hypertensives, those patients with a net decrease of 5 mm of intraocular pressure after topical epinephrine showed a greater tendency for later field defects, preventable by topical epinephrine (see article by Becker and Shin). — Ed. ◄

**Study of Dark Adaptation in Ocular Hypertensives.** Studies of differences in dark adaptation between normal and glaucomatous eyes are difficult to compare because the test methods used are not standardized. D. Goldthwaite, R. Lakowski and S. M. Drance[9] (Univ. of British Columbia) used a new method of dark adaptation testing with chromatic stimuli to permit greater differentiation between rod and cone function during adaptation. Studies were done in 18 normal subjects with a mean age of 57.8 years and 19 ocular hypertensives with a mean age of 59.7. All the latter had good acuity, open angles, normal discs, full visual fields and normal foveal differential thresholds. All had repeated intraocular pressure measurements of 21 mm Hg or above. Dark adaptation curves were obtained for blue-green and for yellow preadaptation and test lights by use of a modified Goldman-Weekers Adaptometer. An 11-degree centrally fixated test patch was used for the separate blue-green and yellow test conditions. All preadaptation and threshold test-

(9) Can. J. Ophthalmol. 11:55–60, January, 1976.

ing was done binocularly with natural pupils. Thresholds were measured by using a continuous method of limits.

Both the blue-green and yellow thresholds were higher in ocular hypertensives than in normal subjects. Blue-green differences were usually greater than yellow differences. All glaucomatous thresholds lay above the mean thresholds of both normal subjects and ocular hypertensives. The 2.8-minute difference in mean curve crossover time between normal subjects and ocular hypertensives was significant. No significant increase in threshold variability was detected over 13 minutes of yellow ocular hypertensive adaptation or of blue-green or yellow normal adaptation. Variability of the blue-green ocular hypertensive mean dark adaptation threshold curve increased significantly over 13 minutes; the largest increase occurred just before the mean crossover time (8.8 minutes).

Retinal changes must be present in ocular hypertensives. Central vision is clearly impaired on dark adaptation measures, although perimetry indicates that no field defect is present at the time of testing. The dysfunction may be associated with processes ultimately resulting in field and disc changes. A longitudinal study will show whether dark adaptation measures can predict subsequent field damage.

**Response to Topical Epinephrine: Practical Prognostic Test in Patients with Ocular Hypertension.** In a long-term follow-up of 19 patients with ocular hypertension treated in one eye with topical epinephrine, glaucomatous field defects developed in 32% of the untreated eyes and in no treated eye. Bernard Becker and Dong H. Shin[1] (Washington Univ.) carried out a retrospective analysis of a larger group of ocular hypertensives from which the study group was drawn to determine the prognostic importance of the response to topical epinephrine.

Data on 80 patients with spontaneous bilateral ocular hypertension of over 20 mm Hg who were homozygous responders to 0.1% dexamethasone were reviewed. All were tested in one eye with 1 or 2% topical epinephrine twice daily. A decrease of over 5 mm Hg in the treated eye, corrected for change in the untreated eye, was considered a response.

(1)  Arch. Ophthalmol. 94:2057–2058, December, 1976.

All patients had at least one eye untreated for 5 – 10 years of follow-up.

Twenty patients (25%) acquired glaucomatous field defects in their untreated eye during follow-up. Thirty-four patients (43%) were responders to topical epinephrine, including 85% of those who acquired field defects and 28% of those who did not acquire field loss. The incidence of field defects was 50% in epinephrine responders and 6.5% in non-responders. Two of 3 patients who failed to respond but acquired field defects had diabetes. Insignificantly more patients with field defects had initial intraocular pressures above 27 mm Hg.

The topical epinephrine test is safe and easy to perform. It appears to be a remarkably sensitive and reasonably specific test for the development of glaucoma in patients falling into the homozygous-ocular hypertensive group. Heterozygotes are less responsive to topical epinephrine than are homozygotes and the test should be applicable generally to all patients. A large-scale, long-term study of tested patients is needed. At present it appears reasonable to advise treating with epinephrine those homozygous ocular hypertensives who respond noticeably to topical epinephrine. Fortunately those homozygotes who respond poorly to topical epinephrine appear to have a much better prognosis and can be followed without treatment.

**Automatic Perimetry in Glaucoma Visual Field Screening: Clinical Study.** Anders Heijl[2] (Univ. of Lund) compared fully automatic computerized perimetry with manual selective perimetry for detection of field defects in 181 eyes of 100 patients at a glaucoma clinic. Eyes with known very large field defects and those with visual acuity below 0.4 were excluded. The median patient age was 64 years. Both patients treated for an ocular pressure of 22 mm Hg or higher and untreated patients with pressures over 21 mm Hg were included.

The computerized perimeter used had 64 static test points, 56 of them in concentric circles at 5, 10 and 15 degrees eccentricity, and 8 test points at 20 and 25 degrees from the fixation point. The stimuli can be lit at 16 intensity

(2)   Albrecht von Graefes Arch. Klin. Ophthalmol. 200:21 – 37, 1976.

levels, the ratio between two consecutive levels always being 1:2. Testing begins at four test points at 10 degrees eccentricity; the threshold values are used to compute intensity levels for further testing. One pathologic paracentral test point was enough for the result not to be accepted as normal.

For the manual test, Armaly's selective perimetry was used.

Forty-seven of the 181 eyes were judged to have pathologic visual fields. All 47 eyes were pathologic by the automatic test. Five of 6 pathologic fields with less than 6 defects initially had reproducible defects on rescreening. One pathologic field was missed on manual selective perimetry. Initially, the automatic test gave 29 false positive results (16% of eyes); the rate was much reduced by rescreening. The false positive rate for manual perimetry was 21.5% of eyes. Test time was shorter for the automatic method. The blind spot was missed in 7.5% of automatic fields. Twenty of the 47 eyes with field defects had previously been classified as normal.

The automatic glaucoma visual field screening technique gives results very like those obtained with optimal manual selective perimetry. The results are unequivocal, and the test is rapid. It will probably prove to be superior to conventional routine perimetry. The introduction of automatic perimeters with built-in rechecking devices into clinical practice may bring about an improvement in the general quality of perimetry.

**Ocusert, New Drug Delivery System for Treatment of Glaucoma.** In earlier reports K. Heilmann[3] (Technical Univ., Munich) discussed the principle of continuous and constant medication, as applied to glaucoma. The first studies compared the ocular pressures, pupillary narrowing and myopic effects of Ocusert Pilo-20 and Pilo-40 controlled pilocarpine delivery system and pilocarpine eye drops in 13 ambulatory patients with chronic wide-angle glaucoma during 5 weeks. The intraocular pressure was decreased around the clock for at least 7 days; the ocular pressure effect of Ocusert Pilo-20 was comparable to that of 2% pilocarpine 4

(3)   Klin. Monatsbl. Augenheilkd. 167:534–542, October, 1975.

times daily; the pupillary narrowing and myopic effect of Ocusert were significantly less than with pilocarpine drops; and miosis and accommodative myopia were constant.

The present report covers a 15-month study during which each patient was controlled once a week. The anterior ocular segments and the fundi were particularly examined and side effects were noted.

No serious complications occurred in any patient treated with Ocusert. Foreign-body sensation was minimal and generally perceived only after the membrane was inserted. Seven of 17 patients reported no instance of loss of the Ocusert from the eye during the entire period, 7 patients lost it fewer than 3 times and 3 patients more than 3 times, all during sleep or while dressing. Deformation of the Ocusert, i.e., twisting of its longitudinal axis in the shape of a figure 8, was frequent, although the device remained functional, if to a lesser degree. The transition from the elliptic shape to that of a figure 8 with partially overlapping membrane may lead to reduction of the active surface by about one third of the original elliptic form.

Unanswered is whether it is necessary to create a permanently uniform tissue level in order to achieve an adequate pressure level. Also, it must be considered whether the continuous drug supply might be harmful to intraocular structures and eventually lead to pathologic alterations. These questions may be clarified only by precise long-term studies, and final judgment on this new type of drug dispenser must be deferred at present.

**Possibility of Isoproterenol Therapy with Soft Contact Lenses: Ocular Hypotension without Systemic Effects.** Giambattista Bietti, Michele Virno, Josè Pecori-Giraldi, Nando Pellegrino and Ettore Motolese[4] studied the effects of low concentrations of isoproterenol, applied by insertion of presoaked soft contact lenses, on intraocular pressure and cardiovascular function in rabbits and in 20 patients with ocular hypertension. The Soflens lenses were soaked at least 24 hours in sterile saline before use. They were totally immersed in isoproterenol sulfate for varying periods. Concentrations of 0.05 – 2% were used in animal

---

(4)    Ann. Ophthalmol. 8:819– 829, July, 1976.

studies and a 0.2% concentration in the patients. Animals were also treated with lenses immersed in 1% propranolol and 1% isoproterenol plus 1% propranolol. Nineteen patient eyes had open-angle chronic simple glaucoma, 3, absolute glaucoma and 2, hypertensive uveitis. Lens wearing times ranged from 1 to 2 hours.

The mean intraocular pressure in rabbit eyes fell about 40% with 0.05% isoproterenol-exposed lenses, with no significant changes in heart rate or arterial pressure. The 0.1% solution reduced intraocular pressures by 54% after 1 hour; the heart rate rose 18% and the arterial blood pressure fell by 7%. With 2% isoproterenol the intraocular pressure fell 40%, the heart rate increased 23.7% and the arterial pressure fell 12.2%. The isoproterenol-propranolol combination resulted in a 54.5% fall in intraocular tension with no significant changes in heart rate or arterial pressure.

Optimal hypotensive responses were seen in chronic simple glaucoma and absolute glaucoma, but no fall in pressure occurred in the patients with hypertensive uveitis. In half the eyes the maximum hypotensive effect lasted over 8 hours. No significant changes in heart rate or arterial pressure were noted and there were no subjective effects. Slight conjunctival hyperemia was noted in some patients. In 1 patient, insertion of a lens soaked in 0.2% isoproterenol resulted in a 33% fall in ocular tension without cardiovascular changes, whereas instillation of 2.4% isoproterenol eyedrops resulted in a 30% fall in ocular tension a 7% fall in arterial pressure and a 20% increase in heart rate.

Marked ocular hypotension can be obtained using soft lenses presoaked in a mixture of isoproterenol and propranolol.

**Loss of Acute Pilocarpine Effect on Outflow Facility Following Surgical Disinsertion and Retrodisplacement of the Ciliary Muscle from the Scleral Spur in the Cynomolgus Monkey.** Contraction of the ciliary muscle by voluntary accommodation or cholinergic drugs in primates causes an acute increase in aqueous humor outflow facility, attributed to mechanical deformation of the trabecular meshwork. The facility-increasing action of adrenergic drugs may well be due to a direct action on the endothelial cells of the meshwork or Schlemm's canal, or both, and there is some evidence that pilocarpine may also act at these sites. Paul L. Kaufman and Ernst H. Bárány[5] (Univ. of Uppsala) report on a technique for disinserting and retrodisplacing the ciliary muscle from the scleral spur over 360 degrees in cynomolgus monkeys and the subsequent, essentially complete loss of the acute facility-increasing effect of pilocarpine.

An ab-interno goniotomy-like operation was done to disinsert the ciliary muscle from the scleral spur. After postoperative miotic and steroid therapy, the eyes did well clinically and the muscle reattached to the sclera posterior to the spur. Total iridectomy simplified the disinsertion procedure done in 25 cynomolgus monkeys. Outflow facility and intraocular pressure were mildly reduced. Aqueous drained via the conventional outflow routes and blood flow to the ciliary body was observed. The outflow facility-increasing effects of intravenous and intracameral pilocarpine were nearly totally eliminated.

These findings suggest that the ciliary muscle was permanently disconnected from the trabecular meshwork in these studies. The trabecular meshwork and Schlemm's canal remained relatively normal structurally and functionally. These eyes may prove useful for testing the functional effects of drugs directly on the conventional outflow channels, independent of drug actions on the ciliary muscle.

**Effects of Dipivalyl Epinephrine on the Eye.** Dipivalyl epinephrine (DPE) is an analogue of epinephrine, which theoretically should be more lipophilic than epinephrine and should penetrate the corneal barriers more readily. Animal studies suggest that DPE is less toxic systemically than epinephrine but more potent as an ocular hypotensive agent. Martin B. Kaback, Steven M. Podos, Thomas S. Harbin, Jr., Alan Mandell and Bernard Becker[6] (Washington Univ.) studied the mechanism of action of DPE and its effects on intraocular pressure and pupil size in human eyes. Single-dose studies were done with 0.005–0.5% DPE in 10 patients with symmetric ocular hypertension. Multiple-dose studies were done with 0.1% DPE, placed in one eye twice

(5)  Invest. Ophthalmol. 15:793–807, October, 1976.

(6)  Am. J. Ophthalmol. 81:768–772, June, 1976.

daily, in 10 similar patients. Mechanism studies were carried out in rabbits.

Dipivalyl epinephrine significantly reduced intraocular pressures in the single-dose studies, in concentrations of 0.025–0.5%. Concentrations of 0.1 and 0.5% significantly dilated the pupil. In multiple-dose studies, 0.1% DPE significantly reduced intraocular pressure at days 2 and 31. The maximum effect was reached in 4–8 hours and persisted for 12 hours after the first and second instillations. Patient responses were variable in time. Most patients had a pupillary response, but this was unrelated to the pressure reduction. Changes in facility of aqueous outflow in DPE-treated eyes were insignificant. No side effects were observed. In the rabbit studies, 0.025 and 0.1% DPE significantly activated the cyclic adenosine monophosphate system, and dose-response relations were demonstrated.

The epinephrine analogue DPE significantly reduces intraocular pressure in concentrations as low as 0.025%. Theoretically, alteration of the parent compound by addition of pivalic acid groups should enhance the ability of the molecule to penetrate the cornea. Use of this low-dose epinephrine compound should minimize or eliminate dose-related extraocular side effects. Epinephrine compounds reduce intraocular pressure by decreasing inflow of aqueous and by enhancing the coefficient of aqueous outflow; DPE appears to act similarly.

**6-Hydroxydopamine in Treatment of Open-Angle Glaucoma.** Ideal treatment for open-angle glaucoma should simultaneously decrease the production of aqueous and facilitate outflow from the anterior chamber. Holland introduced the norepinephrine congener 6-hydroxydopamine for the treatment of chronic simple glaucoma. This agent produces a highly selective but reversible degeneration of the adrenergic nerve terminals, possibly through the finding of a metabolite with the biologic membrane of the storage granule in the nerve terminal. The end result is, in effect, a chemical sympathectomy. James G. Diamond[7] (Univ. of Illinois Eye and Ear Infirm.) evaluated the subcon-

---

(7)   Arch. Ophthalmol. 94:41–47, January, 1976.

junctival administration of a buffered 6-hydroxydopamine solution in patients with open-angle glaucoma.

Eleven eyes of 10 patients were treated for intraocular pressures above 30 mm Hg; 8 eyes had pressures above 38 mm Hg while on maximal standard treatment. All eyes showed endstage glaucoma. An injection of 1-5 mg 6-hydroxydopamine was given in an ascorbic acid-water mixture subconjunctivally after the pupillary response to the agent was determined and denervation hypersensitivity was monitored by instilling 1:1,000 epinephrine.

Consistent conjunctival injection followed the administration of 6-hydroxydopamine; it appeared to be dose-related. Most patients had lower intraocular pressures 2–3 hours after the injection. All pupils were hypersensitive to 1 drop of 1:1,000 epinephrine, given in 3 doses at 5-minute intervals, after 2–3 weeks. All eyes responded negatively to 1% hydroxyamphetamine. Intraocular pressures in some patients began to return to pretreatment levels at weeks 12–16. The average mean pressure throughout the long-term phase of the study (14–90 days) was 27 mm Hg. Outflow facility changed significantly during the long-term phase. All eyes responded similarly to a second subconjunctival injection of 6-hydroxydopamine, given after about 90 days.

These findings indicate the feasibility and effectiveness of subconjunctivally administered 6-hydroxydopamine in the treatment of open-angle glaucoma. Contralateral ocular pressure effects, though present, were not significant, and systemic adrenergic effects were not noted in the present patients. Repeated injections of small doses of 6-hydroxydopamine, such as 1 mg every 3d day for 2 or 3 times, might enhance the degree of sympathectomy.

**"Black Cornea" Secondary to Topical Epinephrine.** Eleven cases of "black cornea" in patients treated with topical epinephrine for a disrupted, irregular corneal surface have been reported. Presumably the pigment plaque that forms rapidly consists mainly of adrenochrome, a partial oxidation product of epinephrine. Rodney W. McCarthy and Raymond LeBlanc[8] (McGill Univ.) report the first case of

(8) Can. J. Ophthalmol. 11:336–340, October, 1976.

black cornea secondary to topical epinephrine therapy in which the pigmented plaque was analyzed biochemically.

Woman, 48, had had bilateral cataract extractions 10 years before, complicated on the right side by a flat anterior chamber, synechiae and secondary glaucoma. A blind, mildly painful right eye was present, with marked bullous keratopathy and extensive corneal vascularization, and the angle was completely closed. Acetazolamide relieved the pain, and 1% epinephrine twice daily was required to control chronic open-angle glaucoma in the left eye. A central, flat, dark, corneal plaque was seen in the right eye and became more distinct in time; the patient had been using epinephrine drops in both eyes. A large black plaque was present the next year, and the right eye was enucleated. The pigment stained for melanin and with the diazo reaction for phenolic groups, and it bleached with potassium permanganate. Infrared absorption studies suggested that the plaque material consisted of melanin.

A disrupted corneal epithelium, usually secondary to bullous keratopathy, favors pooling of epinephrine beneath the epithelium, where it oxidizes to an insoluble compound now known to be an animal-like melanin. The remarkable rapidity of plaque growth is unexplained, but binding of epinephrine to melanin is a possibility. The mechanism of melanin drug binding is obscure. Possibly the effect of light on undeteriorated epinephrine in the region of the palpebral fissure produces hypersensitivity. The plaque in this case conformed to the region exposed by the palpebral fissure, although mechanical factors cannot be excluded.

**Aqueous Humor Dynamics in Glaucomatocyclitic Crisis.** The glaucomatocyclitic crisis is characterized by recurrent attacks of unilateral ocular hypertension associated with mild cyclitic symptoms. Outflow facility is reduced during the attacks but controversial results have been obtained regarding alteration in the rate of aqueous humor formation. Prostaglandins have been found in high concentration in aqueous humor during attacks of the syndrome. Shigetoshi Nagataki and Saiichi Mishima[9] (Univ. of Tokyo) calculated the transfer coefficients of fluorescein in the anterior chamber by flow and by diffusion through analyzing concentrations in the anterior chamber, pupillary aqueous and serum ultrafiltrates after intravenous

(9)   Invest. Ophthalmol. 15:365–370, May, 1976.

injection. Aqueous humor dynamics were examined in 8 patients with glaucomatocyclitic crisis, 6 men and 2 women aged 21–65. Aqueous dynamics were determined in the early period of attacks before treatment and during remission at least 2 months after the cessation of medication.

In 7 patients, the coefficients determined during attacks averaged $1.23 \times 10^{-2}$ min$^{-1}$ for flow and $3.51 \times 10^{-3}$ min$^{-1}$ for diffusion in the involved eye and $0.91 \times 10^{-2}$ and $1.36 \times 10^{-3}$, respectively, in the fellow eye. Differences in coefficients between the 2 eyes were significant. In 6 patients studied during remission, differences in coefficients between the 2 eyes were not significant. In 5 patients the determinations were repeated during attacks and remission and the differences in the coefficients between both phases were significant in the involved eye.

This study showed increases in transfer coefficients by both flow and diffusion during attacks of glaucomatocyclitic crisis. Increases in diffusion coefficients were more marked than those in flow coefficients. During remissions, both coefficients did not differ significantly from normal values. The findings are in accord with animal observations in which prostaglandin E was found to increase blood-aqueous barrier permeability and ultrafiltration, leading to sustained intraocular pressure elevation. The ocular hypertension is apparently due to a decreased outflow facility and also to an increase in aqueous humor formation. The relationship of the outflow facility reduction to an increase in prostaglandin E in aqueous humor remains to be investigated.

**Management of Glaucoma in Nanophthalmos.** Nanophthalmos (from "nanos" meaning "dwarf") connotes a pure type of microphthalmos in which a small but otherwise normal eye is found. This relatively rare condition represents arrested development of the globe in all directions after closure of the embryonic fissure and is usually bilateral; a strong hereditary factor either dominant or recessive is apparent. The eyes are deeply set, with narrow palpebral fissures and examination shows marked hyperopia, small corneas, shallow anterior chambers and occasionally macular hypoplasia. Late glaucoma is a frequent occurrence. F. Phinizy Calhoun, Jr.[1] studied the records of 6 patients with

(1) Trans. Am. Ophthalmol. Soc. 73:97–122, 1975.

TABLE 1. – Clinical Signs of Nanophthalmos

Extreme hyperopia with generally good corrected vision
Small corneal diameter
Shallow anterior chamber, with "vesuvio" pupil
Gonioscopically "slit" or grade I angle
Wide pulse pressure on tonometry
Occasional macular hypoplasia
Tendency to glaucoma in middle age

TABLE 2. – Clinical Characteristics of Glaucoma Occurring in Nanophthalmos

Slow, painless and progressive elevation of intraocular pressure in middle age
Paradoxical response to medical treatment
Failure of conventional glaucoma surgery
Tendency to serious posterior segment complications after anterior segment surgery

bilateral nanophthalmos; 9 of the 12 eyes had various stages of glaucoma.

The clinical features of nanophthalmos are summarized in Table 1, and those of glaucoma occurring in nanophthalmos in Table 2.

Typically these patients develop a slow, painless impairment of vision in one eye or are found to have elevated intraocular pressure on routine examination, when angle-closure and peripheral anterior synechiae are observed. The glaucoma soon becomes refractory to miotics and carbonic anhydrase inhibitors. None of 5 eyes subjected to peripheral iridectomy had acute postoperative malignant glaucoma. Filtering procedures were done in only 2 eyes, with satisfactory results in 1.

▶ [This paper was ably discussed by Drs. Shaffer, Brockhurst, Shoch and Moses. In summary, these dwarf eyes have a short A-P diameter by ultrasonography, high hyperopia, small cornea, shallow anterior chamber, normal-sized lens and probably a thickened sclera. As the patient grows older, a chronic angle-closure glaucoma develops, probably as a result of pupillary block by a normal lens in a small anterior ocular segment. The glaucoma responds poorly to miotics. Surgery consists of iridectomy and the use of atropine postoperatively to avoid ciliary-block "malignant" glaucoma. Only one half of these eyes respond well to surgery, one serious complication being uveal effusion, choroidal and secondary retinal detachment (see the 1976 YEAR BOOK, p. 202). This complication should not be treated by posterior sclerotomy or retinal detachment surgery, but rather by steroids systemically. – Ed.] ◀

**Intraocular Surgery in Advanced Glaucoma.** There is an established view that intraocular surgery may result in obliteration of the central visual field subserving macular function when this is threatened by glaucomatous field loss. E. J. O'Connell and A. G. Karseras[2] (Welsh Natl. School of Medicine) determined the incidence of postoperative loss of central vision in glaucomatous patients having drainage procedures or cataract extraction.

There were 24 eyes with a residual central island, with or without a temporal island of vision, and 22 in which an arcuate scotoma approached to within 5 degrees of central fixation and also extended to the peripheral field to cause a nasal quadrantic defect. An additional arcuate scotoma was occasionally present. Cataract extraction was performed on 13 eyes, and 46 drainage operations were performed. Postoperative follow-up was in 6 months.

Two patients lost central visual field possibly as a result of surgery. Maculopathy complicated 3 drainage operations and 4 of the 13 cataract extractions. A total of 30% of the drainage procedures induced deterioration of visual acuity of lenticular origin to a level normally requiring cataract extraction. Trabeculectomy proved less likely to cause this sequela than was the Scheie procedure. Ten of 25 trabeculectomies resulted in progression of lens opacities, but preoperative opacities were present in 9 of these cases. Five of 12 Scheie operations were associated with progressive postoperative cataract; preoperative lens opacity was present in 1 instance. Satisfactory improvement in vision followed cataract extraction in 77% of the cases.

Loss of visual field subserving macular function is rare after intraocular surgery in patients with advanced glaucoma. Abrupt changes in refractive error, lens opacity and suppression must be carefully excluded before macular fixation is considered lost in these patients.

▶ [In a rather lengthy discussion of the literature, these authors find alternative explanations for data which suggest a reduction or wipe-out of central vision following filtering operations for late glaucoma. Many of these cases of postoperative reduction of macular vision may be the result of refractive change, progressive cataract which reduces vision greatly in a patient with a small visual field or postoperative cystoid macular edema.

(2) Br. J. Ophthalmol. 60:124–131, February, 1976.

These changes may be more frequent if a cataract extraction has been done, or following operations with greater filtration and perhaps temporary hypotony (e.g., trephination, posterior lip sclerectomy, Scheie's thermal sclerectomy) than after trabeculectomy. — Ed.] ◄

**Glaucoma Surgery in Nigerian Eyes: Five-Year Study.** Glaucoma is a major cause of blindness in the sub-Sahara regions of West Africa and will assume more relative importance as infectious and parasitic diseases are controlled more effectively. Benjamin Kietzman[3] (Kano, Nigeria) regards glaucoma in Kano as almost entirely a surgical disease. Review was made of 419 sclerectomies and 612 trabeculectomies followed over 5 years.

Tenon's capsule was routinely excised at sclerectomy. A thin strip of inner sclera 3 mm long was excised from the posterior lip internally and a peripheral iridectomy made as near the vertical meridian as possible. Tenon's capsule was also excised at trabeculectomy. A half-thickness limbal-based scleral flap about 3 × 6 mm in size was raised in the upper nasal or temporal quadrant and the inner half of the sclera was excised over almost the entire width of the scleral incision. A peripheral iridectomy was done as close to the vertical meridian as possible. Depomedrol was injected subconjunctivally at the end of both operations.

Posterior lip sclerectomy gave more frequent good pressure control than trabeculectomy 4 months to 5 years postoperatively (84% compared with 74%, respectively) but comparable numbers of patients had poor or no control after the two operations. Complications included 3 cases of buttonholing of the conjunctival flap at sclerectomy. Hyphema occurred after 5% of the trabeculectomies and 2% of the sclerectomies. Anterior chamber shallowing lasted over a week in 4.4% of the trabeculectomy patients and in 10.5% of the sclerectomy patients; most of the sclerectomy patients required posterior sclerotomy and air injection. Protracted or recurrent iritis followed 3% of the trabeculectomies and 5% of the sclerectomies. Intraocular pressures were elevated in 3.4% of the eyes having trabeculectomy; most patients with pressures below 40 mm Hg had resolution at follow-up. Late postoperative complications included 17 cases of recurrent or persistent iritis, 3 excessively large blebs after scle-

(3)   Ophthalmic Surg. 7:52–58, Winter, 1976.

rectomy and 7 ruptured blebs with endophthalmia after sclerectomy. One sclerectomized eye developed sympathetic ophthalmia after endophthalmitis.

Pressure control after trabeculectomy in this series was about the same as in English eyes reported by Ridgeway, but not as good as those reported by Cairns or by Watson and Barnett.

**Demonstration of Aqueous Outflow Patterns of Normal and Glaucomatous Human Eyes through Injection of Fluorescein Solution in the Anterior Chamber.** O. Benedikt[4] (Univ. of Graz) presents the results of studies on 200 eyes, including normal eyes, those with open-angle glaucoma and those after iridectomy, iridencleisis, Elliot's trephination and trabeculectomy.

The anterior chamber is reached by a diagonal corneal puncture within the left lower quadrant, using a small, straight discission needle. The anterior chamber is filled with a 0.2% fluorescein Ringer's solution using a 1-ml injection syringe; about one third of the aqueous humor is replaced by the dye solution because this amount flows out during puncture and filling. The eyes are examined using a blue filter slit lamp, a sketch is made of each eye and a protocol is made for the temporal course of all outflow phenomena. About 20–30 minutes are required for each examination. Patients later receive antibiotic drops, 5–6 times daily, for 1–2 days; a bandage is not required. Complications are rare; among 200 eyes examined, iridocyclitic phenomena were observed only in 3 instances and subsided easily with treatment. Lenticular injuries did not occur.

In normal eyes, at physiologic intraocular pressure, 1–9 aqueous veins were found, with a mean of 4.6. Their distribution was usually irregular, with those of largest caliber in the lower nasal quadrant. With few exceptions, the aqueous veins originated 1–2.5 mm peripheral from the limbus and joined the episcleral veins after a short course. The venae recipients were characterized by a straight and deep course.

In eyes with open-angle glaucoma the average number of aqueous veins was increased as compared to normal eyes. However, their caliber was smaller and distribution more

---

(4)   Albrecht von Graefes Arch. Klin. Ophthalmol. 199:45–67, 1976.

uniform. Eyes after iridectomy did not differ from normal eyes in the mechanism of aqueous outflow. After iridencleisis and trephination, the transport of aqueous humor from the anterior chamber is achieved through a filtration bleb, including transconjunctival, by bulk flow through lymphatic vessels and diffusely through lymphatic vessels or veins. In most instances different transport mechanisms were combined. There was a definite relationship between the size of the filtration bleb and the development of draining lymphatic vessels.

After trabeculectomy the following drainage mechanisms were observed: subconjunctival outflow (Fig 23), with further drainage in such cases achieved primarily through the lymphatic vessels; direct transport of aqueous humor into the surgical area through newly incorporated veins and lymphatic vessels; and drainage through still functioning aqueous veins (Fig 24).

In eyes with well-regulated intraocular pressure and clin-

**Fig 23.**—Trabeculectomy. Starting at surgical site, richly branched, small-calibered network of lymphatic vessels appears in superficial connective membrane layers. (Courtesy of Benedikt, O.: Albrecht von Graefes Arch. Klin. Ophthalmol. 199:45–67, 1976; Berlin-Heidelberg-New York: Springer.)

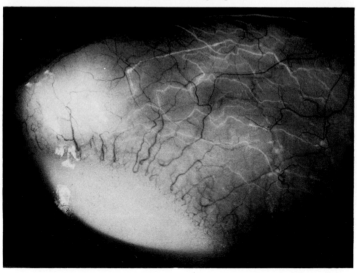

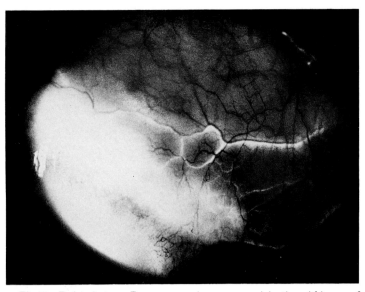

**Fig 24.** – Trabeculectomy. Two aqueous veins are seen, originating within area of scleral flap; course is almost parallel to limbus. (Courtesy of Benedikt, O.: Albrecht von Graefes Arch. Klin. Ophthalmol. 199:45 – 67, 1976; Berlin-Heidelberg-New York: Springer.)

ical absence of a filtration bleb, lymphatic vessels or newly incorporated veins were generally well developed, whereas subconjunctival outflow remained small. The function of an external fistula is not dependent on the size of a filtration bleb but on the possibility of prompt transport of aqueous humor by the vessels present in the area. Other transport mechanisms did not seem important to intraocular pressure regulation. Only in 3 cases could it be assumed that by surgery an opening was achieved between the anterior chamber and Schlemm's canal. Although trabeculectomy must be classified as a fistula-building operation, its degree of effectiveness makes it superior to the old types of filtering operations.

▶ [Injection of fluorescein into the anterior chamber demonstrates the aqueous veins well. The veins are more numerous and smaller in glaucoma. After filtering operations, aqueous drainage may occur transconjunctivally via lymphatic vessels or aqueous veins. – Ed.] ◀

**Cataract Surgery and Trabeculectomy in One Session.** P. Brégeat[5] (Univ. of Cochin) discusses the various means of simultaneously treating these frequently coexisting conditions. These include cataract surgery and drug therapy for the glaucoma, operative management of the glaucoma and later cataract surgery or cataract and glaucoma surgery as one procedure. Since the introduction of trabeculectomy, this combined surgery is based on simultaneous lens extraction and treatment of the glaucoma by "protective filtration." Sixty-five patients have been treated in this manner, among them 11 diabetics; 91 eyes have been observed during a 2-year period after surgery.

After a conjunctival flap is created (lateral-diagonal outward bound), the scleral flap is formed and after trabeculectomy a lateral keratotomy (Castroviejo scissors) is achieved. This is followed by a triphase total basal iridectomy (or peripheral basal iridectomy followed by sphincterotomy). Cryoextraction of the lens, depending on the individual patient, is done with or without zonulysis; 2–3 silk sutures are made on both sides of the keratotomy, one at the upper corners of the scleral flap. The latter are kept rather loose in order to serve their purpose of "protective filtration." The anterior chamber is restored with the help of an air bubble or synthetic aqueous humor. The conjunctival flap is then carefully resutured with individual sutures.

The main indications for this technique are an increased intraocular pressure (regardless of etiology) resistant to medication and associated with cataract and cataract with drug-controlled or noncontrolled chronic increase of intra-

COMPARISON OF PRESSURE REGULATION AFTER TRABECULECTOMY AND OTHER
FISTULATING PROCEDURES IN COMBINED SURGICAL TREATMENT
OF GLAUCOMA AND CATARACT*

| OCULAR PRESSURE | MIOTICS | ELLIOT | LAGRANGE | SCHEIE | VERZELLA | TRABECULECTOMY |
|---|---|---|---|---|---|---|
| Regulated | Without | 33 | 50 | 54.5 | 66.6 | 76 |
| | With | 33 | 12.5 | 27.2 | 16.6 | 22.5 |
| Not Regulated | | 33 | 37.5 | 18.1 | 16.6 | 1.5 |

*All results are per cent.

(5) Klin. Monatsbl. Augenheilkd. 167:505–515, October, 1975.

ocular pressure. Most observed postoperative complications, such as hyphema, vitreous hemorrhage and prolapse, pupillary block or postoperative rise of intraocular pressure, are not severe and do not influence the desired decrease of intraocular pressure.

This combined procedure is the most effective of those known to date (table), given careful monitoring of the patient's vascular state and exclusive use of the surgical microscope in performing the trabeculectomy.

**Histologic and Physiologic Studies of Cyclocryotherapy in Primate and Human Eyes.** Cyclocryotherapy has been a valuable mode of treatment of otherwise inoperable glaucoma. Harry A. Quigley[6] (Johns Hopkins Hosp.) examined the effects of cyclocryotherapy on primate and human eyes at intervals up to 3 months after treatment. Temperatures of the cryoprobe and in the pars plicata of the ciliary were correlated in anesthetized primates and in enucleated human and owl monkey eyes. A cryoprobe and temperature potentiometer with microminiature thermocouple and an operating microscope were used. Monkey eyes were treated with a 2-mm probe tip with the anterior edge 3 mm from the limbus at six spots (one-half circumference) at temperatures of $-60$ to $-70$ C for varying times of $30-60$ seconds. Two human eyes were treated just before enucleation for uveal melanoma. Cryotherapy was also carried out in single patients with total hyphema due to trauma, bullous keratopathy complicated by secondary glaucoma and neovascular glaucoma due to proliferative diabetic retinopathy.

In both human and primate eyes, the epithelial and capillary elements of the ciliary processes were destroyed and replaced by fibroblast-like cells. The trabecular meshwork and Schlemm's canal were histologically altered, and damage to the angle structures impaired aqueous outflow. However, the meshwork and endothelium of Schlemm's canal were normal, after 1 month, although the canal remained more narrow. The loss of ciliary epithelium resulted in breakdown of the blood-aqueous barrier and accounted for chronic aqueous flare. Correlation of the cryoprobe and ciliary pars plicata temperatures in monkey eyes demonstrat-

(6)   Am. J. Ophthalmol. 82:722–732, November, 1976.

ed that uveal blood flow attenuates the effect of cryotherapy on the ciliary body.

Damage to the angle structures from cyclocryotherapy may partially counteract the favorable effect of cryotherapy on intraocular pressure. Although cryotherapy considerably decreases aqueous inflow, it also diminishes outflow facility, leading to a less stable intraocular pressure equilibrium.

▶ [These results show that treatment of monkey and human eyes with the anterior edge of the 2 mm cryoprobe 3 mm from the limbus for 60 seconds at −70C destroys the ciliary processes and also damages the trabeculum (which regenerates) but leaves the canal of Schlemm smaller and reduces inflow and outflow. Ferry confirmed in human eyes that there is no regeneration of ciliary processes (Trans. Am. Acad. Ophthalmol. Otolaryngol., 1977). This might explain the temporary lowering of intraocular pressure in many cases. It may be that associated damage to the drainage pathways might negate the reduction of aqueous production. Placing the probe further posteriorly may destroy the pars plana and peripheral retina but not the secreting ciliary processes (ibid.). Therefore in this procedure, the necessary simultaneous damage to both ciliary processes and drainage angle would suggest that the ophthalmologist apply cyclocryotherapy in areas where the angle is already damaged by firm PAS, and possibly avoid treating the entire circumference but re-treating the same area, if necessary.−Ed.] ◀

**Mode of Action of Trabeculectomy** was determined by O. Benedikt[7] (Univ. of Graz) by clinical investigation of 370 eyes after such intervention, particularly by injection of fluorescein into the anterior chamber in 90 of these eyes. Cairns' (1968) technique of trabeculectomy was designed to achieve pressure regulation by natural drainage of the aqueous humor over existing pathways, based on the idea that excision of a tissue segment from the chamber inlet would open Schlemm's canal and the pathologically altered resistance is localized in front of Schlemm's channel rather cumvented. This concept presupposes that this increased resistance is localized in front of Schlemm's channel rather than in it or within the area of its outgoing cannulae and that the cut ends of the channel remain permanently open after surgery.

Because neither the pathogenesis of all forms of glaucoma nor the reactions of the drainage system of glaucomatous eyes to surgery has been unequivocally established, clinical investigation is relied on to evaluate the effect and mode of

(7)   Klin. Monatsbl. Augenheilkd. 167:679–685, November, 1975.

action of antiglaucomatous intervention. Among the many
test results in evaluating the mode of action of trabeculectomy, the most significant are the postoperative status of
intraocular tension of the pressure-regulated eyes (mean
values); preoperative and postoperative C values of pressure-regulated eyes; gonioscopic control of the operation
site; type of bleb; and results of fluorescein filling of the
anterior chamber.

In the present study the following drainage mechanisms
of the aqueous humor were observed: outflow through newly developed aqueous veins (trabeculectomy veins); bulk-
flow through lymphatic vessels; diffuse resorption into the
subconjunctival connective tissue; and outflow through normal aqueous veins. Outflow through normal veins is generally of minimal quantitative significance; only in 3 instances
did outflow seemingly take place in this manner exclusively
and in these cases pressure regulation presumably was
achieved by a functionally open Schlemm's canal. However,

Fig 25.—After fluorescein filling of anterior chamber, simultaneous representation of subconjunctival bleb, lymphatic vessels originating at operation site and
trabeculectomy vein *(arrow)*. This combination of outflow mechanisms is frequent.
(Courtesy of Benedikt, O.: Klin. Monatsbl. Augenheilkd. 167:679–685, November,
1975.)

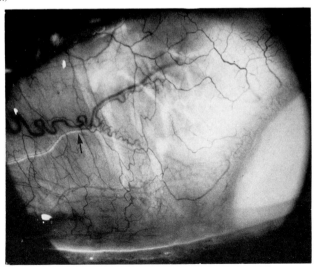

in most instances a combination of several drainage possi-
bilities was found (Fig 25); the respective part in the total
outflow of each of these may be established only on the basis
of the investigator's experience. With few exceptions, trabeculectomy does not lead to opening of Schlemm's canal or
its outflow cannulae and absence of a visible bleb does not
speak for any particular outflow mechanism.

# The Lens

INTRODUCTION

In recent years there has been a considerable advance in cataract surgical technique, including PhacoEmulsification and lens implant surgery. During this same time span there has also been an exciting expansion of our knowledge of the basic biochemistry and physiology of the lens itself and of the changes that occur in cataract formation.

The young lens is composed of low molecular weight proteins, united by covalent linkages and weak noncovalent bonds. These low molecular weight protein aggregates allow transmission of visible light with little scattering. With aging, the percentage of covalent bonding increases and the low molecular weight aggregates are transformed into large protein aggregates and insoluble protein. This occurs primarily in the central region in nuclear sclerotic cataracts, and the concentration of high molecular weight protein increases 10-fold between age 20 and 60. Since the lens appears unable to modify the protein damage that accompanies aging, these large proteins, which are of sufficient size and irregularity to cause light scattering, accumulate and may be responsible for cataract formation. Newer techniques, such as optical mixing spectroscopy, allow study of intact excised lenses and hopefully will be adapted to in vivo measurements in patients. With this technique the possible effects of medical therapy on cataract formation in patients can be studied.

It is well known clinically that the aging lens becomes increasingly yellow. This yellowing occurs in the high molecular weight protein fraction and is due to atypical fluorescence. One of the fluorescent compounds appears to arise from a normal lens constituent and may be involved in the formation of the large molecular weight aggregates which lead to opacification.

Research is currently underway on the biochemical analysis of lens components. A decrease in glutathione in cataractous lenses suggests the loss of glutathione peroxidase may permit toxic accumulation of peroxidase within the lens. Also, as cataracts develop and mature the sphingolipids increase in the lens up to 10-fold and bound cholesterol increases. In vitro, the incubation of lenses with lysophosphatidylcholine, a normal constituent of the aqueous humor, leads to the development of posterior subcapsular cataracts. This is the first demonstration that lens changes can be accentuated by naturally occurring aqueous humor phospholipids. It is possible that this compound may also potentiate the toxic effect of corticosteroids on the lens. If suitable compounds are found, which are nontoxic in vivo and can inhibit this reaction, they might possibly be used to prevent the development of steroid-potentiated posterior subcapsular cataracts in patients on systemic steroids. Similarly, aldose reductase inhibitors have been used to prevent the formation of cataracts in diabetic animals.

In diabetic animals, glucose is converted into sorbitol by the enzyme aldose reductase which is normally present in the lens. This sorbitol accumulates in the lens and leads to opacification. Several aldose reductase inhibitors have been successfully used in diabetic animals to prevent this accumulation of sorbitol and cataract formation. This raises the possibility that such compounds may be used in the future in human diabetic patients to prevent the lens changes that occur. Thus, basic biochemical studies may be expanded and applied to the prevention of disease in humans.

Meanwhile, many elderly patients with visual loss from cataracts are now receiving rapid and almost complete visual rehabilitation with intraocular lenses. The excitement over lens implantation has resulted in an expanding flood of papers on all aspects of this procedure, but only a few of these papers deal with long-term results. There is therefore a sound emphasis on conservative indications and proper concern for the careful elucidation and study of complications, both short- and long-term. Fundamental improvements in surgical technology are already beginning to benefit all patients undergoing anterior segment surgery, and the new order of magnitude of surgical skills, techniques, exactitude and analysis which lens implantation has imposed may be one of its most long-lasting and therefore fundamentally important surgical contributions.

This promises to be one of the most exciting eras in ophthalmology for all of us.

Robert C. Drews, M.D.
Stephen R. Waltman, M.D.
Washington University

► ↓ The introduction to this chapter and the following three articles are testimony that biochemists are active in determining various mechanisms by which cataracts can be produced and, *miserabile dictu* for surgeons, naturally seeking ways to prevent these pathologic reactions. A loss of glutathione peroxidase may permit the toxic accumulation of peroxidase, and any lens opacification may be accentuated by naturally occurring phospholipids in the aqueous which also may potentiate the toxic effect of steroids on the lens (see the Introduction to this Chapter). Other mechanisms have been investigated and reviewed by Ruth van Heyningen in the next article. These include: (1) absence of the enzyme aldose reductase, resulting in the accumulation of sorbitol in the lens of diabetics (review of Kinoshita's work), and the lack of the enzyme mannosidase leading to the lysosomal storage of mannose-rich oligosaccharides in lens and other tissues leading to a Hurler's-like syndrome (see Arbisser et al.); (2) tryptophan deficiency leading to lack of maturation of lens fibers (von Sallman et al., 1956); (3) ingestion of naphtholene which is oxidized to produce toxic naphthoquinones (see article by van Heyningen); (4) proteolysis by activated peptidases and accumulation of peptides (Kinoshita) or loss of normal peptides through the lens capsule permitting the proteolysis of lens proteins; and (5) low ionized calcium and high phosphate in a patient undergoing hemodialysis with formation of a tetany cataract (Koch et al.). — Ed. ◄

**Experimental Studies on Cataract** are summarized by Ruth van Heyningen[8] (Oxford Univ., England). The human lens differs in important ways from lenses of the animals studied most frequently, the cow, rabbit and rat. The human lens grows in the eye throughout life at a slowly decreasing rate, whereas animal lenses grow fast at first and then slow down, increasing little in weight in the second half of life. Only the human and primate lens is thought to alter its shape in accommodation. The human lens is pale yellow in color, perhaps partly because of certain tryptophan deriva-

---

(8)   Invest. Ophthalmol. 15:685–697, September, 1976.

tives which are absent from the lenses of other species. Only human and primate lenses contain 3-hydroxykynurenine glucoside and develop brown nuclear senile cataract.

The similarity in appearance between naphthalene cataract and some types of senile cataract is striking. The absence of polyphenol oxidase (tyrosine oxidase) from the lens protects it from the formation of quinones in situ. The evidence that sorbital in the lens is responsible for the increased rate of cataract extraction in diabetics is impressive. In all types of cataract the lens eventually loses protein. Bovine lens contains a proteinase that will hydrolyze $\alpha$-crystallin. Presumably the enzyme is tightly bound to its substrate, $\alpha$-crystallin, in such a way that proteolysis of crystallin by the enzyme is prevented, and the products of autolysis inhibit enzyme activity, possibly by binding at the active site. In early cataract formation, binding between enzyme and both breakdown products and $\alpha$-crystallin may be weakened once there is some "leakage" from the lens, and peptides escape through the capsule, allowing proteolysis to proceed. There may then be no mechanism to repair the damage.

Tryptophan-deficiency cataract is the only authenticated and reproducible experimental cataract caused by a dietary deficiency. Further studies are needed to determine whether the fluorescent tryptophan derivatives, found only in the lens of man and higher primates, are involved in the development of brown nuclear cataract.

**Ocular Findings in Mannosidosis.** Mannosidosis is a lysosomal storage disorder clinically resembling Hurler's syndrome. $\alpha$-mannosidase is deficient, and mannose-rich oligosaccharides accumulate in the tissues and urine. Amir I. Arbisser, A. Linn Murphree, Charles A. Garcia and R. Rodney Howell[9] (Houston) reviewed the ocular findings in 11 cases of mannosidosis. Similar lenticular opacities were found in 3 patients with typical features of mannosidosis and deficient $\alpha$-mannosidase activity. Corneal opacities were absent. Chamber-angle and striking ophthalmoscopic anomalies were found in 2 young patients who had normal electroretinograms. Two patients had strabismus. Conjunctival

---

(9)   Am. J. Ophthalmol. 82:465–471, September, 1976.

biopsies confirmed the lysosomal nature of the disorder. The most severely affected patient had the most prominent cataract. One patient exhibited progress of wheellike lenticular opacities between examinations. The least affected patient had cataracts not readily visible by direct ophthalmoscopy.

The cataract appears to be a common and distinctive feature of mannosidosis. Strabismus is a nonspecific finding in many storage disorders. Mannosidosis bears some resemblance to the mucopolysaccharidoses, although the ocular findings are apparently distinct and may aid in its clinical differentiation from other disorders. These patients lacked corneal opacities, and their vascular abnormalities appeared to be limited to the retinal vascular system. The ocular changes are superficially similar to those seen in $\alpha$-galactosidase deficiency (Fabry's disease). Mannosidase in the lens may not be of lysosomal origin, but lens fraction mannosidase has not yet been assayed in a patient with mannosidosis. Because mannose and mannosidase are located in the lens, local metabolism may contribute to formation of the cataract.

**Cataract during Intermittent Hemodialysis: Role of Hypocalcemia in Development of Opacities** was investigated by H. R. Koch, K. Siedek, P. Weikenmeier and U. Metzler[1] (Univ. of Bonn). Although intermittent dialysis has considerably prolonged the life expectancy of patients with terminal renal disease, several associated conditions have been observed more frequently, either complications of the basic condition, becoming manifest through this prolonged life expectancy, or side effects of the treatment itself. Twenty uremic patients on intermittent hemodialysis were observed for lenticular changes over a period of 4–53 months. Patients underwent dialysis twice weekly for 12 hours initially, later 3 times for 8 hours and then 10 hours per week.

Occasional opacities of varied form and degree were seen in several patients, but these were comparable to those seen in a normal group of a similar age distribution. Punctate opacities of the cortex were relatively frequent. However, in 1 patient, aged 22, with megaloureters and megalocystis,

(1) Klin. Monatsbl. Augenheilkd. 168:346–353, March, 1976.

bilateral anterior and posterior subcapsular cataracts developed and were felt to be a result of the treatment. The morphology of these cataracts was comparable to that of fresh hypocalcemic opacities, the patient having had a diminished serum calcium level over a prolonged period of time. Hypocalcemia is a fairly frequent finding in the uremic patient; this condition is usually present before the onset of dialysis because of disturbed intestinal calcium resorption.

Experimental studies have shown that aside from the calcium level, the calcium-phosphate ratio has a role in the development of tetanic cataracts, high phosphate concentrations causing a diminished ionized calcium portion. This quotient may be even more disturbed in the dialyzed patient due to increased phosphate accumulation. Another influence is exerted by pH values; increased pH values during the phase of dialysis will also lead to alterations between bound and ionized calcium. Despite an increased serum calcium level, the elimination of acidosis may reduce the ionized calcium content in dialysis patients.

Considering these observations, meticulous control of the calcium and phosphate levels, through timely administration of vitamin D or AT-10, of aluminum hydroxide and a sufficient supply of calcium, will diminish the risk of lenticular opacities.

**Surgery and Results Following Traumatic Cataracts in Children** are reported by David A. Hiles, P. Harold Wallar and Albert W. Biglan[2] (Pittsburgh). Traumatic cataract in childhood is often accompanied by a threat of visual loss due to amblyopia. Such trauma is unfortunately not uncommon.

The goals of cataract surgery after lens injury in children are to remove the injured lens cortex and nucleus and to minimize fibrotic and inflammatory responses in the eye. In acute cases, the cataract is best removed after surgical restoration of the anterior segment. A controlled cataract aspiration is done, preferably through a superior limbal incision. The Phacoemulsifier will remove lens cortex in the presence of formed vitreous without cutting it. An iridecto-

---

(2)   J. Pediatr. Ophthalmol. 13:319–325, Nov.–Dec., 1976.

my is always done after the lens is aspirated. If the anterior chamber remains distorted after closure of the perforating wound or hemorrhage or fibrinous clot persists, delayed surgery may be carried out. If a traumatic cataract forms some time after injury, routine aspiration may be done without undue complications.

Ninety eyes operated on for traumatic infantile cataract were reviewed. About one third of the patients were aged 6 or under; most were boys. Posterior capsular rupture occurred in 22 eyes and vitreous loss in 17. Primary discissions were done on 28 eyes and secondary discissions were completed on 40 eyes. Seventy-five capsular operations were performed. Contact lenses were fitted in 52 eyes; 13 children failed to wear the lens successfully. Intraocular lenses were implanted in 17 patients. Strabismus occurred in 9 eyes. Significant corneal opacity was present in 26 eyes. Glaucoma occurred in 6 eyes, detached retina in 5 and phthisis bulbi in 2. Eight eyes had no light perception postoperatively; 6 of them had retinal detachments associated with trauma and 2 underwent phthisis bulbi.

In this series, 29 cataract extractions occurred in children aged 6 years or less. Six eyes had final vision of 20/30 or better, and all 6 occurred in children over 4 years of age. Six eyes had final vision of 20/40-20/80; 2 had 20/100-20/200; 11 had 20/200 or less, and 4 had no light perception. Sixty-one cataracts occurred in children over 7 years of age; of which 33 eyes had final vision of 20/30 or better; 3 had 20/40-20/80; 2 had 20/100-20/200, 19 had less than 20/200 and 4 eyes had no light perception. In the entire series of 90 eyes, 42% had final vision of 20/30 or better and 12% had final vision of 20/40-20/80.

▶ [This article contains many details of the management of the difficult problem of monocular perforating injuries and traumatic cataract in children. The final visual result was of course dependent on the severity of the injury and secondary complications. Prevention of amblyopia was attempted by placing a contact lens 3–6 weeks following cataract surgery or 2 weeks after secondary capsular surgery; an increase in 1.5 diopters over the distance correction being given to preschool children. After the child was acclimated to the contact lens or a clear visual axis developed after acrylic lens implantation, complete occlusion of the normal eye was done for 1–3 weeks, examination was performed, and additional occlusion continued until maximum visual improvement occurred, or the contact lens was no longer worn for one reason or another (13 of 54 cases). As shown in the article, the age of the patient was important in the final result. Unfortunately, there is no information concerning the outcome of those children in which an intraocular lens was implanted. Certainly, this is an ideal way to eliminate anisemetropia if the lenses would be tolerated sufficiently long to prevent irreversible amblyopia. — Ed.] ◄

**"Contralight Vision" as Aid in Indication for Cataract Surgery** was used by Ch. Junker[3] (Univ. of Freiburg) in a comparative study of 84 eyes with cataracts of varied severity and type of clouding. The well-known fact was confirmed that a cataract will diminish vision against the light, particularly in case of posterior cortical clouding. A vision test chart is presented in front of a window, with the patient gazing against the incoming daylight (Fig 26); pupillary status is not altered by medication. In all cases of cataract, there was a marked reduction of visual acuity against the light. A control group of 30 patients, aged 50–75, without lenticular clouding was similarly tested, revealing no differ-

**Fig 26.** — Presentation of vision test chart for examination of "contralight vision." Patient uses his hand as shield to demonstrate glare effect. In actual examination this protection against glare is not used. (Courtesy of Junker, Ch.: Klin. Monatsbl. Augenheilkd. 169:348–351, September, 1976.)

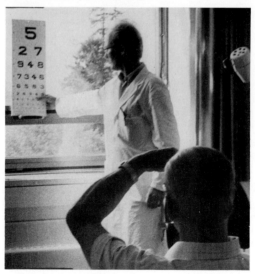

(3)   Klin. Monatsbl. Augenheilkd. 169:348–351, September, 1976.

ence in visual acuity or "contralight vision" under optimal test conditions.

This "contralight vision test" is helpful in all types of cataracts where the indication for surgery is not clearcut.

**Critical Evaluation of Current Concepts in Cataract Surgery** is presented by Arthur Gerard DeVoe[4] (Columbia Univ.). Forty years ago, extracapsular cataract extraction was widely preferred over intracapsular extraction, partly because it was a question whether an intracapsular operation would result in a great increase in the number of retinal detachments. Cystoid macular edema had not yet been recognized, and the entity of delayed visual loss after cataract extraction either did not occur or was not recognized. It may be asked just how much better the current extraction procedure is with respect to final visual results than the procedure of nearly a hundred years ago.

Cataract surgery at present is in a transitional state, making it difficult for the young surgeon to know where the best interest of his patient lies. Microsurgery has not basically changed the orthodox cataract operation. Lay publicity surrounding the newer procedures has not helped their acceptance by conservative surgeons. Removal of lens material by aspiration is not new; it has been the procedure of choice for congenital and soft cataracts for many years. Phacoemulsification by ultrasonography with the sophisticated Kelman unit gives excellent short-term results when performed by a surgeon trained in this technique; the first 50 operations performed being associated with a higher rate of complications before a surgeon masters the technique. Long-term results are not available. The small wound resulting is of less importance now that suturing methods of closing the wound are so satisfactory that the patient can be discharged a day or so after intracapsular cataract extraction. Optimally, a patient is hospitalized the day before surgery for general examination and discharged a day or so after intracapsular cataract extraction to make certain there is no infection. Outpatient surgery carries general systemic risks for old patients and those in poor physical condition. Delayed hemorrhage occurring at home should be no more of

(4) Am. J. Ophthalmol. 81:715–721, June, 1976.

a problem than that which occurs while the patient is still hospitalized.

The virtues of a small wound with phacoemulsification is negated if enlarged to permit introduction of an intraocular lens. Because secondary discissions are so often necessary after phacoemulsification, some surgeons perform a discission at the time of operation, thus negating the virtue of isolation of the anterior chamber from the posterior chamber. After extracapsular extraction, irritation from retained lens material can be a problem. There is no evidence that extracapsular extraction is less likely to be followed by retinal detachment than intracapsular extraction and the incidence of cystoid macular edema after each type of operation is still *sub judice.*

Unquestionably, the optics of the intraocular methyl methacrylate lens are superior to those of spectacle or contact lenses. However, the long-term effects of intraocular lenses are unknown. Most of Barraquer's 400 intraocular implants did not have to be removed until 4–5 years postoperatively because of chronic irritation. Even an inert foreign body such as glass can cause endothelial disturbance and iritis years after intraocular implantation. Whether the present iris and lens capsule supported lenses are better tolerated than the angle-supported lenses used by Barraquer cannot be determined as yet. Development of a more physiologic contact lens which can be worn continuously will probably make the intraocular lens obsolete. Nevertheless, it is fair to say that now there is enough benefit from the intraocular lens in selected cases to justify the additional risk. Any deviation from an orthodox approach increases the risk of malpractice suits although everyone knows that any operation can be followed by complications. It is possible that biochemists will produce an enzyme that can be injected with a fine hypodermic needle into the lens capsule to produce complete liquefaction of the lens cortex and nucleus which could then be aspirated and refilled with optically clear fluid.

▶ [As another older conservative, I like the critical evaluation of current methods of cataract extraction expounded in this George K. Smelser Lecture. For the present, there probably should be special indications and training of the surgeon for either phacoemulsification or lens implantation (see article by Jaffe), and the patient should be aware in writing that lens implantation is a new procedure with certain visual advantages but with uncertainty about long-term results. — Ed.] ◀

**Tranexamic Acid (AMCA) and Late Hyphema: Double-Blind Study in Cataract Surgery.** Ocular trauma is often accompanied by hemorrhage in the anterior chamber; secondary bleeding or rebleeding may occur 3–6 days after injury and may result in a blind, painful eye. Because of a postulated relationship between intraocular posttraumatic fibrinolysis and secondary bleeding, T. Jerndal and M. Frisén[5] (Univ. of Göteborg) studied the effects of an antifibrinolytic drug, tranexamic acid, on the incidence of secondary hyphema in human eyes after a standardized trauma — that induced by routine cataract extraction.

A double-blind study was made in 244 patients, those with vascular or hematologic diseases being excluded. All patients had blood pressure below 190/100 mm Hg, thrombocyte counts above 200,000/cu mm and a serum creatinine not exceeding 1.5 mg/100 ml. They were randomly allocated to placebo or active treatment with 2 tablets of tranexamic acid, 0.5 gm each, 3 times daily, for a total of 21 gm.

Rebleeding occurred in 20 of the 122 placebo-treated and 6 of the 122 tranexamic acid-treated patients, the difference being significant at the 5% level. Among the patients given tranexamic acid, 4 had gastrointestinal disturbances that were not serious, 1 had marked fatigue, and 1 had dysuria due to cystitis, which was considered coincidental. No thrombotic complications occurred. Three placebo patients had gastrointestinal disturbances, and 1 each had giddiness, syncope and urticaria.

Treatment with tranexamic acid, 1 gm, 3 times daily, after cataract extraction resulted in a significant reduction in the rate of late hyphema. The drug probably acts by inhibiting local fibrinolytic activity in the eye. Tranexamic acid may be suggested as conservative therapy in postoperative patients with intraocular rebleeding and as a prophylactic measure after ocular surgery.

▶ [Tranexamic acid inhibits tissue enzymes which activate plasminogen in serum and secondary aqueous to form plasmin which causes lysis of fibrin clots. It has been used in many other systemic conditions associated

(5) Acta Ophthalmol. (Kbh.) 54:417–429, August, 1976.

with bleeding. Although anterior chamber hemorrhage after cataract extraction is relatively rare today and usually harmless, the same cannot be said for recurrent hemorrhage after blunt injury to the eye. The results reported in this article appear encouraging. — Ed.] ◄

**Marginal Ulceration after Intracapsular Cataract Extraction.** Marginal ulcerations after routine cataract extraction are uncommon; only 1 known case has been described. Juan J. Arentsen, John M. Christiansen and A. Edward Maumenee[6] (Johns Hopkins Hosp.) recently encountered 2 patients with this condition, and a review of files at the Wilmer Institute of Ophthalmology revealed 2 other cases.

Man, 75, had an uncomplicated intracapsular cataract extraction in the right eye. A limbal-based flap and three preplaced 6 – 0 silk sutures were used. A slight "exudate" was present 2½ weeks postoperatively, when the corrected acuity was 6/9. Redness in the right eye was noted 3 months postoperatively, and a small crater-like ulcer was seen at the 12 o'clock position, which became progressively deeper and larger. Cultures yielded *Staphylococcus albus*. Four months postoperatively, visual acuity in the operated on eye was 6/18. Slit-lamp study showed a marginal, furrowed ulceration present superiorly, anterior to the limbal scar (Fig 27). There was a trace of aqueous ray, without cells. Subsequently, a lamellar corneoscleral transplant was carried out. The ulcer had healed 2 months later, but a month after this it had recurred at the 12 o'clock position. Two similar operations were later performed, both unsuccessfully. The eye became blind and painful and was enucleated.

Multiple factors responsible for marginal ulceration after cataract extraction may have been present in these 4 patients. By damaging tissues in the limbal area, trauma could initiate an immune reaction that would affect the epithelium and stroma. A transient ischemic reaction, resulting from interruption of the conjunctival and episcleral vasculature, might be a factor in some marginal ulcers. A neurotrophic cause, resulting from loss of corneal sensation after the limbal incision, is another possibility.

Two patients did well with conservative management, whereas the eye of the third patient was eventually enucleated, and 1 patient had a recurrence after aggressive

(6)   Am. J. Ophthalmol. 81:194 – 197, February, 1976.

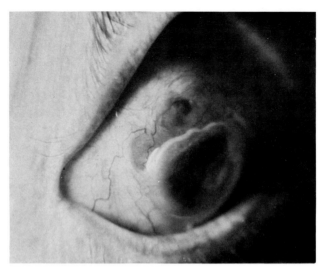

**Fig 27.** — Marginal ulceration 4 months after cataract extraction of the right eye. (Courtesy of Arentsen, J. J., et al.: Am. J. Ophthalmol. 81:194–197, February, 1976.)

treatment with a conjunctival flap and keratectomy, and then peritomy and cryotherapy.

**Phacoemulsification Procedure: I. Effect of Intraocular Irrigating Solutions on the Corneal Endothelium.** Bernard E. McCarey, Frank M. Polack and Walter Marshall[7] (Univ. of Florida) evaluated corneal endothelial function and structure in rabbits after exposure to various intraocular irrigating solutions, particularly Plasma-lyte (balanced salt solution). The corneal tissue was also evaluated after phacoemulsification with Plasma-lyte irrigation. Isolated corneas were maintained in vitro at 34 C with 15 mm Hg intraocular pressure, and perfused with glutathionebicarbonate Ringer's (GBR) solution, Tis-u-Sol, Travenol Ringer's Injection Solution, Travenol Sodium Chloride or Plasma-lyte-148 solution. Corneas excised after phacoemulsification were examined by scanning electron microscopy.

The irrigating solutions caused an immediate corneal

(7)   Invest. Ophthalmol. 15:449–457, June, 1976.

swelling of $67 \pm 5$ $\mu$m per hour, a response not modified by previous stabilization perfusion with GBR. With Plasma-lyte solution corneal swelling began after 20 minutes but did not occur for 60–75 minutes if the cornea was perfused after a GBR stabilization period. Endothelial intercellular junction separations appeared after more than an hour of corneal swelling, except with the calcium-containing Travenol Ringer's Solution. Complete phacoemulsification with Plasma-lyte or irrigation with ultrasound did not cause endothelial cell damage similar to that occurring with prolonged in vitro irrigation. Endothelial cells were traumatically damaged to varying degrees by the surgical manipulations.

Cell junction rupture can be attributed to a lack of calcium in irrigating solutions. Corneal swelling and endothelial cell changes can be reversed when a physiologic maintenance medium (GBR) is supplied to the corneal endothelium. Plasma-lyte solution appears to be adequate for anterior chamber irrigation for a limited period.

**Unusual Presentation of Phacoanaphylaxis Following Phacoemulsification.** Phacoanaphylactic endophthalmitis is a specific form of lens-induced inflammation after operative or other trauma to the lens capsule. More cases might be expected with the increasing popularity of a new form of extracapsular extraction, phacoemulsification. Ronald E. Smith and Peter Weiner[8] (Univ. of Southern California) report a case of phacoanaphylactic endophthalmitis following phacoemulsification, which emphasizes the importance of anterior chamber tap in the diagnosis of such cases.

Woman, 75, underwent extracapsular cataract extraction in the right eye, with 20/30 vision and minimal residual cortical material resulting. The left eye underwent phacoemulsification 5 months later. Moderate postoperative inflammation was treated with topical steroid drops for several weeks. Some residual lens material was present. Redness and photophobia appeared 3 months postoperatively and a yellowish mass was seen in the anterior chamber of the left eye. Vision was light perception and poor projection and the anterior chamber had marked flare and cell, large keratic precipitates and a yellowish exudate. The pupil was bound down by extensive posterior synechiae. Pressure was 26 mm Hg in the left

(8) Ophthalmic Surg. 7:65–68, Fall, 1976.

eye and 18 mm Hg in the right. The patient had been taking moderate doses of systemic prednisone for bullous pemphigoid. An anterior chamber tap revealed large numbers of polymorphonuclear cells and pigment granules but no fungi or bacteria; cultures gave negative results. Antibiotic therapy did not lead to improvement over 3 days and irrigation and aspiration of the remaining anterior chamber material were then carried out. Residual lens material was surrounded by large numbers of neutrophils and eosinophils, epithelioid cells and macrophages were also present. Depo-Medrol was given by subtenon's injection and prednisone was given in a dose of 100 mg daily and tapered to 30 mg on alternate days over 2 weeks. Hourly topical steroid drops and intensive mydriatic therapy were also used. Some improvement in vision occurred and the eye remained quiet.

Phacoanaphylactic endophthalmitis is presumably due to liberation of lens proteins into the eye after damage of the lens capsule. The present case is unusual in that the onset was delayed until 11 weeks after surgery. The clinical picture suggested a fungal endophthalmitis. Management includes the removal of residual lens material and long-term topical and systemic steroid therapy. Phacoanaphylactic uveitis may follow phacoemulsification. Careful cytologic study of an anterior chamber aspirate may lead to the diagnosis.

**Indications and Contraindications** for intraocular implant lens surgery are discussed by Norman S. Jaffe[9] (Univ. of Miami). Generally this type of surgery is restricted to the elderly, is usually restricted to one eye and is performed on patients not likely to benefit from a contact lens. The elderly adapt poorly to aphakic spectacles and contact lenses. Most patients with pseudophakic vision can manage well with one eye even if the opposite eye is nearly blind. Theoretical or special indications include surgery in ranchers, miners and divers and the prevention of amblyopia in patients aged 3–8 with traumatic cataracts. Specific indications for lens implantation include an elderly patient with an advanced cataract in one eye and 20/40–60 vision in the other, the same indication in slightly younger patients with various infirmities, elderly patients with disabling cataracts in both eyes, patients with bilateral senile macular choro-

(9) Trans. Am. Acad. Ophthalmol. Otolaryngol. 81:93–96, Jan.–Feb., 1976.

idal degeneration who have advanced cataracts in both eyes and elderly patients who have long worn a contact lens for unilateral aphakia and are faced with a nearly mature cataract in the second eye.

Some of the contraindications to pseudophakos implantation are a lack of patient motivation, axial myopia greater than 7 diopters, a poor result in the first eye with an implant, vision in only one eye, a young patient, lack of the possibility of postoperative follow-up, senile macular choroidal degeneration without a nearly mature cataract in both eyes, endothelial corneal dystrophy, proliferative diabetic retinopathy, inadequately controlled glaucoma, previous retinal detachment, congenital cataracts, especially of the rubelliform type and cataract associated with other abnormalities such as recurrent iritis or atopic dermatitis.

A conservative approach to indications and contraindications for intraocular implant lens surgery can reasonably be expected to be in the best interests of patients.

▶ [These conservative indications and contraindications for intraocular lens implant surgery should be considered seriously. Perhaps most of us have received the memo of March 1, 1977, from David M. Link of the FDA who stated that at the present time no intraocular lens implants have been approved by the FDA and that all lenses will have to be approved before marketing. He cites the need for supervision as illustrated by evidence of contamination and infection in two separate batches of lenses in 1975 and 1976. These lenses had been sterilized in NaOH and neutralized by sodium bicarbonate. He states: "If the solution upon visual examination appears to be cloudy or the sterility date has expired, do not use these lenses unless explicit instructions have been provided by the manufacturer."

Although there is much sentiment that the FDA is overly cautious about the approval of certain drugs and appliances, the increasingly widespread use of acrylic intraocular lenses and presumably from many new companies jumping on the bandwagon necessitate approval of both the materials used and method of manufacture. — Ed.] ◀

**Pseudophakia: Why Extracapsular Surgery?** C. D. Binkhorst[1] (Zeeland, Netherlands) points out that intracapsular removal of the complete lens leaves the eye with a mobile vitreous and a floating iris diaphragm. The iris is the last foothold for fixation of an intraocular lens in this eye. The corneal endothelium may sometimes be touched with some lens designs and the anterior chamber tends to shal-

---

(1)  Am. Intra-Ocular Implant Soc. J. 2:4 – 6, October, 1976.

lowness in the prone position, which could also promote corneal endothelial contact.

Extracapsular surgery fits the eye with a capsular membrane that steadies the vitreous behind it and to some extent also the iris in front of it. Fixation is independent of pupil size and iris atrophy is ruled out. The capsular membrane is suitable for holding implant material, and dislocation of implants is less frequent than after iris-fixation types. Extracapsular surgery leaves the separation of the anterior and posterior segments intact and prevents the mixing of their contents and its deleterious effects. The long-term fate of the eye is more favorable after extracapsular than after intracapsular surgery. Retinal complications such as macular edema are much less frequent after extracapsular surgery in the author's experience. Extracapsular surgery is the only technique that is practicable in young patients and in many cases of traumatic cataract. The risk from extracapsular surgery is low. Surgical and postoperative accidents are less likely to occur even in less favorable circumstances of anesthesia or nursing.

Capsular fixation does not take place in every case. Visualization of the anterior lens capsule is not always easy; sophisticated capsulotomies or capsulectomies may be helpful. The pupillary area is not always as clean postoperatively as is desirable and secondary procedures such as aspiration of loose cortex or removal of fibrillar material may be necessary. These procedures are likely, when the posterior lens capsule is damaged, to neutralize to at least some extent the superiority of extracapsular surgery over intracapsular surgery, especially with respect to protection of the retina. Extracapsular surgery is more difficult than intracapsular surgery, particularly with the availability of enzymatic zonulolysis and cryoprobes. Study and training for extracapsular extraction are necessary, as they were for intracapsular extraction.

**Sato Needling for Pupillary Membranes.** Sata (Am. J. Ophthalmol. 34:1136, 1951) described a technique for discission of capsular remains in which a needle is passed from limbus to limbus to pick up the capsule, lift it off the vitreous and provide fixation. Then a Sato discission knife is introduced about 3–6 mm from the point of needle entry to cut the tented capsule parallel to and beneath the fixation needle. This avoids the traction of the capsule on adjacent ocular structures occurring with the single knife technique and lessens the chance of damage to the hyaloid membrane of the vitreous.

Theodore Krupin and Michael E. Starrels[2] (Washington Univ.) reviewed 65 eyes of 52 patients who had had this operation, with good pupillary membrane openings produced in 63 of the 65 eyes. Complications included hyphema in 10 eyes, a broken vitreous face in 9, re-formation of the membrane in 5, cystoid macular edema in 2 and acute glaucoma in 1. All hyphemas cleared by the 4th postoperative day. Four of 5 eyes requiring 3 discissions maintained clear pupillary openings. In 2 eyes, since the membrane was too thick to be cut with the discission knife, iridocapsulectomy was performed. The technique is not difficult, the anterior chamber is usually maintained, and no long-term surgical complications have occurred.

(2)  Arch. Ophthalmol. 94:969–971, June, 1976.

# The Uvea

This year I have picked what I consider an important principle in the treatment of toxoplasmic retinochoroiditis. This principle is that these patients should not be treated with corticosteroids alone but should be covered with specific therapy against *Toxoplasma gondii.* For years ophthalmologists have observed that the retinochoroiditis of toxoplasmic etiology responds to corticosteroids but shows little or no response to specific therapy. For this reason, many ophthalmologists have given up the use of antibiotic therapy. In most instances they can get by with this maneuver but occasionally the patient, apparently with poor T cell type immunity, will do poorly because *Toxoplasma gondii* proliferate unrestrained. As pointed out by O'Connor and Frenkel[1] there is a general tendency among ophthalmologists to treat all forms of uveitis with corticosteroids. Patients are treated with steroids first and investigated later. These patients are subjected to investigation as to the cause of the uveitis only when the corticosteroids fail to control the disease. Since corticosteroids are the major agent helpful in uveitis cases this attitude is understandable but is not to be condoned. For example, every patient receiving corticosteroids should have a tuberculin skin test and, if positive, the patient should be covered by isoniazid therapy when taking corticosteroids in order to prevent the development of ocular or systemic tuberculosis while they are being treated with steroids.

The body's major defense against the toxoplasmic parasite is a cellular response in which immune competent lymphocytes participate. Treatment in the future may be directed more toward enhancing the body's T lymphocyte immunity than toward the use of antiparasitic agents. It is, therefore, logical to avoid or be careful about the use of immune suppressive agents and antilymphocytic serum in patients with toxoplasmosis. Since we are unable to tell with certainty whether any one lesion is due to hypersensitivity or to infection it is safer to use both corticosteroids and "specific" therapy if the disease process is severe enough or close enough to the macula to warrant it.

We use prednisone, 50–150 mg with breakfast every other morning and/or a sub-Tenon's injection of steroids such as methylprednisolone acetate (Depo-Medrol) over the lesion every 1 to 6 weeks. Of the two routes, the depot route seems the more effective. Although the dangers of such potent and possibly immunosuppressive therapy have been pointed out,[1] I feel it is the most effective therapy we have and is relatively safe if covered by specific treatment.[2] There are four types of specific therapy most readily available and commonly used:

1. Tetracyclines. A loading dose of 2,000 mg is followed by 250 mg, four times daily, for a period of 3–4 weeks. Chlortetracycline (Aureomycin) is probably the most effective tetracycline.

2. Pyrimethamine (Daraprim). For malaria the prophylactic dose is one 25 mg tablet once weekly. For toxoplasmic retinochoroiditis we use pyrimethamine, 100 mg, twice the first day and 25 mg twice daily thereafter. Pyrimethamine is an antagonist of dihydrofolic acid reductase. Since intestinal absorption tends to be poorer in children they should receive proportionally more. Since pyrimethamine acts only on actively dividing *Toxoplasma gondii,* there is no good evidence that treating inactive cases is worthwhile. In blacks one should look for a glucose 6-dehydrogenase abnormality before using pyrimethamine. The supplemental administration of folinic acid (leucovorin, 1 ml [3 mg]) intramuscularly once a week, in my experience, will prevent excessive thrombocytopenia and leukopenia from pyrimethamine without interfering with its therapeutic action. Folinic acid cannot be utilized by *T. gondii* but can be used by humans to prevent megaloblastosis. One should check to make sure that the patient is not taking folic acid, present in some vitamin preparations, since folic acid is a direct

antagonist to pyrimethamine. If excessive thrombocytopenia (platelet count less than 100,000) develops while the
patient is on pyrimethamine and corticosteroids, the corticosteroids should not be stopped since corticosteroids are of
help in treating the purpura which often develops.

Since the platelet count is the most sensitive indicator of
bone marrow suppression, a complete blood count is not necessary. All that is necessary is a platelet count once weekly.
If the platelet count falls to 100,000, Daraprim should be discontinued or reduced and folinic acid, 6 mg (Leucovorin),
given intramuscularly and repeated several times a week
until the platelet count reaches a safe level. Treatment with
pyrimethamine (Daraprim) should be continued for at least
2 weeks.[3] I routinely use Daraprim for 6 weeks or until activity subsides.

3. Sulfadiazine. I use sulfadiazine in the form of a triple
sulfa in a dosage of 2 (500 mg) tablets 4 times daily. We
usually prescribe this along with some other agent such as
Daraprim, Aureomycin or Cleocin (clindamycin).

4. Clindamycin (Cleocin). Clindamycin, a 7-chloro derivative of lincomycin is an inhibitor of protein synthesis at the
ribosomal level. Tabbara, Nozik and O'Connor[4] have shown
that this drug, administered by periocular and intramuscu-
lar injection has a curative effect on experimentally induced
toxoplasmic lesions in rabbit eyes. It has been demonstrated
by Tabbara and O'Connor[5] that extremely high levels of
clindamycin can be produced in the rabbit eye by a single
subconjunctival injection. There is some indication that clindamycin penetrates the encysted forms of *Toxoplasma gondii.* Also, clindamycin should work synergistically with sulfonamides since sulfonamides interfere with nucleic acid
synthesis in protozoa while clindamycin affects protein synthesis at the ribosomal level. Neither oral or subconjunctival clindamycin has been approved by the FDA. If used, this
fact must be explained to the patient. If the oral form is
used, 2 (150 mg) capsules are prescribed every 6 hours and
the patient is warned that about 10% (0% – 22.2%)[6] of people
will develop diarrhea and a small percentage develop colitis,
which can be serious. If the patient has four or more bowel
movements a day more than normal for them, they should

stop taking clindamycin. Unfortunately, diarrhea may not start until 10 days after the last dose of clindamycin.[7]

Theodore F. Schlaegel, Jr., M.D.
Indiana University

REFERENCES

1. O'Connor, G. R., and Frenkel, J. K.: Editorial: Dangers of Steroid Treatment in Toxoplasmosis. Arch. Ophthalmol. 94:213, 1976.
2. Nozik, R. A.: Results of Treatment of Ocular Toxoplasmosis with Injectable Corticosteroids. Trans. Am. Acad. Ophthalmol. Otolaryngol. In Press.
3. Report of a WHO Meeting of Investigators: Toxoplasmosis, Treatment. WHO Tech. Rep. Ser. 431:24, 1969.
4. Tabbara, K. F., Nozik, R. A., and O'Connor, G. R.: Clindamycin Effects on Ocular Toxoplasmosis in the Rabbit. Arch. Ophthalmol. 92:244, 1974.
5. Tabbara, K. F., and O'Connor, G. R.: Ocular Tissue Absorption of Clindamycin Phosphate. Arch. Ophthalmol. 93:1180, 1975.
6. Friedman, G. D., Gerard, M. J., and Ury, H. K.: Clindamycin and Diarrhea. J.A.M.A. 236:2498, 1976.
7. Axelrod, M., Allon, O., Felton, M., and Goldfinger, M.: Clindamycin-Associated Colitis with Toxic Megacolon. J.A.M.A. 233: 419, 1975.

**Indocyanine Green Fluorescence Angiography of the Choroid.** Flower and Hochheimer (1973) described a method of indocyanine green (ICG) fluorescence angiography in which the arterial and capillary dye phases could be seen. Flower (1974) developed a camera that simultaneously records fluorescein, ICG absorption and ICG fluorescence angiography. A. Craandijk and C. A. Van Beek[3] (Eye Hosp., The Hague) assessed the potential clinical usefulness of ICG fluorescence angiography.

A Zeiss fundus camera fitted with an exciter filter (interference filter with a peak at 777.5 nm) in front of the flash tube was used. The barrier filter (interference filter with a peak at 854.9 nm) fitted in a Zeiss 30-degree conus in front of the film so that the camera body was attached over the conus. Kodak high-speed infrared-sensitive black and

(3) Br. J. Ophthalmol. 60:377–385, May, 1976.

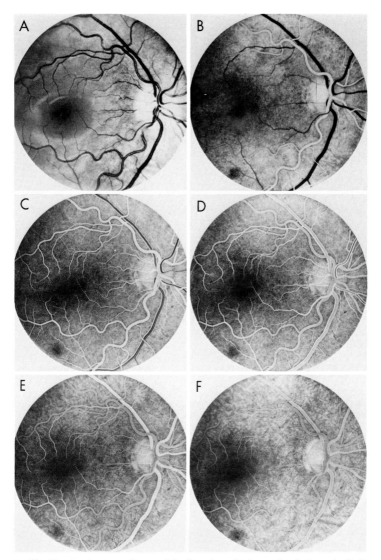

**Fig 28.** — Angiograms of normal fundus. **A,** orthochromatic photograph. **B–F,** fluorescein (7"3, 9"5, 11"3, 14"9 and 36"6, respectively). (Courtesy of Craandijk, A., and Van Beek, C. A.: Br. J. Ophthalmol. 60:377–385, May, 1976.)

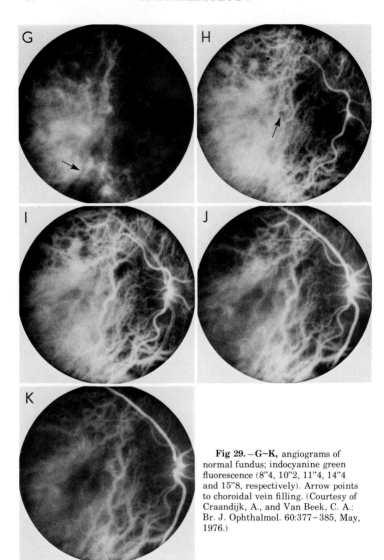

**Fig 29.**—**G–K,** angiograms of normal fundus; indocyanine green fluorescence (8"4, 10"2, 11"4, 14"4 and 15"8, respectively). Arrow points to choroidal vein filling. (Courtesy of Craandijk, A., and Van Beek, C. A.: Br. J. Ophthalmol. 60:377–385, May, 1976.)

white film (HIE-135-20) was used. The camera fired at a rate of 1 frame/0.7 seconds, starting 8 seconds after intravenous injection of 25 mg ICG in 2 ml aqueous solvent.

The findings are shown in Figures 28 and 29. The ICG filling begins at the macula and the optic disc does not fluoresce, in contrast with fluorescein angiography. The ICG angiography of the choroid provides better visualization of the choroidal vessels than does fluorescein angiography. Detachment of the pigment epithelium seemed larger on ICG than on fluorescein angiograms and pigmented lesions were more clearly delineated.

Orth, et al. (1976) found differential leakage of fluorescein and ICG dyes in certain cases of neovascularization. Interpreting ICG angiograms takes far longer than fluorescein angiograms, partly because relatively little is known about the normal choroidal circulation. The ICG angiography does not require a very expensive camera adaptation; it can be done in a few minutes and can be followed by fluorescein angiography by changing the camera body and the syringe. More clinical studies are needed before the clinical usefulness of ICG fluorescence angiography is proved.

▶ [Infrared pictures to reduce interference by the retinal pigment epithelium of indocyanine green fluorescence in the choroid are improving (see the 1971 YEAR BOOK, p. 231 and the 1973 YEAR BOOK, p. 242); simultaneous pictures of fluorescein angiography are also possible (see the next article). The ICG pictures do not outline as clearly the choroidal circulation as fluorescein does the retinal vessels. This is probably because of scattering of the fluorescence by choroidal pigment and the several layers of vessels. ICG filling of choroidal vessels (unlike fluorescein, without leakage) begins at the macula and spreads toward the disc along the pattern of the short posterior ciliary arteries, and quickly empties into the choroidal veins. The optic disc does not fluoresce. The sharp blocking out of choroidal fluorescence by nevi, and the larger areas of choroidal leakage in maculopathies than are visible in fluorescein angiography are illustrated in the above article. — Ed.] ◀

**Indocyanine Green Dye Fluorescence and Infrared Absorption Choroid Angiography Performed Simultaneously with Fluorescein Angiography.** R. W. Flower and B. F. Hochheimer[4] (Johns Hopkins Univ.) observe that indocyanine green (ICG) dye overcomes the defects of fluorescein with respect to choroid angiography. Nearly all ICG is bound to serum albumin, preventing significant leakage

(4)   Johns Hopkins Med. J. 138:33–42, February, 1976.

from the choroid vasculature, and the absorption and fluorescence spectra of ICG are in the near-infrared region, where the pigmented tissues of the eye are more transparent to light energy. Indocyanine green choroid angiograms represent a relatively complex, three-dimensional, multilayered vascular network. A Zeiss fundus camera was modified so that fluorescein and ICG fluorescence angiograms and ICG infrared absorption angiograms could be made simultaneously. The retinal fluorescein filling patterns would serve as a reference for the sequence of choroid filling events. The excitation and barrier filters and dichroic beamsplitters of the standard fundus camera were modified. A mixture of ICG and sodium fluorescein dyes was injected antecubitally and followed by a normal saline flush.

The multispectral fundus camera produces a set of three simultaneous angiograms every 0.7 second. The three-dimensional, spongelike choroid is composed of multiple layers of anastomosing vessels that fill with dye in a direction essentially parallel to the optical axis, i.e., toward the camera. A significant limitation to the resolution of choroid structures appears to result from anatomical features. Specifically, pigment in the pigment epithelium and in the cho-

**Fig 30 (left).** — Indocyanine green fluorescence angiogram of patient with chloroquine retinopathy.

**Fig 31 (right).** — Indocyanine green fluorescence angiogram of patient with segmental loss of pigment epithelium and overlying choriocapillaris.

(Courtesy of Flower, R. W., and Hochheimer, B. F.: Johns Hopkins Med. J. 138: 33–42, February, 1976.)

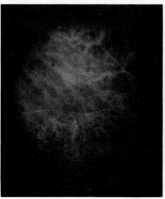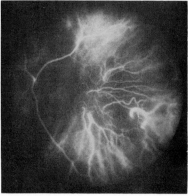

roid interstices causes significant scattering of the light emitted by the fluorescing dye. This phenomenon is illustrated in Figures 30 and 31. The optical components of angiography have been so refined that resolution of choroid vascular structures is limited by properties inherent in the eye itself, rather than by those of the camera. Choroid angiography should be used to study the choroid circulation in both normal eyes and eyes with known disease.

**Fluorescein Angiographic Picture of Sympathetic Ophthalmia** is described by M. Spitznas[5] (Univ. of Essen), as seen in a patient with onset at the posterior pole. The acute phase is an exudative process with numerous progressively enlarging subretinal hyperfluorescent dots and some dye pooling; the retinal vascular system remains unaffected.

Man, 50, had a corneal perforation of the left eye at age 2 during the course of a corneal abscess, with subsequent loss of vision in that eye. In 1952 he underwent an undetermined surgical procedure with the purpose of improving visual acuity in the left eye; the attempt was unsuccessful. Twenty-three years later the left eye was bruised by a hoe handle. Two months later he reported diminution of vision in the right eye. On examination the left eye showed dense white clouding of the superficially vascularized cornea and central corneal ulcer; the connective membrane was largely unremarkable and light perception was only temporal. In the right eye the anterior segment was unremarkable. There were no cells in the anterior chamber or vitreous. There was a flat, pigmented, papilla-sized area in the fundus above the papillomacular bundle. Immediately adjoining there was a pear-shaped, sharply delineated zone with an extremely flat subretinal effusion, tapering out toward the papilla. Because of a suspicion of choroid nevus with incipient malignancy, fluorescein angiography was performed (Fig 32). In the arteriovenous phase numerous small dotlike fluorescein overflows were seen within the entire posterior pole and above the papilla. Subsequently enlargement and partial confluence of the leakage points and staining of the suprapapillar subretinal effusion were noted.

The diagnostic criterion of a true sympathetic ophthalmia remains the histologic demonstration of intact lens in the initially diseased eye. The present case is of interest because the sympathetic reaction had its onset at the posterior pole, with signs of an iridocyclitis appearing only later. In the

---

(5)   Klin. Monatsbl. Augenheilkd. 169:195–200, August, 1976.

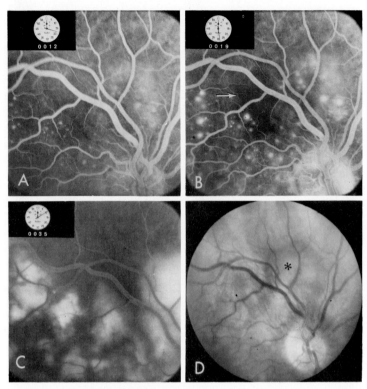

**Fig 32.** — Sympathetic ophthalmia; acute phase. **A–C,** angiographic series shows multiple fluorescein leakage points on fundus; papilla is unremarkable. **D,** fundus film shows clear edema and sharp papillar edge. *Asterisk,* subretinal effusion; *arrow,* choroid nevus. (Courtesy of Spitznas, M.: Klin. Monatsbl. Augenheilkd. 169:195–200, August, 1976.)

healing phase a transitory involvement of the optic nerve head was observed, whereas the cicatricial phase was characterized by a coarsening of the pigment pattern of the fundus. Aside from the fluorescein angiogram, the degree of transitory hyperopia was an excellent indicator of the pathologic activity in the present patient.

▶ [In spite of the history in the left eye of a perforated ulcer 48 years ago, a surgical procedure 23 years before and a blunt injury 2 months previously, there does not appear to be any histologic proof that this represents a posterior sympathetic ophthalmia in the right eye. However, suspicion of a malignant melanoma of the choroid was allayed by fluorescein angiography which showed a widespread spotty leakage of fluorescein in the deeper layers of the retina. — Ed.] ◄

**Choroidal Abiotrophies.** Ronald E. Carr, Rainer N. Mittl and Kenneth G. Noble[6] (New York Univ. Med. Center, New York) classified 138 patients with various diseases of the choroidal vasculature on the basis of central, peripapillary and generalized involvement, with hereditary and acquired variants within each of the three main groups. The hereditary generalized choroidal diseases included choroideremia and gyrate atrophy.

All patients were readily classified into one of the three groups. The rather nonspecific ophthalmoscopic changes present in the early stages of both central areolar choroidal dystrophy and choroideremia may not be appreciated until a family history is obtained. If this does not clarify the diagnosis, fluorescein angiography will show loss of choriocapillaris in early central areolar choroidal dystrophy. Electroretinography will show generalized retinal degeneration in early choroideremia. Angiographic findings may be similar in the "acquired" and hereditary variants; however, in some cases an inflammatory disorder may be responsible for such changes. The peripapillary entity of helicoid peripapillary degeneration may in some cases be of inflammatory nature.

Fluorescein angiography has become increasingly important in classification of these diseases, in all of which the associated loss of pigment epithelium leads to some confusion as to the etiologic site. Abnormalities of the pigment epithelium or Bruch's membrane, or both, do not lead to abnormalities of the choriocapillaris. The loss of pigment epithelium in severe disorders of the choriocapillaris appears to be a secondary change. Angiography can show the true state of the retinal vasculature and assist in defining the primary site of an abnormality. The only disorder in which convincing proof of choriocapillaris loss following pigment epithelial atrophy has been obtained is fundus flavimaculatus, in which the finding of atrophic-appearing areas scattered through the retina and a history of autosomal recessive disease will help clarify the diagnosis.

---

(6)   Trans. Am. Acad. Ophthalmol. Otolaryngol. 79:796–816, Nov.–Dec., 1975.

## Immunosuppressives in Uveitis: Preliminary Report of Experience with Chlorambucil.

Hersh et al. (1966) reported improvement of uveitis in patients given methotrexate but most had recurrences. Mamo and Azzam (1970) first reported use of chlorambucil, obtaining encouraging results in 11 patients with Behçet's disease; others also have reported good results with this drug in cases of Behçet's disease. W. J. Dinning and E. S. Perkins[7] (Univ. of London) gave chlorambucil to 14 patients seen over the past 2 years with uveitis not responding to steroids or with unacceptable steroid side effects. Three early patients received 10 mg chlorambucil daily but later patients received 5 mg daily at first and 5 mg every other day after several months. Attempts were made to reduce the amount of steroid at the same time. Two patients were treated for 4 months and the rest for about 9 months.

The results are summarized in the table. All 5 patients with Behçet's disease had had very poor vision for several years before chlorambucil therapy; the most impressive results were obtained in this group. Anemia did not occur; only 2 patients were leukopenic and 1, thrombocytopenic. Five patients benefited from treatment; judgment is being reserved in 2 cases. Two of 10 patients had chromosomal changes of doubtful significance.

Only in Behçet's disease does a clearer role for immunosuppressive therapy seem to emerge but it is too early to say whether treatment will alter the course of the disease permanently. Chlorambucil is probably one of the least dangerous immunosuppressive agents but its long-term side effects

RESULTS OF TREATMENT OF UVEITIS

| Diagnosis | Total | Improved | No change | Worse |
|---|---|---|---|---|
| Chronic generalized uveitis | 3 | 2 | 1 | |
| Uveitis with retinal vasculitis | 3 | 1 | 1 | 1 |
| Behçet's disease | 5 | 3 | 2 | |
| Vogt-Koyanagi-Harada disease | 1 | 1 (temporary) | | |
| Sympathetic ophthalmitis | 1 | 1 (probably) | | |
| Pars planitis | 1 | | | 1 |

(7) Br. J. Ophthalmol. 59:397–403, August, 1975.

are unclear and it should not be used indefinitely or in repeated courses. Treatment for 6 months probably would have sufficed at the dose used in most of these patients.

► [This is a cautious report, giving the rationale of using immunosuppressive agents in diseases suspected of formation of antibodies to common tissue antigens, the immune complex causing vascular damage and subsequent inflammation. From a review of the literature and their own experience, it appears that only Behcet's disease with recurrent hypopyon and severe uveitis, aphthous lesions of the buccal mucous membrane, ulceration of the genitalia and systemic involvement of vessels, central nervous system, skin and joints, responds well to the use of immunosuppressives. Sympathetic ophthalmia not responding to steroids may be another indication for this treatment. The authors state that, "we should remind ourselves that these drugs have only recently masqueraded under the title of 'immunosuppressives.' They were once known as antimetabolites and cytotoxic agents." Apparently, chlorambucil is one of the least toxic. – Ed.] ◄

**Comparison of Ocular Prostaglandin Synthesis Inhibitors.** Many ocular inflammatory responses may be mediated by prostaglandins. Steven M. Podos (City Univ. of New York) and Bernard Becker[8] (Washington Univ.) compared the topical effects of a large number of inhibitors of prostaglandin synthesis on the intraocular pressure elevation produced by arachidonic acid in rabbits. Eyes of awake rabbits were treated with a solution or suspension of each drug or with diluent, followed in 30 minutes by exposure to two drops 5% arachidonic acid in peanut oil, placed on the corneas. Studies were also done with removal of aqueous humor 30 minutes after arachidonic acid application. The drugs were tested in concentrations of 0.01 – 2.0%.

The peak elevation of intraocular pressure occurred 30 minutes after arachidonic acid application. Indomethacin, flurbiprofen, clonixin and meclofenamic acid in 1 and 2% concentrations produced at least 65% inhibition of the arachidonic acid effect. At the 0.1% concentration, only flurbiprofen was this active. The effect of indoxole was appreciably enhanced by adding polysorbate 80; near complete inhibition of the arachidonic acid effect occurred with a 1% concentration. Dose-response curves were not linear, but the drug concentration needed to half inhibit the arachidonic acid-induced ocular hypertension could be derived from linear portions of the curves. Indoxole-polysorbate, flurbipro-

(8)   Invest. Ophthalmol. 15:841 – 844, October, 1976.

fen, meclofenamic acid, indomethacin and clonixin were the most effective, in decreasing order of potency. Similar results were obtained with respect to inhibition of the aqueous humor protein response to arachidonic acid.

This study showed several nonsteroidal anti-inflammatory drugs to be effective topically in inhibiting the intraocular pressure response to arachidonic acid in the rabbit eye. This is a good model of prostaglandin-mediated inflammation. The results may not, however, be applicable to human eyes. Other mediators of inflammation besides prostaglandins exist, many of them susceptible to the effects of corticosteroids.

**Intraocular Effects of Pimaricin.** An increase in intraocular fungal infections as well as mycotic keratitis has occurred in recent years. Arthur C. Ellison and Emanuel Newmark[9] (Univ. of Texas, San Antonio) evaluated direct intraocular injections of pimaricin in the infected and normal rabbit eye, because of problems of systemic toxicity and the apparent failure of this agent to penetrate the cornea well. Groups of pigmented Dutch rabbits received intracameral injections of spores of *Aspergillus fumigatus* in one or both eyes, followed in 24 hours by the intracameral injection of pimaricin in a concentration of 250 or 500 $\mu$g/0.1 ml. The eyes were enucleated from 24 hours to 2 weeks after treatment. Other animals received only pimaricin. Duration of drug pimaricin levels were determined after intracameral injection.

Increasing the intracameral level of pimaricin increased the severity of the ocular reaction. Drug residue was seen as a precipitate on the pupillary margin at doses of 250 $\mu$g and above. Conjunctival chemosis, severe ciliary injection and marked corneal edema were noted when 1,000 $\mu$g were injected intracamerally into the normal rabbit eye and the effects persisted at 96 hours. Fungistatic drug levels had a half-time of about 6 hours for the lower doses and about 8 hours with the higher dose levels. Tissue drug levels at 48 hours were generally below those needed to inhibit most pathogenic or saprophytic fungi. About half the eyes treated with 250 $\mu$g pimaricin intracamerally never developed

(9) Ann. Ophthalmol. 8:987–995, August, 1976.

infection, and most of those treated with 500 μg were not infected.

In cases of fungal endophthalmitis involving the anterior segment that will lead to ultimate loss of the eye, an injection of 250 μg pimaricin might preserve useful vision. This dosage was well tolerated by the infected and normal animal eye and therapeutic ocular drug levels were maintained for over 24 hours. Higher doses resulted in irreversible damage to ocular structures in the infected eye.

**Light Coagulation in Central and Paracentral Choroiditis** is discussed by A. Heydenreich, L. Lemke, A. Jütte and R. Krautwald[1] (Univ. of Jena). This study includes 108 eyes with varying morphologic types of choroiditis treated with the Zeiss photocoagulator, localization of the active areas being made by fluorescein angiography staining. As compared with a control group treated by drugs, photocoagulation shortened the duration of the acute inflammation, decreased the frequency of recurrences by about 40% and improved the visual prognosis (final vision of 0.8 compared with the control group of 0.5).

**Juvenile Uveal Xanthogranuloma in an Adult.** A. Hamburg[2] (Utrecht) discusses this ophthalmologic disease which is often misdiagnosed and is recognized only on histopathologic investigation. The clinical symptoms of this essentially benign lesion are misleading and will often occasion radical intervention even with the use of modern diagnostic methods. It is precisely the strikingly rapid growth which contraindicates malignancy as shown in the present patient.

In this man, aged 22, the right eye was removed because of a rapidly growing iridic tumor (Fig 33); fluorescein angiography and isotope examinations had shown signs of malignancy. However, later histopathologic investigation revealed a juvenile xanthogranuloma, a benign granulomatous process of unknown etiology occurring almost exclusively in young children and associated with corresponding skin alterations.

The "tumor" is mainly composed of histiocytes, at times with multiple giant cells, and contains numerous delicate

(1)  Klin. Monatsbl. Augenheilkd. 167:645–651, November, 1975.
(2)  Ophthalmologica 172:273–281, 1976.

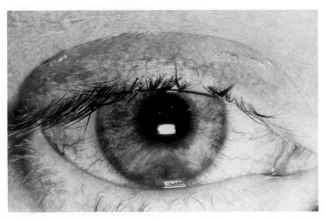

**Fig 33.** — Tumor-like lesion protruding from iridocorneal angle at 6 o'clock. (Courtesy of Hamburg, A.: Ophthalmologica 172:273–281, 1976.)

blood vessels which may give rise to spontaneous hyphema, an important clinical sign. Secondary glaucoma may occur, which makes timely recognition and treatment essential. The granulomatous tissue responds well to irradiation. According to Maumanee and Longfellow a single dose of 200 R is often sufficient. Corticosteroids may also be tried. Given the "self-limiting" nature of the condition, smaller lesions may disappear in time even without treatment.

**Diagnosis of Tumor-Like Fundus Changes by Combination of Echography, Infrared Photography and Fluorescein Angiography** is discussed by H. Freyler[3] (Univ. of Vienna). This combination was used to study 100 patients with suspected tumors during 1969–75. The following diagnoses were established: malignant melanoma of the choroid (12), melanocytoma of the optic nerve (2), choroidal metastases (7), choroidal nevi (24), disciform degeneration of the macula, (29), serous detachment of the pigment epithelium (4), subpigment epithelial hemorrhages (3), subretinal hemorrhages (4), serous or exudative choroidal detachment (2), hemorrhagic choroidal detachment (3), pigment epithelial hyperplasia (2), serous retinal detachment (4) and intramural foreign bodies (3).

---

(3) Klin. Monatsbl. Augenheilkd. 167:555–570, October, 1975.

Echography allowed exact measurement of the prominence and provided a means of tissue differentiation in lesions exceeding 1.1 – 1.5 mm. The results of infrared photography were unaffected by the height of the lesion; infrared
penetration of amelanotic melanomas of the choroid membrane was 2 mm at most. In strongly pigmented melanomas
of the choroid reflection and absorption of infrared light occurred at the surface of the tumor.

With infrared photography, the normal fundus appears in a
yellow to yellowish green color tone; the arteries are yellow
and papillary veins and their larger branches are brownish
yellow. Melanin-containing tissue is a purplish brown. Lipo-
fuscin deposits appear in the form of yellow patches. In superficial localization and thin layers the blood stain shows
up yellow; greater thickness (more than 0.5 mm in the echogram) produces various nuances of light to darker yellowish
brown. In a layer of 0.5 – 1.5 mm in the echogram and choroidal localization hemosiderin produces a yellowish brown, in
a layer more than 1.5 mm an increasingly bluish brown
color tone appears (this bluish tone is seen also in all nonfo-
cused areas). Connective tissue in the subretinal or subpigment epithelial space is seen as white to bluish white. Intramural metallic foreign bodies contrast as black, sharply delineated patches against the yellowish brown of the blood-
soaked tissue. The clear marking of piment-containing tissue against the normal environment allows precise statements regarding alterations in the expanse of pigmented
processes.

Fluorescein angiography visualizes the vascular pattern
and permeability of tumor or pseudotumor vessels. Results
of echography and angiography are influenced by the height
of the lesion with the accuracy of echographic findings increasing with greater prominence and the reliability of fluorescein angiography decreasing in similar proportion. Infrared light penetrates the retina and pigment epithelium,
as well as the inner layers of the choroid membrane; the
largest penetration of living tissue is at a wave length between 720 and 800 m$\mu$. Infrared color film offers not only
heightened contrast (as compared to normal color photography) but the characteristic color changes allow determination of pigment type, localization and layer thickness of the

COMPARISON OF BENIGN AND MALIGNANT TUMORS OF CHOROID MEMBRANE BY VARIOUS INVESTIGATIVE METHODS

| DIAGNOSIS | INVESTIGATIVE METHODS | | |
|---|---|---|---|
| | Echography | Infrared Photography | Fluorescein Angiography |
| Malignant melanoma | Characteristic picture starting at 1.5 mm | Patchy yellowish brown to dark brown, imprecise delineation | Finely granular early arterial peripheral fluorescence; patchy, in late phase diffuse staining |
| Choroid metastasis | Generally higher degree of reflection than in melanoma | Absence of melanin, yellowish white to brownish yellow | All transitional phases from absence of fluorescence to typical melanoma angiogram |
| Melanocytoma | Melanoma echogram starting at 1.5 mm | Dark brown | Shadowy |
| Hemangioma | Blood lacunae demonstrable from 3.5 mm on | Patchy brownish yellow | Early arterial coarse patchy staining, diffuse fluorescein impregnation in late phase |
| Degenerative pseudotumor | To be differentiated from melanoma from 1.1–1.5 mm onward | White to bluish white | Slow fluorescein inhibition in late phase |
| Choroidal nevus | Not diagnosable | Dark brown, sharply delineated | Shadowy; rarely melanoma-like angiogram |

pigment-containing tissue. Hemangiomas of the choroid (table) can be differentiated by the yellow to light brown patchy image they produce. Differentiation between malignant melanoma and choroid metastases, although not possible by means of angiography, is aided by the infrared image, establishing the absence of melanin, which would indicate metastasis. Combination of these three investigative techniques gives best results in avoiding enucleation due to erroneous assumption of an intraocular tumor.

**Clinical Experience with Presumed Hemangioma of the Choroid: Radioactive Phosphorus Uptake Studies as Aid in Differential Diagnosis.** In contrast to choroidal melanoma and tumors metastatic to the choroid, choroidal hemangioma has a good visual prognosis if the correct diagnosis is made early and proper treatment is instituted. William H. Jarrett II, William S. Hagler, James H. Larose and Jerry A. Shields[4] (Philadelphia, Pa.) reviewed 27 case reports of patients with presumed hemangioma of the choroid, with reference to the importance of the $^{32}$P uptake test in making the differential diagnosis. The patients were among more than 400 patients referred for evaluation of a choroidal mass, most of whom proved to have malignant melanoma. Men outnumbered women by nearly 3:1. Most cases occurred in the 5th and 6th decades of life. Hemangioma was suspected clinically in every case, but in most cases the possibility of amelanotic melanoma was also considered.

The $^{32}$P test was negative in all patients with suspected choroidal hemangioma. The hemangiomas usually appear as subtly elevated mass lesions in the posterior choroid, varying in size from 4 to 8 disc diameters. Hemangiomas do not cause a transillumination defect. Fluorescein studies yield fluorescences in the prearterial phase of angiograms, but this is not of differential diagnostic value. Fifteen hemangiomas were located close to the optic disc, and the others were adjacent to the macula. A serous retinal detachment usually accompanies a choroidal hemangioma, and frequently it involves the macular region, even though the tumor itself is on the nasal side of the disc. Two patients had bullous secondary retinal detachments inferiorly, and 1 had

(4)   Trans. Am. Acad. Ophthalmol. Otolaryngol. 81:862–870, Sept.–Oct., 1976.

cystic macular changes that cleared after treatment. None had evidence of secondary glaucoma or cataract. Twenty-two patients were treated by xenon or argon laser photocoagulation. Ten required two or more treatment sessions before the detachment cleared. In several instances, ablatio fugax occurred transiently after treatment. Visual improvement was prompt and dramatic in several patients.

Histologic confirmation of choroidal hemangioma was lacking in these cases, but no patient to date has shown growth of the lesion or reaccumulation of subretinal fluid after treatment.

**Malignant Melanoma Arising in Choroidal Magnacellular Nevus (Melanocytoma).** Only one case of malignant change occurring in a melanocytoma has previously been reported. Ann E. Barker-Griffith, P. Robb McDonald and W. Richard Green[5] (Johns Hopkins Med. Inst.) report another such case.

Man, 55, noted reduced vision and distortion of objects on the right and was found to have a pigmented lesion in the macular region of the eye, which appeared to enlarge over 3 months. Acuity was 20/40 on the right and 20/20 on the left. Ophthalmoscopy showed a 3–4-disc diameter tumor in and above the right macular area. A crescent-shaped, yellowish-orange lesion was seen in the upper part of the tumor. Fluorescein angiography indicated malignant melanoma; the orange pigment crescent blocked fluorescence. The lesion was thought to enlarge over 2 months and the eye was then enucleated. The patient is well 8 years after enucleation.

Sections from the lower part of the lesion showed a densely pigmented choroidal tumor, diagnosed as melanocytoma of the choroid. Spindle-shaped cells appeared at the nasal edge of the lesion and in the center in serial sections and eventually constituted all the tumor. Both spindle-A and spindle-B melanoma cells were observed. Pigment-containing cells were present in the subretinal space. Moderate uveal pigmentation was also noted, as was a flat retinal detachment. The malignant tumor cells exhibited mild pleomorphism and rare mitoses. The bulk of the tumor was a malignant melanoma of spindle-A and spingle-B type, arising in a choroidal melanocytoma.

The orange yellow pigmentation seen over some choroidal

(5) Can. J. Ophthalmol. 11:140–146, April, 1976.

melanomas is believed to represent a response of the retinal pigment epithelium to the gradual encroachment of a lesion on the choriocapillaris. The origin of the pigmented cells in the present patient is not known but they probably originated both from macrophages and the retinal pigment epithelium. The cells showed autofluorescence typical of lipofuchsin pigment.

**Changing Concepts of Prognosis and Management of Small Malignant Melanomas of the Choroid** are discussed by Lorenz E. Zimmerman and Ian W. McLean[6] (Armed Forces Inst. of Pathology). It was once generally assumed that all malignant melanomas of the uvea carried a poor prognosis and that immediate enucleation of the tumor-containing eye was indicated. However, uveal melanomas exhibit greater cytologic variation than cutaneous melanomas, which can be correlated with the prognosis. Factors other than vascular invasion are important in determining the outcome. Melanomas of the anterior uvea can often be successfully resected while preserving useful vision. Melanomas of the posterior uvea differ strikingly in prognosis according to their size. Useful vision may be retained by an eye harboring a small melanoma. Even when the tumor is near the macula and visual acuity is reduced, the rest of the retina may be unaffected.

Analysis was made of 217 small tumors and 7 factors were found to be closely correlated with the outcome. These were cell type, pigmentation, size, mitotic activity, transscleral extension, optic nerve invasion and the position of the anterior border of the tumor (the more anterior, the worse the prognosis). A mathematical expression of the chance of a fatal outcome was derived from the largest tumor diameter, cell type, mitotic activity and transscleral extension. However, there were some striking exceptions to the ability to predict the outcome after enucleation. Nonsurgical treatment methods might produce less mechanical trauma to the eye and allowing some devitalized but still antigenic tumor tissue to remain for a time might have a beneficial immunologic effect on tumor cells that have escaped into the circulation.

(6) Trans. Ophthalmol. Soc. U.K. 95(Pt.4):487–494, 1975.

It will be some time before the long-term results of surgical resection of choroidal melanomas are evaluable. Photocoagulation appears generally unsuitable for melanomas that are elevated more than 2 mm. Irradiation may be similarly restricted. Diathermy and cryotherapy have also been tried but have much less appeal. Currently, some clinicians are merely observing patients who have small asymptomatic malignant melanomas in eyes that retain useful vision, especially when growth and progressive intraocular damage have not been documented. Evaluation for over 10 years after diagnosis is needed to compare the results of these treatment approaches with those of enucleation.

► [This is a rational evaluation of the clinical and histologic characteristics of malignant melanomas of the choroid which influence prognosis, plus a rather complete discussion of the various modes of therapy. It appears that more clinicians are only observing small relatively nonprogressive tumors which do not affect vision, and there is much evidence that general immunity is important in prevention of metastases. The trauma of enucleation itself may disseminate malignant cells. Localized irradiation appears to be the best nonsurgical treatment. Photocoagulation should be used only for very flat tumors that are not over 2 mm in elevation. Cryotherapy and diathermy seem to be falling into disuse. The prognosis after local resection of the melanoma is still uncertain. – Ed.] ◄

# The Vitreous

INTRODUCTION

In a relatively short time, vitrectomy, has become a safe and well-accepted procedure. The discovery that the human eye would tolerate the removal of a significant portion of the vitreous led to a proliferation of instruments designed to facilitate this procedure. It was not long before adequate patient data was accumulated to document the beneficial results of this new technique in a variety of clinical situations, and the past year has seen further documentation of gratifying results.[1-4] Thus, Peyman and associates[1] reported visual improvement following pars plana vitrectomy in 68% of eyes with posterior segment opacities, most of these being vitreous hemorrhage. Similar excellent results in diabetic patients with vitreous hemorrhage are reported by Myers and Bresnick[3], and by Mandelcorn and associates[4].

Complications encountered in these recent series are similar to those reported in earlier studies and include retinal dialysis or tear with or without detachment, cataract, increasing rubeosis with hemolytic glaucoma, hemorrhage and corneal edema. Certain complications can be minimized fairly easily, for example, by carefully selecting candidates for surgery[4, 5], by appropriate instrument modification[6] and by use of physiologic intraocular irrigating solutions.[7, 8] Other complications are indigenous to the surgery or are dependent on the facility of the surgeon. The complication rate is certainly tolerable and is justified by the potential benefits.

The ophthalmologist who does not perform pars plana vitrectomy must consider this procedure in patients with ocular pathology other than vitreous hemorrhage. Severely traumatized eyes are often candidates for vitrectomy[9, 10] and recent studies have described new techniques and satisfactory surgical results in these cases.[11-14]

When vitrectomy is supplemented with other instruments and techniques — for example, vitreous scissors, foreign body forceps, scleral buckling and sulfur hexafluoride injection — the results have been encouraging. Using these methods in eyes with severe penetrating or perforating injuries, Benson and Machemer[11] reported an overall surgical success rate of 46%, and Hutton et al.[12] achieved significant visual improvement in 64% of eyes similarly treated. These results were achieved in eyes that might have been unsalvageable using more conventional techniques. Significant help may even be afforded eyes harboring a nonmagnetic, nonvisible foreign body,[15, 16] a circumstance which formerly implied a very poor prognosis.

Although open to question, it appears that surgery should be performed early in traumatic cases in an attempt to prevent complications arising from the proliferation of intraocular fibrous tissue. However, even when such proliferation has taken place, vitrectomy may be of benefit. Unfortunately, there are still many traumatized eyes which do poorly, such as those with large corneoscleral lacerations or double perforations. Nonetheless, it would seem appropriate to consider vitrectomy and related techniques in all severely-injured eyes.

Intraocular infection, particularly bacterial endophthalmitis, is another instance in which one should strongly consider vitrectomy, along with intravitreal antibiotic and steroid administration. Forster and his associates[17] have used an aggressive approach in the diagnosis and treatment of endophthalmitis, including vitreous aspiration and culture and intravitreal antibiotic injection. Although many eyes in this series did well, those that harbored virulent pathogens such as pseudomonas and proteus did poorly. Because some of these cases continue to do badly in spite of vigorous therapy, it seems reasonable to consider vitrectomy at times. Accordingly, Peyman and associates[2, 18] recently reported excellent visual results in 3 cases of culture-proven endophthalmitis treated with vitrectomy and intravitreal antibiotic injection. Other reports have also been encouraging.[19]

Because of this recent work, along with past reports,[20] we feel that all cases of culture-positive endophthalmitis may be candidates for intravitreal antibiotic, and possibly steroid, injection. Should a virulent pathogen such as pseudomonas, proteus or staphylococcus aureus be isolated, we would then favor vitrectomy in addition to the above measures. Naturally, these techniques may be supplemented with the simultaneous administration of periocular and systemic antibiotics and steroids, if deemed necessary. If appropriate dosage guidelines are followed,[2, 17, 18, 20, 21, 22] the risks of the above procedures would seem to be justified by the potential rewards.

Vitrectomy has also been used to treat other forms of intraocular infection. Hutton et al.[23] used the Douvas instrument to remove the larval form of the pork tapeworm Taenia Solium from the vitreous of a man, aged 23. Visual acuity of 20/20 was preserved in an eye that probably would have become blind or been lost had other types of treatment been employed.

There are other instances in which vitrectomy has recently been shown to be of therapeutic value in previously desperate situations, for example giant retinal tears[24] and massive vitreous retraction.[25] If these results are borne out by others, a great advance will have been made in dealing with the most significant causes of failure in retinal detachment surgery.

We have only briefly reviewed the significant impact that vitrectomy has had on a wide variety of ocular disorders. For general ophthalmologist and vitreous surgeon alike, it is most rewarding to offer surgery to previously hopeless cases with an excellent chance of success.

Robert W. Herbst, M.D.
Joel A. Kaplan, M.D.
Rush Medical College and
University of Illinois.

## BIBLIOGRAPHY

1. Peyman, G., Huamonte, F., and Goldberg, M. F.: One Hundred Pars Plana Vitrectomies Using the Vitrophage, Am. J. Ophthalmol. 81:263, March, 1976.
2. Peyman, G., Huamonte, F., and Goldberg, M. F.: Vitrectomy Treatment of Vitreous Opacities, Trans. Am. Acad. Ophthalmol. Otolaryngol. 81:394, May–June, 1976.

3. Myers, F. L., and Bresnick, G. H.: Vitrectomy in Diabetic Retinopathy, Trans. Am. Acad. Ophthalmol. Otolaryngol. 81:399, May–June, 1976.

4. Mandelcorn, M. S., Blankenship, G., and Machemer, R.: Pars Plana Vitrectomy for the Management of Severe Diabetic Retinopathy, Am. J. Ophthalmol. 81:561, May, 1976.

5. Tardif, Y. M., and Schepens, C. L.: Closed Vitreous Surgery, Arch. Ophthalmol. 95:235, February, 1977.

6. Peyman, G. A.: Improved Vitrectomy Illumination System, Am. J. Ophthalmol. 81:99, January, 1976.

7. Edelhauser, H., Van Horn, D., Schultz, R., and Hyndiuk, R.: Comparative Toxicity of Intraocular Irrigating Solutions on the Corneal Endothelium, Am. J. Ophthalmol. 81:473, April, 1976.

8. Christiansen, J. M., Killarits, C. R., Fukui, H., Fishman, M. L., Michels, R. G., and Mikuni, I.: Intraocular Irrigating Solutions and Lens Clarity, Am. J. Ophthalmol. 82:594, October, 1976.

9. Coles, W. H., and Haik, G. M.: Vitrectomy in Intraocular Trauma, Arch. Opthalmol. 87:621, 1972.

10. Machemer, R., and Norton, E. W. D.: A New Concept in Vitreous Surgery. 3. Indications and Results, Am. J. Ophthalmol. 74:1034, 1972.

11. Benson, W., and Machemer, R.: Severe Perforating Injuries Treated with Pars Plana Vitrectomy, Am. J. Ophthalmol. 81:728, June, 1976.

12. Hutton, W., Snyder, W., and Vaiser, A.: Vitrectomy in the Treatment of Ocular Perforating Injuries, Am. J. Ophthalmol. 81:733, June, 1976.

13. Coleman, D. J.: The Role of Vitrectomy of Traumatic Vitreopathy, Trans. Am. Acad. Ophthalmol. Otolaryngol. 81:406, May–June, 1976.

14. Hutton, W.: The Role of Vitrectomy in Penetrating Ocular Injuries, Trans. Am. Acad. Ophthalmol. Otolaryngol. 81:414, May–June, 1976.

15. Michels, R. G.: Surgical Management of Nonmagnetic Intraocular Foreign Bodies, Arch. Ophthalmol. 93:1003, October, 1975.

16. Hutton, W., Snyder, W., and Vaiser, A.: Surgical Removal of Nonmagnetic Foreign Bodies, Am. J. Ophthalmol. 80:838, November, 1975.

17. Forster, R. K., Zachary, I., Cottingham, A., and Norton, E. W. D.: Further Observations on the Diagnosis, Cause and Treatment of Endophthalmitis, Am. J. Ophthalmol. 81:52, January, 1976.

18. Peyman, G., Vastine, D., and Diamond, J.: Vitrectomy and

Intraocular Gentamicin Management of Herellea Endophthalmitis after Incomplete Phacoemulsification, Am. J. Ophthalmol. 80:764, October, 1975.
19. Abel, R.: Diagnostic and Therapeutic Vitrectomy for Endophthalmitis, Ann. Ophthalmol. 8:37, January, 1976.
20. Peyman, G., Vastine, D., Crouch, E., and Herbst, R.: Clinical
Use of Intravitreal Antibiotics to Treat Bacterial Endophthalmitis, Trans. Am. Acad. Ophthalmol. Otolaryngol. 78:862,
1974.
21. Peyman, G., May, D., Ericson, E., and Apple, D.: Intraocular
Injection of Gentamicin: Toxic Effects and Clearance, Arch.
Ophthalmol. 92:42, 1974.
22. Meisels, H., and Peyman, G.: Intravitreal Gentamicin in the
Treatment of Induced Staphylococcal Endophthalmitis, Ann.
Ophthalmol. 8:939, August, 1976.
23. Hutton, W., Vaiser, A., and Snyder, W.: Pars Plana Vitrectomy
for Removal of Intravitreous Cysticercus, Am. J. Ophthalmol.
81:571, May, 1976.
24. Machemer, R.: Retinal Tears 180 Degrees and Greater. Management with Vitrectomy and Intravitreal Gas, Arch. Ophthalmol. 94:1340, August, 1976.
25. Machemer, R.: Removal of Preretinal Membranes, Trans. Am.
Acad. Ophthalmol. Otolaryngol. 81:420, May–June, 1976.

**Summing Up–Symposium on the Vitreous.** Michael
J. Hogan[7] (Univ. of California) summarizes current information on vitreous structure and the changes occurring in
ocular diseases. Mucopolysaccharide and collagen formation
by hyalocytes contributes to the rapid increase in vitreous
volume seen in human beings up to age 3. Little is known of
the turnover of vitreous collagen in the human being. The
gel structure of the vitreous appears to be due to the cooperative actions of hyaluronic acid and collagen. There appears
to be a large-molecule pathway through the vitreous, the
hyaluronic acid moving forward into the posterior and anterior chambers. Stability of the gel is constant despite the
loss of hyaluronic acid. In aphakia and myopia the hyaluronic acid content of the vitreous appears to be lower and in
myopia there is also a reduction in the collagen content.

Inflammations of the vitreous lead to coagulation of the
gel and the formation of strands. The coagulation results

(7)  Trans. Ophthalmol. Soc. U.K. 95(pt.3):445–446, 1975.

from blood products interacting with the vitreous protein. Many pigmented cells are characteristically found in the vitreous in patients about to acquire massive vitreous retraction. The effects of trauma on the vitreous depend on the vascular response in adjacent tissues as well as on the presence or absence of hemorrhage. The question of whether diabetes itself affects the vitreous or whether the vitreous changes seen are secondary to diabetic retinal vascular lesions remains open.

The normal vitreous is ultrasonically silent. Contact ultrasonography appears to be the best diagnostic approach. Pars plana vitrectomy is used in anterior segment disease to treat cystoid macular edema; in clearing vitreous opacities due to inflammation and an aphakia with pupillary membranes. In the posterior segment, vitrectomy can be used to remove vitreous opacities of various types. In treating traction retinal detachments in diabetic retinopathy, the general principles are to clear the vitreous, sever the traction bands and insert gas to reattach the retina.

**Physical Structures of the Vitreous** are described by Jürgen Gärtner[8] (Univ. of Mainz). The mammalian vitreous body is a specialized connective tissue which has evolved to serve as a transparent medium and to absorb and redistribute forces applied to the surrounding tissues. The main structural components are collagen fibrils, which are embedded in a so-called amorphous ground substance, and a small amount of cells.

Both the fibroblast-like and the macrophage-like cells of the vitreous originate from the walls of the hyaloid vessels. These cells are believed to be variants whose morphology depends on functional activity. Active fibril-forming cells are found in the whole vitreous cortex of the adult human eye, especially in the region of the disc and within the vitreous base. Fundamentally the vitreous cells have the same general properties as the connective tissue cells. Like fibroblasts in general, the fiber-forming vitreous cells have a phagocytic capability. During senile vitreous detachment the collagen of the vitreous framework undergoes various stages of degradation, which may be best explained by a

(8)   Trans. Ophthalmol. Soc. U.K. 95(Pt.3):364–368, 1975.

combined collagenase-lysosomal theory. In pathologic states, most of the phagocytic cells within the vitreous body are thought to be derived from circulating cells of marrow origin, usually monocytes.

The possibility that the developing lens epithelium and the developing Müller cells of the retina participate in formation of the embryonic vitreous body remains an open question. The vessel wall cells of the tunica vasculosa lentis appear to have the major role in zonule formation in the prenatal and early postnatal rat, rabbit and monkey eyes. In the adult rat and human eye, the source of collagen required for modeling of the ligament of Zinn appears to be the fibril-forming vitreous cells, situated mainly in the area of the pars plana. The protein of the zonular fibrils has been proved to belong to the collagens.

**Inflammation and Its Effect on the Vitreous** are discussed by Michael J. Hogan[9] (Univ. of California). Inflammation of tissues contiguous to the vitreous produce a complex exudate that alters its composition and structure. The products of inflammation in the uveal tissues diffuse through the vitreous to produce inflammation and edema of the macula and optic disc. Migration of monocytes from adjacent vessels is important in the cortical cellular proliferation that leads to fibrosis. The macrophages and polymorphonuclear cells release proteolytic enzymes that are capable of damaging effects, whereas the fibroblasts are active in fibril synthesis. Normal vitreous lacks resistance to the growth of organisms, even saprophytes.

The early effects of inflammation are due to spread from adjacent tissues and are manifest as cellular, fibrinous and proteinaceous vitreous exudate. Intermediate effects include a variable amount of necrosis and coincident repair. Late effects include the absorption of exudate and repair. Macrophage activity at this stage is important in the dissolution of fibrin clots and the phagocytosis of debris. Membrane formation occurs on the inner surfaces of damaged and repaired tissues and in the adjacent vitreous.

Suppurative infections lead to destruction of the interior of the eye unless rapidly controlled. Nonsuppurative infec-

(9)  Trans. Ophthalmol. Soc. U.K. 95(Pt.3):378–381, 1975.

tions tend to last for considerable periods and to eventually result in severe degenerative changes in the vitreous, with membrane formation and liquefaction. Characteristic dust-like vitreous opacities are found in chronic cyclitis. Toxo-plasmic retinitis is characteristically associated with severe vitreous opacification and inflammation. Larvae of *Toxocara canis* and *T. cattis* may produce vitreous disease, with in-flammation and shrinkage usually leading to retinal de-tachment. The growing malignant melanoma leaks plasma into the vitreous and leads to membrane formation. Reticu-lum cell sarcoma is accompanied by severe diffuse opacifica-tion of the vitreous by exudation from the affected retina and ciliary body. Irradiation of such eyes leads to clearing of the vitreous and the retinal lesions but coarse and fine opac-ities persist after healing.

**Use of A-Scan Echography in Clinical Diagnosis of Persistent Hyperplastic Primary Vitreous (PHPV).** W. Schroeder[1] (Univ. of Hamburg) studied 15 patients in whom patterns of rudimentary hyaloid vessels could be detected by this method (in 9 patients up to age 7) although the vessels were seen by an ophthalmoscope in only 1 patient. This is significant because this condition is a major differential diag-nosis for leukokoria of infancy.

In addition to ascertaining visual acuity, position and motility, horizontal and perpendicular corneal diameter and intraocular pressure are measured. Evaluation of anterior segments is done microscopically; fundus examination is by indirect binocular ophthalmoscopy. An echo-ophthalmo-graph is used to determine the axial lengths in both eyes and to examine the vitreous space for reflecting structures. Axial length is the distance from the corneal apex to the ret-inal inner surface at the posterior pole. Once solid and larger vitreous alterations are excluded, detection of a weak par-axial echo is possible by scanning from a bulbus-equatorial direction (Fig 34).

This ultrasonographic finding represents an important contribution to the clinical diagnosis of PHPV, particularly when the monolateral cataract is too dense for observation of other signs (elongated ciliary processes and retrolenticu-

(1)   Klin. Monatsbl. Augenheilkd. 163:210–216, February, 1976.

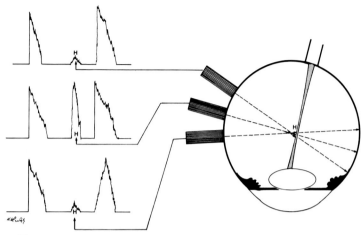

**Fig 34.** — Only when ultrasonic beam hits vitreous vessel perpendicularly on horizontal level as well can less intensive echo *(H)* be demonstrated, in center position, which will nearly or totally disappear when ultrasonic beam leaves this position. (Courtesy of Schroeder, W.: Klin. Monatsbl. Augenheilkd. 163:210–216, February, 1976.)

lar fibrovascular tissue). It could also be demonstrated that lenticular thickness was diminished even in case of a swollen cataract with a flattened anterior chamber. Contrary to expectation, the axial length of the involved bulbus was increased in one third of the patients, whereas a relative microcornea was missing in only 2 eyes.

**Toxicity of Intravitreal Whole Blood and Hemoglobin.** Donald Sanders, Gholam A. Peyman, Gerald Fishman, Joseph Vlchek and Michael Korey[2] (Univ. of Illinois) found that intravitreal injections of 0.3 ml autogenous blood and single injections of 22.4 mg hemoglobin did not produce toxic effects on the monkey retina. Intravitreal injections of over 0.6 ml whole blood or 40 mg hemoglobin produced definite histologic and electroretinographic toxicity. The histologic damage correlated well with the degree of hemosiderin deposition. Explosive lesions produced by xenon arc photocoagulation, inducing moderate vitreous hemorrhage, failed to produce toxic doses of blood in the eye. In humans having

(2) Albrecht von Graefes Arch. Klin. Ophthalmol. 197:255–267, 1975.

vitrectomy, the amount of whole blood recovered from vitrectomy fluid was considered nontoxic, except when the patient had massive vitreous hemorrhage or intraoperative bleeding.

Free hemoglobin was more toxic than the equivalent hemoglobin concentration of whole blood in these studies. Hemosiderin deposition correlated with the histologically apparent damage, indicating that iron may be a factor in blood-induced toxic effects on the retina. At moderately toxic dosages, electroretinography was a more sensitive indicator of damage than was microscopic evaluation. Clinically, when the amount of vitreous hemorrhage cannot be judged ophthalmoscopically and the retina is shown to be attached, serial bright-flash electroretinograms may reveal a blood-induced toxic effect on the retina.

**Principles of Instrumentation** for vitrectomy are summarized by Stephen J. Ryan, Jr.[3] (Univ. of Southern California). Initial instrumentation for the "open-sky" vitrectomy technique proved inadequate for surgery deep in the vitreous cavity near its interface with the retina. Many instruments that use different engineering principles or modifications of the original vitreous infusion suction cutter (VISC) have become available (table). The most important function of any of the instruments is the ability to cut cleanly and without traction in a repeatable manner. Most instruments use a rotating knife powered by an electric micromotor. The single-edged or multiple-edged knives rotate across the port, amputating material aspirated into the port. An adjustable port offers several advantages, large for lens removal and small for better control. The instrument should permit the separation of cutting from aspiration and other functions and should possess a capacity for reflux; infusion is another essential feature. Good visibility is essential. The question of the ideal size and shape of these vitrectomy instruments remains unsettled, but further miniaturization is needed.

There is significant advantage to having a stereoscopic magnified image, as provided by the operating microscope. The two-instrument technique developed by Machemer et al. is being used with increasing frequency. The second in-

---

(3)   Trans. Am. Acad. Ophthalmol. Otolaryngol. 81:352–357, May–June, 1976.

INSTRUMENTS FOR VITRECTOMY
PERSONAL EXPERIENCE

| VITREOUS SURGEON | INSTRUMENT |
|---|---|
| Machemer | VISC |
| Douvas | Roto-extractor |
| O'Malley | Vitritome |
| Peyman | Vitrophage |
| Birretta* | Sukon |

OBSERVED BUT NO PERSONAL EXPERIENCE

| VITREOUS SURGEON | INSTRUMENT |
|---|---|
| Federman | SITE |
| Klöti | Vitreous stripper |
| Schepens et al | Nibbler |
| Krieger et al | Vitrectomy instrument |
| Girard† | Ultrasonic fragmentor |
| Kaufman | Vitrector |

*Although the vitreous surgeon has been arbitrarily mentioned as the developer, the engineer of the Sukon has been given the credit in this case (personal communication).
†Personal communication.

strument can be a 22-gauge 4-cm needle for use in stripping preretinal membranes, or else a knife, scissors, punch or forceps. A whole range of accessory instruments has become available, including a sclerotomy knife and a trochar and cannula. Diathermy has been used to coagulate intravitreal tufts of neovascularization and cryotherapy has been of value in treating retinal holes. Air and sulfur hexafluoride gas have been used for internal tamponade. Use of a scleral buckle remains a useful adjunct to vitrectomy because many patients have retinal detachment as well as vitreous hemorrhage and also because retinal detachment remains a major complication of vitrectomy.

**Optimized Underwater Diathermy for Vitreous Surgery** is described by Charles L. Schepens, Francois Delori, Frank J. Rogers and Ian J. Constable[4] (Boston).

Intraocular blood vessels that must be closed often cause problems to the clinician. Two types of optimized underwater electrodes have been developed, 1 for open-sky vitreous surgery and 1 for closed transscleral vitreous surgery. The former type of surgery is done under an operating microscope with a short focal length. The electrode is mounted on a 60-mm handle at an angle of 35 degrees. The electrode is 38 mm long and 0.5 mm wide, with a tapered tip having an active portion 0.2 mm thick and 0.5 mm long. The insulation is epoxylite. The electrode lead is constructed with a foot switch. The instrument used in closed transscleral vitreous surgery is shown in Figure 35. The probe, about 50 mm long, is mounted in a 19-gauge steel tube connected to a saline reservoir or large syringe. The rate of saline flow under moderate digital pressure is 10 cc/minute, great enough to maintain ocular pressure within normal limits, even under very adverse conditions.

À radio frequency current, about 35–50% higher than is

**Fig 35.**—Simplified cross-section of underwater electrode and handle used in transscleral closed vitreous surgery. The 1.5-mm metal plug closes end of 50-mm 19-gauge steel tube. The 0.5-mm round hole, 3 mm from tip, infuses saline and maintains normal intraocular pressure. Fluid originates in syringe (or saline bottle), penetrates into fluid chamber, up steel tube and into eye. Assembly is easily replaced; system is waterproofed with epoxylite seals *(E)*. (Courtesy of Schepens, C. L., et al.: Ophthalmic Surg. 6:82–89, Winter, 1975.)

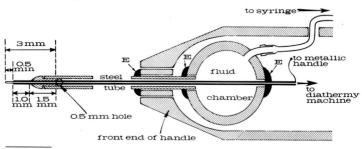

(4) Ophthalmic Surg. 6:82–89, Winter, 1975.

used on dry tissue, is needed to coagulate under water. Charring should be avoided. A trial is done in the conjunctival sac before inserting the electrode into the vitreous cavity. Closure of blood vessels often requires a higher current setting than is needed to coagulate tissue, especially if the vessel is embedded in a scar. Where practical, each sizeable vessel is closed with 3 adjacent applications and the surgeon waits 10 minutes to see if the treated vessels reopen.

Over 150 cases have been treated with underwater electrodes. Newly formed blood vessels not obscured by bleeding were closed successfully in 28 cases by the closed transscleral technique. Minute immediate hemorrhages were frequent but of no clinical consequence. Treated vessels did not reopen during follow-up for up to 2 years. In the last 90 cases of open-sky vitrectomy, immediate effectiveness in closing new vessels was constant but the long-term effect often could not be determined with certainty.

Another potential use of the underwater electrode is for the application of diathermy to a lamellar scleral undermining prepared for scleral buckling of a retinal detachment. In this instance, the electrode tip should be immersed in saline solution. This technique may be useful where it is difficult to dry the surgical field or where the surgeon's assistant is inexperienced.

**Vitrectomy Technique in Anterior Segment Surgery** is described by Ronald G. Michels and Walter J. Stark[5] (Johns Hopkins Hosp.). The concept of excising intraocular tissue a bite at a time while maintaining a "closed eye" with normal or elevated intraocular pressure can be applied to certain disease states of the anterior segment of the eye.

The technique involves the controlled excision of intraocular tissue to create an adequate pupillary space or to remove vitreous from the anterior segment. An operating microscope and a fiberoptic sleeve around the instrument tip are used. The vitrectomy instrument is usually introduced in the superotemporal quadrant through the pars plana, with the cutting port directed anteriorly. Excision of iris tissue is avoided where possible. Where both a dense pupillary membrane and an intact cataractous lens exist, a pars plana

---

(5)  Trans. Am. Acad. Ophthalmol. Otolaryngol. 81:382–393, May–June, 1976.

approach can also be used. A two-instrument technique is used where the pupillary membrane is nonpliable and cannot be aspirated into the cutting port. The vitrectomy instrument tip supports the membrane from behind while a discission knife cuts the membrane from in front. Then the tags of membrane can be removed with the vitrectomy instrument. A two-instrument technique is also used to coagulate large vessels in the pupillary membrane or iris, by positioning the vessel between the 2 instruments and applying diathermy. Formed vitreous that has herniated into the anterior chamber is readily removed by a pars plana approach.

Twelve eyes with dense, fibrotic capsulolenticular membranes were operated on by this technique and all attempts were successful. Three eyes with pupillary membranes after trauma were operated on and an adequate pupillary space was created in each eye. Good results were obtained in 3 eyes with inadequate, updrawn pupils and in 1 with a secluded pupil and iris bombé. An anatomic success was obtained in an eye with persistent hyperplastic primary vitreous. Four eyes with aphakic pupillary-block glaucoma were treated by the pars plana approach. The anterior chamber was deepened in each and visual acuity improved but 2 eyes required cyclocryotherapy for peripheral anterior synechiae. One eye treated for vitreous touch and corneal edema improved postoperatively but cystoid macular edema limited vision after operation.

This approach to selected cases of anterior segment disease offers several advantages over conventional techniques but definite indications for this method are not firmly established.

**Pars Plana Vitrectomy for Management of Severe Diabetic Retinopathy.** Mark S. Mandelcorn, George Blankenship and Robert Machemer[6] (Univ. of Miami) reviewed results of pars plana vitrectomy performed in 100 consecutive patients with late complications of diabetic retinopathy in 1972 and 1973, who were followed for at least 5 months postoperatively. A total of 105 eyes was operated on, and 14 were followed for more than a year after surgery. Median

(6)   Am. J. Ophthalmol. 81:561–570, May, 1976.

follow-up was 7 months. Five patients died before the 6-month follow-up examination. The 65 men and 35 women had a median age of 51 years at operation. Median duration of established diabetes was 20 years, and that of visual symptoms referable to retinopathy in the eye that was operated on was 3 years. Insulin was used by 80 patients. Photocoagulation had previously been performed in 21 eyes. In most eyes, acuity was less than finger counting preoperatively. Most eyes had dense vitreous hemorrhages, and all had some proliferative tissue. Pars plana lensectomies were performed in 67 of 83 eyes. The two-instrument technique was used to remove preretinal blood from 44 eyes and to peel preretinal membranes in 27 (see the next article by Machemer).

Dialyses and retinal holes were produced in 11 eyes. Delayed epithelialization or recurrent epithelial sloughing of the cornea occurred in about one fourth of eyes. Five eyes had intraocular pressures exceeding 30 mm Hg. Rhegmatogenous retinal detachments developed postoperatively in 6 eyes. Various procedures were combined with vitrectomy to prevent or treat retinal detachment: e.g. cryopexy, injection of air or $SF_6$ mixture, and scleral buckles. Fifteen eyes had no light perception at follow-up. Corneal abnormalities were seen in 31 eyes, apparently related to rubeosis and not to aphakia.

In these severely diseased diabetic eyes, major visual improvement resulted after pars plana vitrectomy in 49% of the eyes, and those with only vitreous hemorrhage did better (71% improved). Those with surgical complications (16%) did poorly (19% had visual improvement), as did those who developed rubeosis or vitreous hemorrhage or both. The prognosis was better in patients over 30 years of age. Ultrasonography and bright flash ERG were better prognosticators than entoptic phenomenon, which was inaccurate.

**Removal of Preretinal Membranes** is described by Robert Machemer[7] (Univ. of Miami). The removal of preretinal membranes requires additional instrumentation when the vitreous infusion suction cutter (VISC) is used. A 22-gauge 4-cm needle is effective; it is bent 80 degrees in

(7)   Trans. Am. Acad. Ophthalmol. Otolaryngol. 81:420–425, May–June, 1976.

such a way that the bent part is not longer than the thickness of the needle. The hooked needle is attached to a handle for easier manipulation. The needle is introduced into the eye through the pars plana at an angle of 90–180 degrees to the VISC. After conventional vitrectomy, the needle is guided toward areas of preretinal proliferation and used to lift off the membranes. When thick connective tissue strands are present, the hooked needle is exchanged for vitreous scissors after enlarging the scleral opening.

Membrane peeling may be used in proliferative diabetic retinopathy and is presently used in about half of all cases. The proliferations usually have several direct connections with the retina, and an attempt is made to isolate these roots and circumcise the areas with the VISC. In massive periretinal proliferation, intravitreal and retrovitreal strands are removed, and the retinal surface is then approached with the hooked needle. It is usually convenient to start close to the disc and work toward the periphery.

The success rate in 32 eyes considered untreatable by conventional buckling procedures was 34%. Eyes with perforating injuries and excessive scar formation in the vitreous and on the retinal surface may also be treated by preretinal membrane removal. Membrane peeling was performed in 17 of 41 cases of severe perforating injury, and 19 eyes had successful surgical results.

**Role of Vitrectomy in Traumatic Vitreopathy** is discussed by D. Jackson Coleman[8] (Columbia Univ.). In traumatic vitreopathy the coagulum of vitreous and blood undergoes fibroblastic change and is organized into a system of membranes that can continue to obstruct vision even after red blood cell clots have disintegrated and can contract and cause the remaining vitreous matrix to detach the retina or suppress the production of aqueous. The irritative or inflammatory response of the vitreous body presumably influences the rapidity of these changes. Surgery would then be necessary either immediately or as soon as the irritative or inflammatory response is suppressed, usually within 3 months after injury.

Wounds with prolapsed vitreous can be used as access

(8) Trans. Am. Acad. Ophthalmol. Otolaryngol. 81:406–413, May–June, 1976.

routes for central vitrectomy or lensectomy, or both, by using a superior ring. The suction cutter is used without infusion to aspirate formed vitreous from the wound. When vitrectomy is used as part of a secondary procedure to sever vitreous traction to the wound, a second incision may be used. The ruptured lens can be removed through the pars plana with the vitrectomy instrument or with an ultrasonic fragmentor or phacoemulsifier. Vitrectomy is indicated if the media are opaque or if the foreign body has become incarcerated in a fibroplastic capsule. Magnetic extraction of the foreign body may be possible. Otherwise a second instrument may be needed to remove the foreign body; a 22-gauge needle is useful for this purpose. When traction on the retina is suspected, clearing of the opaque vitreous can allow the retinal wound to be visualized. Early removal of the vitreous scaffolding that exerts traction on the retina reduces the chance of detachment and allows direct visualization and treatment of the posterior injury.

Debridement of vitreous from perforating injuries can be more effectively carried out using vitreous suction and cutting instruments than with conventional sponge-forceps technique. The earliest possible surgical intervention is recommended in these situations.

**Severe Perforating Injuries Treated with Pars Plana Vitrectomy.** Eyes that have sustained a penetrating or lacerating injury may develop persistent vitreous hemorrhage or fibrovascular proliferation in the vitreous, leading to tractional retinal detachments that are inoperable by standard scleral buckling procedures. Vitrectomy through the pars plana gives good results in such eyes. William E. Benson and Robert Machemer[9] (Univ. of Miami) reviewed the records of 48 consecutive patients who underwent vitrectomy for sequelae of ocular trauma in 1972–74. All had had either a penetrating injury, with the foreign body remaining in or behind the eye, or a laceration, with a resultant full-thickness perforation of the cornea or sclera. Follow-up of 41 patients was possible. Mean interval from injury to referral was 7.6 months. Fifteen patients had had previous surgery other than wound closure. Pars plana vitrectomy was done

(9) Am. J. Ophthalmol. 81:728–732, June, 1976.

with the vitreous infusion suction cutter (VISC), and a posterior lensectomy was done with the VISC if the lens was cataractous. Foreign bodies were removed with forceps under direct illumination from an intraocular fiberoptic illuminator.

Thirteen results (32%) were successful, with improvement of two lines or more on the Snellen acuity chart or preservation of initial good vision. There were 6 (15%) technical successes, with clear media and an attached retina but no improvement in poor vision. There were 4 initial successes, but the retina later redetached. Only 9 of 16 retained foreign bodies could be removed. Twenty-one eyes had hemorrhagic vitreous and intravitreous proliferations, and 2 patients had severe vitritis. Operative complications included retinal dialysis in 12 patients, holes in detached retina in 4 and retinal detachment within a month of vitrectomy in 3. Retinal detachment developed in 4 patients 4 weeks to 6 months postoperatively. In each the detachment was due to proliferative tissue.

Nearly half the patients in this series had at least technically successful pars plana vitrectomy for sequelae of severe perforating injuries. The main cause of failure was intravitreous proliferation of fibrous tissue.

**Pars Plana Vitrectomy for Removal of Intravitreous *Cysticercus*.** Intraocular cysticercosis usually results in blindness unless the parasite is surgically removed from the eye. William L. Hutton, Albert Vaiser and William B. Snyder[1] (Texas Retina Associates, Dallas) report a case in which pars plana vitrectomy, with use of an operating microscope and intraocular fiberoptics, provided a controlled, safe means of removing an intravitreous *Cysticercus* without removal of the clear lens.

Man, 23, a Latin American, noticed blurred vision and redness of the right eye about 10 days after leaving Mexico, where he had eaten indigenous foods, including pork. Acuity was 20/60 in the right eye 2 weeks after onset of symptoms, and a 4- or 5-mm, undulating, translucent cyst was present in the posterior vitreous cavity, moving freely during eye movements. Light stimulation resulted in contraction and eversion of the scolex. An area of elevated, whitish retina was present nasal to the optic nerve. Stools

(1) Am. J. Ophthalmol. 81:571–573, May, 1976.

contained no ova or parasites. After 3 days of prednisolone therapy, a pars plana vitrectomy was performed with the Douvas rotoextractor. The *Cysticercus* was impacted on the probe tip and cut and sectioned from the eye. A subtotal vitrectomy was performed. Microscopic study showed characteristic findings of *Taenia solium*. Systemic steroid therapy was given for 5 days postoperatively. Inflammation was minimal, and acuity was 20/20 2 weeks after operation.

Although rare in the United States, *T. solium,* the pork tapeworm, is prevalent in Mexico, South America and Central Europe. The *Cysticercus,* or larval stage, can involve vital structures. Man is infected from exogenous sources or from reflex peristalsis of eggs from a resident adult worm. All ocular spaces have been sites involved by the *Cysticercus.* The subconjunctival space is the most common site. Destruction of the *Cysticercus* without its removal usually results in release of toxins and loss of the eye. Pars plana vitrectomy proved to be an ideal operation in this patient. Obligatory removal of a clear lens is avoided, and all toxic particles and vitreous debris can be removed when the *Cysticercus* is aspirated, resulting in minimal postoperative inflammation.

**Elevation of Intraocular Pressure after Pars Plana Vitrectomy.** Robert S. Weinberg, Gholam A. Peyman and Felipe U. Huamonte[2] (Univ. of Illinois, Chicago) analyzed this complication in a retrospective study of 115 patients having 118 eye operations in 1974–75. The mean patient age was 45.8. Forty-nine diabetic patients had 51 eye operations. All but one of these patients had vitreous hemorrhage and 24 of the 66 nondiabetic patients had vitreous hemorrhage secondary to trauma, whereas 19 had a secondary membrane after extracapsular cataract extraction or a congenital cataract. Elevated intraocular pressure (IOP) was defined as a rise of at least 10 mm Hg above the preoperative level by applanation tonometry or an IOP above 24 mm Hg in eyes with perforating injury.

A postoperative increase in IOP occurred in 33 eyes (28%), including 25 (49%) diabetic and 8 (12%) nondiabetic eyes. Average increases in pressure were similar in the two groups. Most pressure rises occurred in the first 3 weeks af-

(2) Albrecht von Graefes Arch. Klin. Ophthalmol. 200:157–161, 1976.

ter vitrectomy. Eleven of the 25 diabetic eyes required surgical intervention and 4 were uncontrolled at last examination. Pressure elevations in the nondiabetic eyes were either transient or medically controllable. No nondiabetic eye with perforating injury developed a postoperative rise in IOP. One third of the diabetic eyes with a rise in IOP had hyphema and half of these had preoperative rubeosis iridis. Four other eyes with rubeosis iridis had a rise in IOP without hyphema. Five eyes acquired rubeosis iridis postoperatively; 4 of these had an increase in IOP and the fifth became phthisical. Only one nondiabetic eye with an IOP elevation had a hyphema and none developed rubeosis iridis.

Increased IOP after pars plana vitrectomy is more frequent in diabetic eyes and tends to occur within 3 weeks after vitrectomy. Preoperative rubeosis iridis results in increased IOP postoperatively. Postoperative rubeosis iridis, seen only in diabetics, is associated with more refractory elevations of IOP than is preoperative rubeosis.

# The Retina

This Introduction is a summary of those diseases most frequently seen in which diffuse degeneration of the retinal pigment epithelium and of photoreceptors is found in association with hearing deficiency.

---

## Alström Syndrome

The clinical features of this rare autosomal recessive disease include profound childhood blindness associated with nystagmus, cataracts, optic atrophy and a pigmentary retinopathy of the retinitis pigmentosa-type, moderate to severe progressive neurosensory deafness, obesity that is most evident during infancy, diabetes mellitus (carbohydrate intolerance associated with hyperinsulinemia), acanthosis nigricans, hyperuricemia, hypertriglyceridemia with elevation in the pre-betalipoprotein fraction, and in males, hypergonadotrophic hypogenitalism associated with normal secondary sex characteristics. Goldstein and Fialkow (Medicine 52:53, 1973) emphasized the presence of a chronic nephropathy, characterized in its early stages by aminoaciduria and nephrogenic diabetes insipidus and in its late stage by uremia. The earliest symptom is blindness with an onset within the first 2 years of life, followed in order by obesity (between age 2-10 years), nerve deafness (age 7 years), carbohydrate intolerance (age 22 years) and chronic renal disease (age 26 years) (ibid.). The patients maintain normal intelligence.

## Bardet-Biedl Syndrome

The Bardet-Biedl syndrome is an autosomal recessively inherited genetic disorder characterized by structural and functional abnormalities of organs and tissues of diverse embryonic derivation. Five cardinal features include polydactyly or syndactyly (66%–75%), pigmentary retinopathy (87%), obesity (75%–92%), mental retardation (73%–87%) and hypogonadism or a delay in sexual development (24% –86%). Some affected individuals may also show brachycephaly (50%), short stature (35%), various neurologic disorders, congenital heart disease or kidney disease. Deafness can occur, but probably does so in less than 5% of patients.

Patients generally have visual problems within the first 10 or, in some cases, 20 years of life. Most often, the first complaint is that of poor night vision, which is frequently followed or accompanied by defects in central vision. Nystagmus may also be a common feature. Fundus changes include constricted arterioles, waxy disc atrophy and peripheral pigmentary changes including areas of white deposits, pigment atrophy and bone spicule pigmentation. The last tends to occur between the age 8–10 years. Although only approximately 15% of patients with the Bardet-Biedl syndrome have fundus changes similar to those with typical retinitis pigmentosa, essentially all patients have night blindness and abnormal electroretinogram (ERG) amplitudes. Most patients are legally blind by age 30.

Patients in this group should not be confused with those having the Alström syndrome, in which a pigmentary retinopathy is combined with obesity, perceptual deafness and diabetes mellitus. Polydactyly and mental retardation are lacking. As noted, deafness is infrequently seen in the Bardet-Biedl syndrome.

Regrettably, the term Laurence-Moon-Biedl syndrome has gained acceptance in the literature. The Bardet-Biedl and Laurence-Moon syndromes are separate and distinct genetic diseases with overlapping features. Common to both are retinal dystrophy, mental retardation and hypogenitalism. Spastic paraplegia is the predominant feature in the Laurence-Moon syndrome while polydactyly and obesity, prominent in the Bardet-Biedl syndrome, are not features of the Laurence-Moon syndrome.

## Cockayne's Syndrome

This rare, autosomal recessively inherited disease is characterized by dwarfism, a prematurely senile appearance, microcephaly, a beaked nose, sunken eyes, prognathism, proportionally long limbs (which may appear blue and feel cold), large hands and feet, flexion deformities of the joints, unsteady gait and movement from extrapyramidal and cerebellar lesions, a segmental demyelinating peripheral neuropathy, moderate kyphosis, photosensitive dermatitis leading to scarring and pigmentation, mental retardation, deafness, cataracts, keratitis, retinal degeneration and optic atrophy. Death usually occurs sometime between age 20 and 30 years.

The patients have a latent period during the first 6–12 months of life, during which time they appear normal. A failure to grow then becomes progressively evident, as does kyphosis, mental retardation, loss of weight, and a diffuse loss of subcutaneous fat, which gives them their typical wizened old man's facies. All components of the syndrome are usually well developed in the patient by the age of 5 years. Fundus changes include a widespread fine speckled pigmentation ("salt and pepper") appearance that is unrelated in distribution to retinal vessels and most dense within the macula. The optic discs are pale and the arteries narrowed. The retinal dystrophy is progressive and eventually leads to severe visual loss. The majority of patients also suffer from a progressive sensorineural type of deafness.

## Leber's Congenital Amaurosis

Patients afflicted with this disease are either blind at birth or develop a visual disorder in the first year of life. External signs include wandering nystagmoid ocular movements and an oculodigital phenomenon, in which the fists are rubbed forcibly into the eyes, probably to induce mechanically the sensation of light. Some of the patients are photosensitive.

In infancy, the ocular fundus may show few definite lesions. Some cases may exhibit a salt and pepper appearance to the fundus or a pigmentary retinopathy with bone spicule pigmentation not unlike that seen in retinitis pigmentosa. When present, the bone spicule changes usually become apparent between age 8 and 14 years. Other patients may show either an albinotic fundus appearance or a fundus similar to that of choroidal atrophy. Lens opacities eventually occur in approximately 50% of cases. Although not a frequent or consistent finding, auditory or neurologic abnormalities have been reported by François (Fr. Ophthal. 76:1, 1963) and Dekaban and Carr (Arch. Neurol. 14:294, 1966).

This disease probably represents several autosomal recessive genetic diseases all with the common feature of early and profound visual loss. The ERG recordings in this disease are traditionally nondetectable at an early age and provide an important diagnostic means of identifying a retinal disease and not "cortical blindness."

## Usher's Syndrome

This autosomal recessively inherited syndrome is characterized by the association of a congenital neurosensory hearing defect, which can vary in severity, and retinitis pigmentosa. Associated features may include vestibular deficiency abnormalities demonstrated by caloric testing. These include unsteadiness of gait and postural vertigo. Posterior subcapsular cataracts are also seen. This syndrome is estimated to account for 3% – 6% of profound childhood deafness and approximately 50% of deaf-blindness. The prevalence is approximately 3 per 100,000 people while the prevalence of carriers has been estimated at 1:200 to 1:300 of the general population.

In addition to hearing deficiency, patients initially complain of poor night vision within the first 10 or 20 years of life, which progressively increases in severity. Peripheral fields are constricted and pronounced abnormalities are present on ERG, EOG and dark adaptation testing. In a high percentage of patients, central acuity is eventually diminished to legal blindness by age 40 or 50 years when involvement of the macula generally becomes visible ophthalmoscopically. There appears to be an intrafamilial consistency in expressivity of the ocular disease. The course of the cochlear, vestibular and optic lesions is frequently variable and dissociated. All of these systems are probably affected through the expression of a single polyphenic gene. Although abnormal EOG, dark adaptation and audiometric findings have been implicated as diagnostic for the identification of heterozygotes, there is no uniformity of opinion or consistency of data in this regard. Merin and Auerbach (Acta Genet. Med. Gemellol. (Roma) 23:49, 1974) suggest that this disease may be genetically identical to Hallgren's syndrome in which retinitis pigmentosa is seen not only with deafness but also with vestibulocerebellar ataxia and mental deficiency.

## Hallgren's Syndrome

Hallgren's syndrome includes congenital deafness, vestibulocerebellar ataxia, primary pigmentary dystrophy associated with night blindness, and mental abnormalities. Hallgren (Acta Psychiatr. Scand. 34: suppl. 138, 1959) investigated 177 patients belonging to 102 families. The incidence of this syndrome in Sweden was approximately 3:100,000 people. A single autosomal recessive gene with complete penetrance in both sexes and a pleiotropic effect is thought to be responsible for the syndrome.

The clinical appearance of the primary retinal pigmentary dystrophy is characteristic of that seen in patients with retinitis pigmentosa. Cataracts are also frequently associated. Nystagmus occurs in approximately 10% of patients. All patients suffer from a congenital neurosensory deafness. More than 90% of the clinically deaf have a gait disturbance of vestibulocerebellar type, possibly due to a labyrinthine disorder, since other signs of cerebellar deficiency are not generally found. There is a positive correlation between the degree of hearing loss and vestibulocerebellar ataxia. About 25% of patients show mental retardation and 25% show a psychosis reminiscent of schizophrenia.

The genetic distinction between patients with Hallgren's syndrome and Usher's syndrome is not always apparent in individual cases, as an overlap in signs and symptoms clearly exists. Patients with Usher's syndrome showing profound congenital neurosensory hearing loss can also manifest an ataxic gait, presumably from labyrinthine disease. Within one family with Usher's syndrome, I have seen one family member with and another without clinically apparent ataxia, although both had severe deafness. The presence of mental retardation and psychotic behavior may be a nonspecific response in some patients to a double sensory handicap and not an inherited trait.

## Refsum's Syndrome

This autosomal recessively inherited trait most characteristically includes an atypical pigmentary retinopathy with irregular clumping of pigment or a salt and pepper fundus appearance associated with night blindness and constricted peripheral fields, a peripheral neuropathy with paresis and sensory disturbance, and cerebellar ataxia.

An increase in the fatty acid, phytanic acid, is seen in the blood and tissues of affected patients. Additional signs include increased protein of the cerebrospinal fluid without an increase of cells, weak and atrophic lower extremities and absent deep tender reflexes. Less constant findings include a progressive neurosensory hearing loss in about 50%, hypoactive vestibular responses, ichthyosis-like skin changes, and electrocardiographic abnormalities, especially conduction defects. The ERG findings show moderate to marked reduction in rod and cone functions. In advanced cases, ERG responses are often nondetectable.

If patients are diagnosed at an early age, phytol, a precursor of phytanic acid, should be witheld from the diet. The ultimate effectiveness of early dietary control on retarding neurologic and ophthalmologic changes is yet to be evaluated in a substantial number of patients.

## Kearns-Sayre Syndrome

A rare, sporadic syndrome beginning in childhood, which includes slowly progressive external ophthalmoplegia, pigmentary retinopathy, and disorder of cardiac conduction, was described by Kearns and Sayre in 1958 (Arch. Ophthalmol. 60:280, 1958). In addition to this triad, other deficits may occur with abnormalities of brain wave activity, hearing and an elevation of cerebrospinal fluid protein. The electroencephalographic (EEG) abnormalities include diffuse slow activity. Clinical disorders of the pyramidal, extrapyramidal and cerebellar motor systems, although infrequent, can also be seen.

This disorder first begins within the first 10 or 20 years of life with ptosis and external ophthalmoplegia. Sensorineural deafness is a less frequent and less prominent sign but may also be noted during this period; in some cases it may become severe. Neurologic abnormalities implicating the cerebellar, pyramidal, and extrapyramidal motor systems are initially mild, but may slowly progress during adolescence and early adulthood. The development of mental retardation is less frequent and, when present, is slowly progressive and therefore not recognized early in the disease. Other associated findings include short stature and delayed or absent secondary sex characteristics. Dental anomalies including hypoplasia and a peculiar yellow discoloration may be seen.

The retinal changes are generally not those of typical, primary retinitis pigmentosa but are more characteristic of a primary retinal pigment epithelium-choriocapillaris abiotrophy. Areas of hyperpigmentation and hypopigmentation are seen most notably within the posterior pole and particularly in the peripapillary area. Pigment clumping and migration are most frequently not of the typical bone-spicule type seen in retinitis pigmentosa but rather consist of round clumps. Retinal vessels are attenuated in more advanced stages of the disease. The ERG cone and rod amplitudes are either nondetectable or subnormal in most cases. Visual fields may be normal or show ring scotomas, an enlarged blind spot or peripheral constriction. Most patients do not complain of nyctalopia.

The changes of external ophthalmoplegia are in most cases probably associated with a primary myopathy. Histologic examination of the extracular muscles shows diffuse loss of muscle fibers and an increase in loose connective tissue and fat. Patients may exhibit evidence of systemic muscular involvement and sometimes accompanying signs of facial muscle weakness and depressed limb muscle strength. Diseased muscle tissue is noted histologically where "ragged red" muscle fibers associated with the deposition of fat and presence of increased numbers of abnormally large mitochondria with concentric cristae and crystalloid inclusions are seen. Abnormal mitochondria have also been evident in skin eccrine sweat glands (Karpati et al.: J. Neurol. Sci. 19:133, 1973).

It is of vital importance for the ophthalmologist to recognize the potential association of external ophthalmoplegia and pigmentary retinopathy with cardiac conduction defects, as patients may suffer a sudden and fatal cardiac arrest. Early recognition and the use of an artificial cardiac pacemaker may avert this disaster.

## Syphilitic Retinopathy

A) Acquired Syphilis

Some patients with acquired syphilitic infection may show extensive pigmentary changes within the fundus with the formation of bone spicules not unlike those seen in patients with genetic retinitis pigmentosa. A ring scotoma and the complaint of night blindness may be additional features. The presence of bone spicules is not the most common fundus presentation as patients most frequently exhibit either a localized or diffuse chorioretinitis with patches of atrophy and pigment clumping. Optic atrophy may also occur. Most fundus changes are seen in patients within the second stage of their syphilitic infection. A feature of syphilitic chorioretinitis is the tendency to recurrences after the disease has been dormant for a year or more. The retinal changes can be accompanied by iridocyclitis.

B) Congenital Syphilis

Patients with congenital syphilis can present with a finely pigmented salt and pepper fundus, atrophic chorioretinal areas or large masses of migrated pigment in the form of clumped pigment or bone spicules. As in cases of acquired syphilis, signs of anterior uveitis may also be present.

Additional features of congenital syphilis include the presence of rhinitis or "snuffles," fever, anemia, osteochondritis, flattening of the nose, high arched palate, synovitis of the knee joint (Clutton's joint), lymphadenopathy, hepatosplenomegaly, skin lesions, pneumonitis, wide spacing and notching of the central incisors (Hutchinson's teeth), saber

shins and jaundice. The first permanent molar is also frequently affected in congenital syphilis and shows a characteristic appearance with several small atrophic cusps on the
occlusal surface. This is known as a mulberry molar. Ocular
findings in addition to the chorioretinal changes include an
interstitial keratitis in about 10% to 15% of the cases, chronic iridocyclitis, and secondary cataracts. Pupillary abnormalities (Argyll Robertson pupil), optic atrophy, and eighth
nerve deafness may occur following central nervous system
involvement. Nerve-type deafness was present in 15.6% of
the 175 cases of congenital syphilis studied by Dalsgaard-
Nielsen (Acta Ophthalmol. 17:38, 1939).

## *Mucopolysaccharidosis*
(Hunter's Disease-Mucopolysaccharidosis Type II)

Two forms of Hunter's disease are seen. One, a mild form
with absent or minimal mental retardation and survival
into adulthood, and a severe form with significant mental
retardation, hepatosplenomegaly, gargoyle-like facies, skeletal deformities, growth retardation, deafness, pigmentary
retinal degeneration associated with night blindness, severe
neurologic changes and early death. The presence of deafness, X-linked inheritance, and the absence of lumbar gibbus
and clinically evident corneal clouding differentiate Hunter's disease from Hurler's disease according to Goldberg, M.
F., and Duke, J. R. (Arch. Ophthalmol. 77:503, 1967) and
François, J. (Ophthalmologica 169:345, 1974). Both dermatan sulfate and heparan sulfate are stored intralysosomally
in the visceral tissues and excreted in the urine.

Although the corneas in these patients are typically
transparent clinically, a slight stromal haze may be visible
biomicroscopically. The pigmentary retinopathy seen in
these patients may be associated with either normal or abnormal ERG amplitudes, the latter reflecting diffuse photoreceptor disease. Histologic findings are somewhat similar
to those seen in patients with retinitis pigmentosa
(Goldberg, M. F., and Duke, J. R.: Arch. Ophthalmol. 77:503,
1967). Atrophic changes are seen within the retinal pigment
epithelium and photoreceptors, as well as in bipolar and
ganglion cells. Membranous lamellar vacuoles, probably

composed of glycolipid, were reported in retinal ganglion cells and migrated pigment epithelial cells by Topping and co-workers (Arch. Ophthalmol. 86:164, 1971).

(Sanfilippo's Disease-Mucopolysaccharidosis Type III)

Sanfilippo's disease is characterized by a severe mental retardation and by neurologic signs that include uncoordination of gait, seizures, contractures and deafness. Hepatosplenomegaly and skeletal abnormalities are less conspicuous than in Hurler's disease. Gargoyle-like features are very mild. The disease is inherited as an autosomal recessive trait.

Two clinically similar types of Sanfilippo's disease are seen: Sanfilippo type A shows a defect in the enzyme heparan sulfatase while type B demonstrates a deficiency in N-acetyl-alpha-glucosaminidase. In both types elevated levels of heparan sulfate and small levels of dermatan sulfate are found in the urine. Clinically evident corneal changes are not seen, although mild changes may be evident on biomicroscopy. Fundus changes frequently show a pigmentary retinopathy with subnormal or nondetectable ERG responses. Correspondingly, the patients may complain of night blindness.

## Friedreich's Syndrome

Friedreich's ataxia is an autosomal recessively inherited spinocerebellar ataxia involving symptoms referable to the posterior column, pyramidal pathway, lateral cerebellar tract and cerebellum as well as cranial nerve disorders in the form of eye muscle paralysis and optic atrophy. Deafness and mental deficiency may also be seen in patients with this form of ataxia.

When cases of Friedreich's ataxia are reported with hearing loss and tapetoretinal degeneration, a clear distinction from Hallgren's syndrome is often difficult to make. When patients with Friedreich's ataxia and retinal degeneration without hearing loss are seen, a clear differentiation from cases of Laurence-Moon syndrome is uncertain. Bottermans concludes from his extensive review of the literature that "the combination of true primary pigmentary degeneration with Friedreich ataxia is extremely rare" (cited in Vinken, P. J., and Bruyn, G. W. [eds.]: *Handbook of Clinical Neurology* [Amsterdam: North-Holland Publishing Co., 1972] vol. 13, p. 303).

Gerald A. Fishman, M.D.
University of Illinois Eye and Ear Infirmary

**Visual Cells and the Concept of Renewal.** Richard W. Young[3] (Univ. of California, Los Angeles) observes that rods and cones appear to expend most of their energies not on initiating visual messages, but on the repeated replacement of their own molecules. Awareness of the impermanence of the structural components in visual cells is part of the broad concept that the ingredients of living matter are in a dynamic state of continuous renewal. Ribonucleic acid is rapidly and continuously renewed in rods and cones. Protein is also continually renewed in these cells; the major protein produced in rods is opsin. There is evidence of lipid formation in the myoid region of the inner segment and in the region of the synaptic body. Rods and cones renew their outer segments differently (Fig 36). Aggregation of new protein in growing membranes at the base of the outer segment after administration of labeled amino acids and displacement of labeled membranes along the outer segment are always apparent in rods but have never been observed in cones. The nature of the normally balanced degradative mechanisms is poorly understood.

The growth of rods and cones appears to be independent of stimulation by light, but there is some evidence that renewal mechanisms are influenced by function, though renewal seems to continue whether or not the cells are excited by light. The efforts devoted by rods and cones to renewal mechanisms must greatly exceed what they expend on their visual functions. The goal of renewal processes in rods and cones may be preventive maintenance. No definite age changes have been found in the visual cells of several different species; visual cells "grow old without aging." Several inherited diseases that kill the rods and cones may act by

(3) Invest. Ophthalmol. 15:700–725, September, 1976.

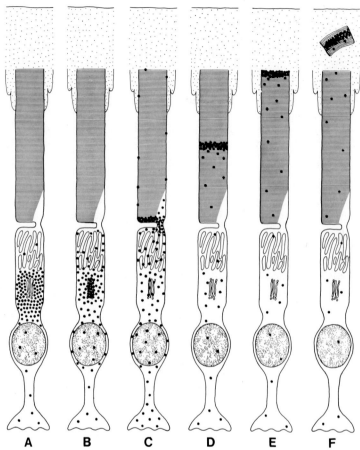

**Fig 36.** — Renewal of protein in rod visual cells as revealed in autoradiograms after administration of radioactive amino acids. New protein is first concentrated at its major site of synthesis, myoid zone of inner segment *(A)*. Protein molecules then scatter throughout cell, many migrating by way of Golgi complex, where they are modified by addition of carbohydrate *(B)*. Much of new protein traverses connecting cilium and is incorporated into growing membranes at base of outer segment. Some protein diffuses from new membranes into outer cell membrane with which they are continuous *(C)*. Detachment of disk-shaped double membranes from outer membrane traps labeled protein within disks. Repeated formation of new membranes displaces labeled disks along outer segment *(D)*. Eventually, they reach end of cell *(E)* from which they are shed in small packets. These are phagocytized by pigment epithelium *(F)*. (Courtesy of Young, R. W.: Invest. Ophthalmol. 15:700–725, September, 1976.)

interrupting renewal pathways. In retinitis pigmentosa and
in the several genetically distinct diseases in which signs of
deteriorating cone function predominate, the abnormal
genes do not prevent development of rods and cones, but
they seriously reduce their longevity, strongly suggesting
that the genetic defects disrupt visual cell renewal systems.
Differential effects on rods and cones may result from intrinsic differences in pathways of preventive maintenance in the
two classes of photoreceptor cells.

▶ [This beautifully illustrated Friedenwald Lecture by a member of the
Department of Anatomy at the University of California, Los Angeles demonstrates the enormous renewal power of the rods and cones, and the
author speculates that some genetic degenerative diseases of the rods
and cones which develop some years after birth might indicate a breakdown in this renewal system. It is unfortunate that all body cells cannot
"grow old without aging"! – Ed.] ◀

**Oxygen Toxicity: Membrane Damage by Free Radi-
cals** is discussed by Lynette Feeney (Univ. of Oregon) and
Elaine R. Berman[4] (Jerusalem). Conversion of oxygen to a
number of transient free radicals, highly reactive substances containing unpaired electrons, makes oxygen a
"two-edged sword." The free radicals are responsible for
producing irreversible damage to such biomolecules as enzyme proteins and membrane lipids and they may also be
causative agents of ubiquitous aging processes. A small part
of cellular molecular oxygen can be reduced through univa-
lent pathways, with the resulting production of free radicals
such as superoxide anion radical ($O_2 \cdot ^-$), hydroxyl radical
($OH \cdot$) and hydrogen peroxide ($H_2O_2$). All oxygen-metaboliz-
ing cells have evolved protective mechanisms that minimize
free radical production or destroy them. One such mechanism involves the enzyme superoxide dismutase (SOD),
which catalyzes the superoxide radical to form $H_2O_2$, and
another involves a battery of enzymes that reduce $H_2O_2$ to
water, including catalase and the peroxidases. Many free
radicals can act on the polyunsaturated fatty acids of bio-
membranes to result in the formation of a lipid free radical
which, in the presence of oxygen, is converted to lipid peroxide radical ($LO_2$), a highly reactive species which results in
autooxidation and membrane damage. Free radical scaven-

(4)   Invest. Ophthalmol. 15:789–792, October, 1976.

gers such as $\alpha$-tocopherol can intercept or terminate the autooxidative chain reaction and protect the membrane.

The lipid peroxide free radical can also decompose to highly reactive fragments such as malonaldehyde and may be converted to hydroperoxide (LOOH), which can enter into the autooxidative chain reaction. A system using glutathione peroxidase inactivates LOOH by converting it to a harmless hydroxy fatty acid, LOH. Oxygen toxicity and light damage may have a common mechanism through which they cause cellular destruction, the production of free radicals. Biochemical damage to the retinal pigment epithelium by light or oxygen, or both, should be re-examined in view of the free radical nature of melanin and its possible role as a biologic electron-transfer agent. Yellowing of human lenses with age is postulated to be due to ultraviolet light-induced free radical alteration of aromatic amino acids of lens proteins, principally tryptophan. Light-induced free radical oxidation of polyunsaturated fatty acids in lens fiber membranes could lead to permeability changes that initiate cataracts. The lens glutathione peroxidase system may protect lens membrane lipids against radiation insults during the long human lifespan.

▶ [Excellent editorials such as this make the clinician marvel at how well destructive forces such as oxygen and free radicals that damage membranes are counterbalanced by good enzymes. — Ed.] ◀

**Visual Functions after Perinatal Macular Hemorrhage** were investigated by Martin Lowes, Niels Ehlers and Ib Krarup Jensen[5] (Univ. of Aarhus). Retinal hemorrhages are known to occur in a large percentage of newborn infants. Of 413 newborn infants delivered by forceps or vacuum extraction in 1969–71, 48 showed retinal or preretinal macular hemorrhage in one or both eyes (11.6%). Delivery was by vacuum extraction in 21 infants, forceps in 6 and both methods in 3, whereas in 8 delivery was normal.

Visual functions were evaluated in 38 children at an average age of 5.5 years. Acuity was equal in both eyes in 35 patients, whereas in 3 a slight difference in acuity of two to three lines was found. Two of these patients had microstrabismus and 1 had normal muscle balance and no signs of strabismus, 2 of these had had a macular hemorrhage in 1

(5) Acta Ophthalmol. (Kbh.) 54:227–232, April, 1976.

eye which later became amblyopic, whereas 1 had had hemorrhage in both maculas. In all 3 patients the macular hemorrhage had resolved by 1 week. None of the patients with persisting hemorrhage developed amblyopia. Three of 58 eyes with macular hemorrhage and none of 18 without hemorrhage had reduced visual acuity; the difference was not significant. No occlusion therapy was necessary. Three patients exhibited a mild heterophoria but were otherwise normal. Ophthalmoscopy was normal in all children. No abnormalities of the macula or fovea were observed.

There is no reason to think that perinatal macular hemorrhages produce organic amblyopia, strabismus or macular scars.

► [This series helps to explode the idea that macular hemorrhage at birth can explain unexplained amblyopia. – Ed.] ◄

**Acquired Arterial Macroaneurysms of the Retina.** Isolated aneurysms of the principal divisions of the central retinal artery are found infrequently in older patients. Richard Alan Lewis, Edward W. D. Norton and J. Donald M. Gass[6] (Univ. of Miami) reviewed the findings in 15 cases of acquired, arterial retinal macroaneurysm. The fluorescein angiographic findings are shown in Figures 37 and 38.

The average age at presentation was 66 years; 9 patients were women. Thirteen patients were or had been hypertensive; 3 of these also had diabetes of adult onset, though none had significant diabetic retinopathy. One patient had bilateral aneurysms. The right eye was involved in 79% of unilateral cases. All aneurysms were temporal to the optic disc and were usually superior to the horizontal raphe. Seven of 17 aneurysms occurred at an arterial bifurcation; 3 others occurred at an arteriovenous crossing point. Observations in 1 case suggested that arterial aneurysms may develop as a result of focal damage to the vascular wall.

Five of 16 eyes were followed without therapy; 3 of these 5 patients had good, stable visual acuity in the affected eye for up to 5 years after presentation. One patient improved spontaneously. Visual recovery after xenon arc photocoagulation was unsatisfactory in 5 instances. Treatment resulted in visual improvement of 2 or more Snellen chart lines in 3 of 5

(6) Br. J. Ophthalmol. 60:21–30, January, 1976.

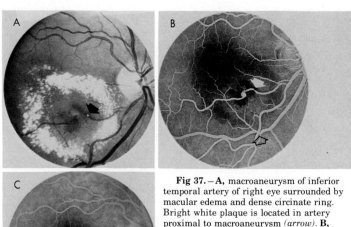

Fig 37. — **A,** macroaneurysm of inferior temporal artery of right eye surrounded by macular edema and dense circinate ring. Bright white plaque is located in artery proximal to macroaneurysm *(arrow).* **B,** midvenous phase of fluorescein angiogram of right eye. Note defect in fluorescein column corresponding to bright plaque *(white arrow).* Disruption of laminar venous flow is present at arteriovenous crossing *(open arrow).* **C,** 2 months later, late venous angiogram shows obstruction of arterial perfusion at macroaneurysm and segmental retrograde filling of distal artery from venous tree. Macular edema is more extensive. (Courtesy of Lewis, R. A., et al.: Br. J. Ophthalmol. 60:21 – 30, January, 1976.)

Fig 38. — **A,** several macroaneurysms *(arrows)* of temporal arteries of right eye with associated exudates. **B,** 15 months later, several macroaneurysms have enlarged and some are obscured by blood. (Courtesy of Lewis, R. A., et al.: Br. J. Ophthalmol. 60:21 – 30, January, 1976.)

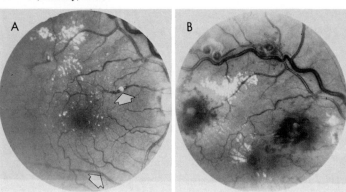

eyes; 3 of 5 eyes treated with argon laser photocoagulation showed this degree of improvement. All treated aneurysms were obliterated ophthalmoscopically and angiographically. Visual improvement was documented an average of 6–8 weeks after photocoagulation.

Photocoagulation may speed visual improvement in patients with macular edema and circinate retinopathy who have not improved spontaneously after 3 months of observation. It is probably indicated if the aneurysm increases in size and if further exudation results in failing visual acuity but more experience is needed to confirm these impressions. Macroaneurysms that do not affect macular function probably do not need photocoagulation.

**Regional Ischemic Infarcts of the Retina.** Robert Y. Foos[7] (Univ. of California, Los Angeles) examined the macroscopic and light microscopic features of regional ischemic infarction of the retina in the eyes of 31 patients autopsied

**Fig 39.** – Macroscopic appearance of ischemic infarct in diabetic woman, aged 72. Lesion is dark, due to enhanced visibility of pigment epithelium through thinned retina, is roughly wedge shaped and extends to horizontal meridian through fovea. Retina shows deep exudates temporal to fovea, residues of cotton wool patches below apex of infarct *(arrow)* and subtle patchy ischemic degeneration; reduced from ×10. (Courtesy of Foos, R. Y.: Albrecht von Graefes Arch. Klin. Ophthalmol. 200: 183–194, 1976; Berlin-Heidelberg-New York: Springer.)

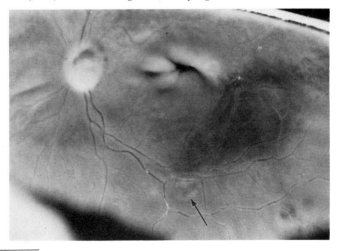

(7) Albrecht von Graefes Arch. Klin. Ophthalmol. 200:183–194, 1976.

in 1971–75. The 18 men and 13 women were aged 16–86 at the time of death. Generalized arteriosclerosis was severe in 10 subjects, moderate in 11 and minimal in 9; 1 subject, aged 16, with sickle cell anemia, had no detectable arteriosclerosis. Infarction of organs other than the eye was noted in 19 subjects, involved two or more organs in 7 and the brain in 9. Thromboembolism of organs other than the eye was present in 6 subjects. Five patients were known to be diabetic and hypertension was a significant problem in 10. Two patients had rheumatic heart disease and 1 each had congenital heart disease, disseminated intravascular coagulation and an orbital tumor.

The typical ischemic retinal infarct was roughly wedge shaped, with its apex toward the optic disc (Fig 39). Most

**Fig 40.** — Microscopic features of infarct. **A,** low magnification shows abrupt thinning of macular retina at margin of infarct, within which there is irregular preservation of inner nuclear layer (causing surface corrugation). Hematoxylin-eosin; reduced from ×50. **B,** higher magnification shows complete loss of inner retinal layers, irregular preservation of inner nuclear layer and well-preserved outer layers of retina. Hematoxylin-eosin; reduced from ×180. (Courtesy of Foos, R. Y.: Albrecht von Graefes Arch. Klin. Ophthalmol. 200:183–194, 1976; Berlin-Heidelberg-New York: Springer.)

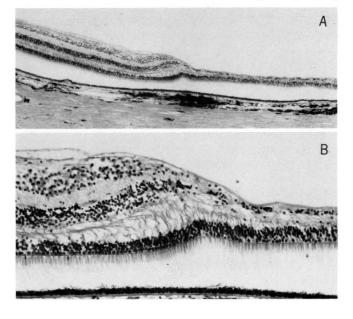

were in the posterior fundus and involved the macula to some degree. In some infarcts the retinal surface was corrugated. Microscopy showed loss of the nerve fiber and inner plexiform layers, ganglion cells and accessory glia in the healed stage (Fig 40). The thickness of the inner nuclear layer was markedly reduced. The larger vessels within the infarcted region may exhibit mural sclerosis and a marked decrease of cells within their walls. Sometimes arterioles adjacent to the lesions showed hyperplastic or sclerotic changes in their walls. Marked acellularity of capillaries and the walls of related arterioles was shown in trypsin-digested retinas. Infarcts were bilateral in 2 of the 31 patients studied and 5 of the 33 positive eyes had two separate lesions. All but 8% of the infarcts were postequatorial. Patchy sparing of the ganglion cell layer was seen centrally in five lesions involving the macula. Definite retinal arteriolar occlusion related to the infarct was noted in only two lesions.

Most patients with ischemic retinal infarction have either primary or secondary vascular disease. The effects of regional ischemic infarcts of the retina on the vitreous are minimal.

▶ [In this study of eyes of patients that had been autopsied, loss of the inner nuclear layer with thinning (area appeared darker because of greater visibility of the pigment epithelium) was associated with both systemic and retinal vascular disease. The authors distinguish these regional ischemic infarcts from background diabetic retinopathy (patchy and less effect on inner nuclear layer), glaucoma (destruction of ganglion cell layer), cotton wool patch or cytoid body (mainly involving ganglion cells), and branch vein occlusion (many more cystic and proliferative changes). – Ed.] ◀

**Fibrin Clots in Choriocapillaris and Serous Detachment of the Retina.** David G. Cogan[8] (Natl. Inst. of Health) remarks that intravascular clotting of blood is a normal reaction to many noxious processes and usually serves a useful purpose. Accumulation of platelets and a fibrin meshwork are observed in the choriocapillary layer of the choroid and ciliary body after injury. Clots tend to form along the inner surfaces of the capillary sinuses when the cause of injury is outside the vessel. The choriocapillaris is also the preferred site in the eye for clots to form when thromboplastin is discharged into the blood from extensive tissue de-

(8)  Ophthalmologica 172:298–307, 1976.

struction or from antigen-antibody reactions. Thrombi were observed in the submacular choriocapillaris and adjacent small vessels in a patient who died with thrombotic thrombocytopenic purpura (TTP) initially related to pregnancy. The ophthalmic complications of disseminated intravascular coagulopathy (DIC) are identical with those of TTP and are similarly attributable to occlusive blockade in the submacular choriocapillaris. When severe enough, the blockade leads to retinal detachment and hemorrhage in the choroid. The appearances in a case of DIC are shown in Fig-

**Fig 41.**—Fibrin clot in case of DIC showing occlusion of choriocapillaris and paracapillary vessel. Note absence of involvement of larger vessels. Periodic acid-Schiff; reduced from ×610. (Courtesy of Cogan, D. G.: Ophthalmologica 172:298–307, 1976.)

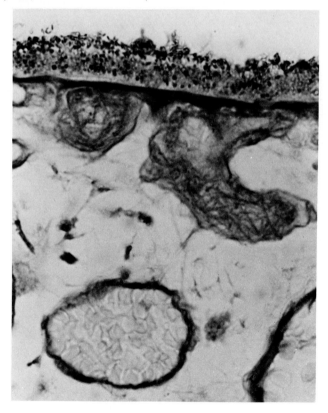

ure 41. The clots in this case consisted of fibrin and platelets and were interpreted as having been of recent origin.

Fibrin clotting in the eye has a predilection for the choriocapillaris, especially for the submacular choriocapillaris. Presumably with extravascular ocular inflammation the choriocapillary wall becomes patent enough for the bloodstream to be exposed to the basement membrane, and the contact of platelets and fibrinogen with extravascular collagen triggers the clotting mechanism. The vulnerability of the submacular region in systemically induced hypercoagulability is presumably due to hemodynamic peculiarities of the circulation in this region. In TTP and DIC, presumed slowing of the circulation in the choriocapillary sinuses may contribute not only to the ocular localization, but to the preferred localization in renal glomeruli. Some patients with a diagnosis of uveal effusion may have inappropriate clotting in the choriocapillaris, accounting for their retinal detachments. It may be reasonable to treat such patients with anticoagulants.

**Ophthalmoscopic Signs of Obstructed Axoplasmic Transport after Ocular Vascular Occlusions** are discussed by David McLeod[9] (Moorfield's Eye Hosp., London). The energy to sustain axoplasmic transport is apparently generated along the length of an axon, probably by oxidative metabolism. When part of an axon is deprived of its blood supply, axoplasmic debris accumulates at each end of the ischemic segment as a result of continued orthograde or retrograde flow. In man, branches of the central retinal artery supply the metabolic requirement of ganglion cells and their proximal axon segments; the posterior ciliary arteries supply the needs of axons at the optic nerve head and, via the cilioretinal arterioles, within a variable area of peripapillary retina.

Central retinal artery occlusion causes ischemic necrosis of ganglion cells and their proximal axon segments and axoplasmic transport in the nerve-fiber layer of the retina ceases. Retrograde axoplasmic transport continues for a short time before ascending degeneration begins, so that axoplasmic debris accumulates in distal axon terminals at the

---

(9) Br. J. Ophthalmol. 60:551–556, August, 1976.

boundary of the ischemic area. The boundary between viable and ischemic axon segments is displaced from the optic nerve head to the edge of the cilioretinal arterial territory where this circulation exists and debris accumulates near the border of viable peripapillary retina. Absence of a visible accumulation of axoplasmic debris soon after central artery occlusion sometimes indicates that there is an associated occlusion of the posterior ciliary supply to the optic disc. In such cases, retrograde axoplasmic transport along the optic nerve is obstructed behind the lamina cribrosa.

Occlusion of the posterior ciliary arteries deprives axons of oxygen and nutrients at the level of the optic nerve head and continued orthograde axoplasmic transport results in massive accumulation of debris at the border of the posterior ciliary territory, causing gross white swelling of the disc, or acute ischemic optic neuropathy. Where associated cilioretinal arteriolar occlusion is present, white debris accumulates in the retina at the boundary between the central retinal and cilioretinal arterial territories. A retrolaminar aggregation of organelles due to obstructed retrograde axoplasmic transport probably contributes to the well-demarcated zone of retrolaminar degeneration seen pathologically in temporal arteritis.

► [The author provides illustrations to support his thesis that a block in retrograde axoplasmic transport of optic nerve fibers occurs at the edge of an ischemic area, resulting in a visible accumulation of axoplasmic debris that looks like edema or exudate at that point. − Ed.] ◄

**Viscosity and Retinal Vein Thrombosis.** Increased blood viscosity is associated with various pathologic states of which vascular thrombosis or occlusion is a feature. C. P. Ring, T. C. Pearson, M. D. Sanders and G. Wetherley-Mein[1] (St. Thomas's Hosp. Med. School, London) examined the role of viscosity and blood flow in the etiology of retinal vein occlusion and the development of capillary nonperfusion. Forty-four unselected patients with retinal vein occlusions, 25 men and 19 women with a mean age of 61.6 years, were studied. Twenty-three were seen within the 1st week of presentation and 15 within a further 4 weeks. Thirty controls with a mean age of 57.9 years were also evaluated. Viscosity

(1)  Br. J. Ophthalmol. 60:397–410, June, 1976.

measurements were made within 7 hours of collection of lithium-heparinized blood.

Significantly higher values of whole blood viscosity, packed-cell volume and yield stress were obtained in patients with capillary nonperfusion than in those not exhibiting this change. Higher whole blood and plasma viscosity values and plasma fibrinogen levels were found in the entire patient group than in the control group. Patients with capillary nonperfusion had a higher packed-cell volume than those without nonperfusion, but abnormal plasma fibrinogen levels in the patients did not correlate with the presence or absence of capillary nonperfusion. Highly significant blood pressure differences were found between the retinal vein occlusion and the control groups; 59% of patients were considered to be normotensive.

Changes in blood viscosity may be of critical importance during episodes of retinal vein occlusion and of etiologic significance in the development of capillary nonperfusion. A strong association of retinal vein occlusion with arterial disease has been observed. There was no increase in blood lipids or uric acid. It seems reasonable to perform a controlled study to determine whether the incidence of further occlusion in patients with retinal vein occlusion who have rheologic abnormality can be modified by various forms of treatment. This might include phlebotomy to reduce packed cell volume, clofibrate to reduce the fibrinogen level and treatment of hypertension if present.

**Cilioretinal Infarction after Retinal Vein Occlusion.** Only 2 cases of retinal infarction in the cilioretinal distribution have been described in association with central retinal vein occlusion. D. McLeod and C. P. Ring[2] (London) report 10 further cases and a case of cilioretinal infarction associated with a hemisphere branch retinal vein occlusion. Fluorescein angiography was performed by injecting 10 or 20% fluorescein solution antecubitally.

The patients noticed sudden visual deterioration in one eye and often a localized scotoma in the central visual field. Funduscopy showed widespread retinal hemorrhages and distention and tortuosity of all tributaries of the central ret-

(2) Br. J. Ophthalmol. 60:419–427, June, 1976.

inal vein. Retinal pallor contiguous with the optic disc and variable swelling of the optic nerve head were also seen. Fluorescein often leaked from veins in the late phases of angiography. Perfusion through the cilioretinal circulation was consistently impaired relative to central arterial perfusion. In 6 cases, advancement of dye along the cilioretinal arterioles was extremely slow, and reversal of flow was seen in 4 cases. There was variable late leakage of dye from the optic disc. Central fixation was preserved except in 1 case. Rubeotic glaucoma developed in 2 patients. The patient with a hemisphere branch retinal vein occlusion exhibited distention and tortuosity of the veins draining the superior retinal hemisphere and swelling of the upper rim of the optic disc. Angiography showed extremely slow perfusion of a dilated capillary bed within the ischemic area. Signs of venous obstruction subsided within a few weeks without treatment.

Central retinal vein occlusion with partial obstruction of the posterior ciliary arteries may explain at least some of these cases, although the relative contributions of reduced ciliary arterial pressure and elevated venous pressure to cilioretinal ischemia probably varied from 1 patient to another. These cases may represent ocular vascular lesions intermediate between acute central retinal vein occlusion and acute ischemic optic neuropathy, which is commonly associated with peripapillary hemorrhages and venous dilatation.

**Fluorescein Angiography and Its Prognostic Significance in Central Retinal Vein Occlusion.** L. Laatikainen and E. M. Kohner[3] (London) undertook a prospective study correlating the fluorescein angiographic findings in central retinal vein occlusion (CRVO) with the final status of affected eyes in 75 eyes of consecutive patients with CRVO. Eyes with associated major retinal vascular disease were excluded. No patient received specific treatment for the occlusion for at least 1 year after presentation.

Initial angiograms showed good retinal capillary perfusion in 15 to 16 eyes with good final visual acuity and small areas of nonperfusion in the periphery in 1 eye. The macular

(3) Br. J. Ophthalmol. 60:411–418, June, 1976.

venules leaked dye in 5 of these 16 eyes. Findings were comparable in 12 eyes with a final acuity of 6/12 to 6/18. Retinal capillary perfusion was good in 11 of 24 eyes with maculopathy. Leakage from macular capillaries was seen in 22 of these eyes, and leakage from the main veins was a regular finding. Central and peripheral capillary nonperfusion was nearly complete in 7 of 13 eyes with thrombotic glaucoma, and extensive nonperfusion was seen in 3 other eyes in this group. In 1 eye with initially good capillary perfusion, the perifoveal arcade was broken. Other complications included proliferating retinopathy in 7 eyes and preretinal fibrosis in 3. All major vessels crossing nonperfused areas leaked fluorescein. In the overall series, nearly all patients with an acuity of 6/12 or better after 1 year had good capillary perfusion and a nearly intact perifoveal capillary arcade, whereas eyes that became blind exhibited large areas of central and peripheral nonperfusion.

The prognosis of CRVO in this series was related to the initial state of capillary perfusion and of the perifoveal capillary arcade. Angiography in the 1st month was of prognostic value only in cases with a poor prognosis, whereas the 3-month angiogram was an accurate indicator of visual outcome in all cases.

**Early Breakdown of the Blood-Retinal Barrier in Diabetes.** José Cunha-Vaz, J. R. Faria de Abreu, António J. Campos and Gabriela M. Figo[4] (Univ. of Coimbra, Portugal) used vitreous fluorophotometry to examine a series of diabetic patients, especially those who failed to show any retinal lesions with other methods of fundus examination. A slit lamp was modified with a photometric detection system to measure the fluorescein concentration in the vitreous. The detection system consisted of a modified eyepiece containing a fiberoptic probe superimposable on any area of the image of the optical cross-section and connected to a photomultiplier tube, an autoranging photometer and either a recorder or an oscilloscope with storage. The instrument registered electrically as it scanned. Fluorophotometry was performed an hour after the intravenous injection of 10 ml of 10% sodium fluorescein, which was immediately followed by flu-

(4) Br. J. Ophthalmol. 59:649–656, November, 1975.

orescence angiography. Studies were done in 30 normal eyes, 30 diabetics with apparently normal retinas and normal acuity and 15 diabetics with different stages of retinopathy.

Marked impermeability of the retinal vessels to fluorescein was confirmed in these studies. Significant breakdown of the blood-retinal barrier was seen in all diabetic eyes and was apparent before any clinically visible lesion was seen in the fundus. Higher fluorophotometry readings were closely correlated with the severity of the vascular lesions. Insulin-requiring patients had higher values of fluorescein penetration through the blood-retinal barrier than those controlled by oral sulfonylureas or by diet alone.

With vitreous fluorophotometry, the extent of the breakdown in the blood-retinal barrier can be measured, permitting comparative and evolutionary evaluations and studies on the effects of drugs and diabetic control on diabetic retinopathy. Disturbance of the blood-retinal barrier appears before microaneurysms or capillary closure can be demonstrated by fluorescein angiography.

**Clinicopathologic Correlations in Diabetic Retinopathy: I. Histology and Fluorescein Angiography of Microaneurysms.** Guillermo de Venecia, Matthew Davis and Ronald Engerman[5] (Univ. of Wisconsin) had an unusual opportunity for clinicohistopathologic correlation when a patient with symptomatic nonproliferative diabetic retinoapthy was seen for a malignant choroidal melanoma.

Man, 56, had had diabetes diagnosed at age 46 and had received insulin since then. Occasional mild insulin reactions but not diabetic coma had occurred. Endarterectomies of the left leg were done at age 54. The blood pressure was 210/75 mm Hg. Acuity was 10/200 on the left. Transient mild epithelial edema was present in the left cornea. A choroidal mass was present about 2 disc diameters inferotemporal to the macula, with serous retinal detachment over the tumor, involving the macula. Diabetic retinopathy of moderate degree was present in both eyes, with several areas of "intraretinal microvascular abnormalities."

The retinopathy was documented by stereoscopic fundus photographs and fluorescein angiograms. After enucleation, the microangiopathies were correlated histologically using

(5)  Arch. Ophthalmol. 94:1766–1773, October, 1976.

the retinal trypsin digest technique. Four types of micro-aneurysms were seen and believed to represent stages in development of this lesion. Most thin-walled aneurysms that were tightly packed with erythrocytes did not fluoresce. Those that were hypercellular and those with thick walls showed early and late fluorescence. Intraretinal microvascular abnormalities were hypercellular dilated channels; those originating from terminal arterioles are believed to represent attempts at neovascularization.

Some red dots in the fundus are erythrocyte-filled micro-aneurysms that may fail to perfuse on fluorescein angiography. Presumably, proliferation of endothelial cells results in a thin-walled microaneurysm, which eventually becomes thick-walled and finally hyalinized and completely obliterated. Some intraretinal microvascular abnormalities appear to be attempts at new vessel formation.

► [The original article gives an excellent pictorial correlation of clinical appearance, fluorescein angiography and trypsin digestion preparation of microaneurysms in a case of nonproliferative diabetic retinopathy. – Ed.]

**Insulin-Induced Immunogenic Retinopathy Resembling Retinitis Proliferans of Diabetes.** Commercial insulin has many antigenic properties, and the increased incidence of blindness from diabetic retinopathy has paralleled the use of insulin. Alan L. Shabo and David S. Maxwell[6] (Univ. of California, Los Angeles) attempted to determine whether insulin can initiate or potentiate the development of proliferative ocular disease, superimposed on the background retinopathy inherent in diabetes. Fifteen adult Rhesus monkeys were sensitized to insulin by injection of three 1-cc weekly doses of crystalline beef insulin in complete adjuvant intradermally, and 0.1-0.5 units of sterile crystalline beef insulin in saline intravitreally. One unsensitized animal received three 10-unit injections of insulin intravitreally over 10 days.

Injection of small intravitreal doses of insulin in sensitized animals led to the preferential involvement of optic nerve head vessels. Marked vascular tortuosity and venous "beading" were followed by glial sheathing of the vessels. With repeated injections of small doses, proliferative tissue extended forward from the optic disc and was associated

(6) Trans. Am. Acad. Ophthalmol. Otolaryngol. 81:497–508, May–June, 1976.

with vessel tortuosity. Injection of relatively large doses of 2–5 units led to perivascular cuffing by inflammatory cells and accumulations of red blood cells in the inner retinal layers. These findings are similar to those in which bovine serum albumin is used as an antigen. No fundus lesions developed in the unsensitized animal given large doses of intravitreal insulin. No retinal or optic nerve changes were seen in a sensitized animal given sterile saline by intravitreal injection.

Presumably, abnormally "leaky" vessels within the eye allow antigen to enter. The characteristics of insulin-induced immunogenic ocular inflammation are similar to those of the retinitis proliferans of diabetes, warranting consideration of the hypothesis of an immunologic pathogenesis for this form of diabetic retinopathy.

► ↓ Photocoagulation of diabetic retinopathy was reviewed previously by Herbst and Kaplan (1976 YEAR BOOK, p. 235). In their review they discussed the cooperative study of the Diabetic Retinopathy Study Research Group (see next article). The results in this cooperative study were considered so conclusive that specific recommendations were made for treatment. The xenon arc photocoagulator produced somewhat greater reduction in vision and visual field loss than the argon laser. The series by Koerner et al. treated by xenon arc also produced good results, although the macular lesions did not improve if the patient was over age 60 years and had systemic hypertension (see article by François and Cambie). In their series, using the argon laser, François and Cambie reported undesirable sequelae: increase in macular edema and hemorrhages after perimacular photocoagulation, neovascularization following inadequate treatment of avascular zones and heavily leaking areas and retinal and vitreous hemorrhages following feeder-vessel treatment without previous peripheral ablation. — Ed. ◄

**Preliminary Report on Effects of Photocoagulation Therapy: The Diabetic Retinopathy Study Research Group**[7] presents an analysis of findings obtained to date in the Diabetic Retinopathy Study, begun in 1971 as a randomized, controlled trial involving over 1,700 patients at 15 medical centers. Analysis was limited to effects of photocoagulation on visual acuity and visual field. Patients with diabetic retinopathy in both eyes and either proliferative change in one or both eyes or severe nonproliferative changes in both eyes were included in the trial if visual acuity was 20/100 or better in both eyes.

---

(7) Am. J. Ophthalmol. 81:383–396, April, 1976.

One eye of each patient was treated by xenon arc or argon laser. Best-corrected visual acuity was measured by "masked" techniques at 4-month intervals after treatment. Fundus photographs were graded by a modified version of the Airlie classification, in which "mild" new vessels on the disc are of lesser severity than is shown in Figure 42. Cumulative event rates were calculated, as were z values, or observed differences between the proportions of events in the treated and untreated groups divided by the standard error of the difference. Of 1,727 evaluable patients, 858 were treated with the argon laser and 869 with the xenon arc technique.

Visual acuity less than 5/200 at 2 or more follow-up visits occurred in 9.4% of untreated eyes and in 4.1% of treated eyes for a reduction of 57% in occurrence of severe visual loss in treated eyes. Losses of 2–4 lines of visual acuity occurred in 18% of xenon-treated eyes compared with 8% in untreated controls. This small loss of visual acuity did not occur in argon-treated eyes. Visual field scores were comparable in

**Fig 42.**—Standard photograph 10A modified Airlie classification of diabetic retinopathy. (Courtesy of Diabetic Retinopathy Study Research Group: Am. J. Ophthalmol. 81:383–396, April, 1976.)

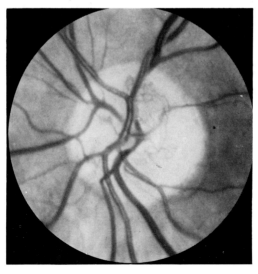

the argon-treated and untreated eyes (500 degrees or more), whereas about 44% of xenon-treated eyes had scores in the range 240–500 degrees. The 2-year event rate in eyes with new disc vessels was reduced 66% in treated eyes. In eyes with mild new disc vessels and no hemorrhage, the rate was reduced 70% in treated eyes.

Extensive "scatter" photocoagulation with focal treatment of new vessels appears to be of benefit in preventing severe visual loss over a 2-year follow-up period in eyes with proliferative diabetic retinopathy. In the future, photocoagulation treatment will be considered for eyes with moderate or severe new vessels on or within 1 disc diameter of the optic disc; mild new vessels on or within 1-disc diameter of the disc and fresh hemorrhage; or moderate or severe new vessels elsewhere if fresh hemorrhage is present.

**Diabetic Retinopathy Study: Preliminary Results from 215 Patients Treated Uniocularly with Photocoagulation** are reported by Fritz Koerner (Univ. of Bern), Dieter Schlegel and Ursula Koerner[8] (Univ. of Tübingen). Of the 215 patients, 80 had nonproliferative and 135 had proliferative diabetic retinopathy. Maximum follow-up was 6 months to 6 years.

Only one eye was treated in each patient. The second eye was treated only when the results obtained in the first eye were overwhelmingly positive. Treatment was generally on an outpatient basis, with use of the Zeiss photocoagulator and retrobulbar anesthesia. For most treatments, a field size of 3 degrees and intensity settings of green 1–3 were used. As many retinal lesions as possible were directly coagulated, but neovascularizations from the disc were not treated directly. Severe macular edema was treated by a series of burns placed temporally 180 degrees around the macula at a distance of 1–1½ disc diameters, often combined with scattered treatment of the midperipheral retina.

Improvement in intra- and epiretinal new vessel formation was much more pronounced in treated eyes; about three times as many untreated as treated eyes deteriorated. Photocoagulation did not seem to protect the eye against development of new-vessel formation on the disc. Treated eyes

(8)　Albrecht von Graefes Arch. Klin. Ophthalmol. 200:99–111, 1976.

showed less development of peripheral preretinal new vessel formations, but the difference between treated and untreated eyes was significant only for the first 2 years. The frequency of vitreous hemorrhage was significantly less in extensively treated eyes after 1–3 years of follow-up. Macular deterioration was more rapid in the untreated eyes of younger diabetics (under age 60), and the difference between treated and control eyes increased with duration of follow-up. No such difference was seen in patients over age 60 years. Visual acuity remained stable in treated eyes of younger patients, whereas that of untreated eyes fell significantly after 3 years of follow-up. Patients over age 60 showed a progressive fall in acuity in both treated and untreated eyes.

Photocoagulation may protect the macula, perhaps for a considerable time, in younger diabetics, preserving useful visual acuity. Photocoagulation reduces retinal new vessel formation and also prevents to some extent development of intra- and epiretinal neovascularization. In patients with preretinal new vessel formations, extensive photocoagulation reduces risk of vitreous hemorrhages.

**Further Vision Deterioration after Argon Laser Photocoagulation in Diabetic Retinopathy** is more frequent than is generally thought. J. François and E. Cambie[9] (Univ. of Ghent) examined 222 unselected eyes of 125 diabetic patients, followed for 6–42 months, that had clear media. Progressive visual deterioration with objective changes of diabetic retinopathy was observed in 66 eyes (30%). After photocoagulation, 29% of the eyes improved and 41% remained the same. Patients were treated with a coherent radiation argon laser mounted on a Zeiss slit lamp after topical anesthesia, through the Goldmann three-mirror contact lens. From 50 to 500 applications were given in one session. Focal photocoagulations were given with a peripheral barrage or partial ablation to destroy avascular zones, leaking areas and neovascular tufts. Spot sizes of 500 $\mu$m were used for the barrage and of 50 or 100 $\mu$m for focal treatments.

Vision deteriorated by at least 2/20 in study patients. The most common complication was a rapid increase in pre-

(9) Ophthalmologica 173:28–39, 1976.

viously existing macular edema due to extensive and heavy perimacular treatment. Another complication was an increase in neovascularization due to inadequate treatment of avascular zones and heavily leaking areas and to the growth of a neovascular tuft after feeder-vessel treatment without previous peripheral ablation. Retinal and vitreal hemorrhages were frequent in these cases. Fibrous tissue formation and vascular pseudopapillitis were less frequent complications.

Macular edema is an overlooked complication of diabetic retinopathy; when associated with diffuse leakage it becomes worse. Arterial hypertension is associated with the progression of postoperative macular edema in older patients. Large coagulations outside the macular area (peripheral ablation) are necessary to destroy zones of borderline nutritional supply, which are probably closely related to new-vessel formation. The feeder-vessel technique should not be used without peripheral ablation, although it may be of great help in destroying prepapillary or large neovascularization.

**Massive Congenital Ocular Toxoplasmosis.** Massive intraocular involvement by congenital toxoplasmosis, producing extensive posterior-segment disorganization leading to total retinal detachment, is not commonly found in the neonatal or early childhood period. Milton C. Pettapiece, David A. Hiles and Bruce L. Johnson[1] (Univ. of Pittsburgh) report data on 2 neonates with early, massive congenital ocular toxoplasmosis. The patients exhibited filling of the posterior segment by a detached and disorganized retina and anterior-segment inflammation. One patient who presented with leukocoria had enucleation for a tentative diagnosis of retinoblastoma.

The ocular lesions present in the neonatal period are typically in the posterior pole, especially the macular area, but peripheral regions of the retina may also be involved and the lesions may occur in only one eye. The typical active lesion is a focal necrotizing retinitis. The anterior segment of the eye may become secondarily inflamed. The present patient who had routine autopsy exhibited microphthalmus,

(1)   J. Pediatr. Ophthalmol. 13:259–265, Sept.–Oct., 1976.

corneal stromal infiltration, cataract, angle-closure glaucoma, retinal necrosis, total retinal detachment and choroidal infiltration. A necrotizing encephalitis with encysted toxoplasma organisms present was also found at autopsy. The other patient presented at age 6 weeks with bilateral leukocoria and had enucleation to rule out retinoblastoma. Anterior-segment inflammation, cataract, diffuse retinal necrosis, complete retinal detachment and chronic choroiditis were observed. Serologic study confirmed toxoplasmosis in this case.

Toxoplasmosis should be considered in infants presenting with leukocoria. Massive congenital ocular toxoplasmosis must be more common than is thought. A high suspicion and serologic testing of patients with leukocoria are indicated to identify unsuspected cases of congenital toxoplasmosis.

**Ocular Toxocariasis in Adults.** The larva of the nematode *Toxocara canis* may produce a variety of ocular lesions, including localized retinal granulomas, endophthalmitis and papillitis. Nearly all reported cases have been in children; clinical reports of retinal lesions in adults are few. E. R. Raistrick and J. C. Dean Hart[2] (Bristol, England) report the ocular findings in 3 patients aged 20–29 who reported a relatively sudden uniocular visual loss. All had posterior polar retinal lesions and positive toxocaral fluorescent antibody tests. The ophthalmoscopic findings closely resembled those of proved toxocaral granulomas in children.

Woman, 20, noted deteriorating vision in the left eye over 4 weeks and intermittent left frontal headaches. Corrected acuity was less than 6/60 on the left and 6/5 on the right. The left fundus exhibited a raised pigmented lesion involving the macula and a few small, deep retinal hemorrhages nearby with edema of the surrounding retina. A dense central scotoma was present on the left. Vision had improved spontaneously, 5 months later, to 6/12 although the retinal lesion appeared more extensive. Left-sided vision subsequently fell to 6/18. A short trial of systemic steroids failed to ameliorate the symptoms. Finger-counting was present on the left 9 months later and the lesion appeared as a raised white swelling. A toxocaral fluorescent antibody test was positive and the patient admitted close contact with a dog a few months before the onset of symptoms. The retinal lesion flattened somewhat and retinal scarring later was seen that involved the macula. Fluores-

(2)   Br. J. Ophthalmol. 60:365–370, May, 1976.

cein angiography initially showed masking of choroidal fluorescence at the site of the pigmented lesion. Repeated angiography showed changes of pigment epithelial clumping and atrophy localized at the posterior pole, with minimum uptake or leakage of dye.

Retinal hemorrhages produced by the passage of larvae through the vessel wall adjacent to the macula could cause initial visual disturbances in these cases. Retinal function may improve transiently as the parasite becomes less active but eventually the larva dies and disintegrates, causing an intensified tissue response with focal disruption of the neural layers of the retina and disturbance of the pigment epithelium. Increased vascularity near the mass is expected during this active inflammatory stage.

Toxocariasis should be considered in adults presenting with these symptoms and signs. Toxocaral antibody tests were positive in all the present cases.

**Morphology of Posterior Segment Lesions of the Eye in Patients with Onchocerciasis.** A. C. Bird, J. Anderson and H. Fuglsand[3] (Kumba, United Cameroon Republic) studied the morphology of posterior segment lesions attributable to onchocerciasis in 244 patients seen in the Sudan savanna and rain forest zones of the United Cameroon Republic in 1974–75. Sixty-seven patients had received treatment with suramin or diethylcarbamazine citrate (DEC), or both, under medical supervision, and many others had taken variable amounts of DEC on their own initiative. The male-female ratio was about 5:1.

Lesions of differing appearance were commonly seen in the same fundus. Atrophy of the retinal pigment epithelium ranged from an area of uneven thinning of the pigment epithelium to a well-defined area of confluent atrophy. Atrophy of the choriocapillaris occurred in areas of pigment epithelial atrophy. Ill-defined pale swelling at the level of the choroid and pigment epithelium occurred in areas of diffuse disease in 5.7% of patients. These lesions were highly vascular. Subretinal fibrosis with widespread atrophy of the retinal pigment epithelium and choroid was seen in 8.6% of patients. Hyperpigmentation at the level of the pigment epithelium was common to all forms of atrophy of the pigment

(3) Br. J. Ophthalmol. 60:2–20, January, 1976.

epithelium and choriocapillaris; it was never seen in isolation. It presented as brown or mauvish-brown spots or discs distributed uniformly throughout the area of choroidoretinal atrophy, or as irregular hyperpigmentation in any part of the lesion. The posterior retina was edematous in 3 patients who had severe uveitis with a cellular reaction in the aqueous and vitreous. Fluorescein angiography showed dye leakage into the retina from the retinal capillaries and veins in these cases.

Inflammation alone appears to be responsible for fundus lesions in onchocerciasis. Optic nerve disease, alone or in the presence of choroidoretinal changes, is responsible for a large percentage of the blindness due to posterior-segment lesions in onchocerciasis. It was responsible for 87.6% of cases in the present series.

▶ [This infection by the microfilaria of *Onchocerca volvulus* is an important cause of blindness in the tropics. The cornea is involved frequently, and the aqueous, vitreous, and in this report, the temporal fundus and optic nerve. The fundus lesions apparently involve the choriocapillaris and retinal pigment epithelium and they may vary from fine pigment mottling to large areas of chorioretinal atrophy and pigmentation. Because these organisms are not very antigenic, the inflammatory reaction may be minor and only detected by leakage on fluorescein angiography. – Ed.] ◀

**Herpesvirus Hominis Encephalitis and Retinitis.** *Herpesvirus hominis* (HVH) type I is a common cause of fatal encephalitis in adults in this country. Don S. Minckler (Armed Forces Inst. of Pathology), Edward B. McLean, Cheng Mei Shaw and Anita Hendrickson[4] (Univ. of Washington) report data on a previously healthy man who died 3 weeks after the simultaneous onset of encephalitis and retinitis.

Man, 44, presented with a 3-day history of malaise, headache, chills, myalgia and a left superior field defect. Acuity was 20/15 on the right and 20/40 on the left. Iritis, mild vitreous clouding, perivenous retinal sheathing and flame-shaped hemorrhages were noted in the left eye and a superotemporal defect was confirmed. Vision deteriorated rapidly to no light perception and an exudative retinal detachment developed nasally. Retrobulbar and systemic steroids and antibiotics were given. The patient became intermittently disoriented and a right temporal hemianopsia was demonstrated. No localizing neurologic signs were present 10 days after

(4)   Arch. Ophthalmol. 94:89–95, January, 1976.

the onset of symptoms. Papilledema appeared in the right eye, with flame hemorrhages in all quadrants and an exudative detachment in the posterior pole. Pyrexia, seizures and progressive cerebral dysfunction ensued and, despite cytarabine therapy, the patient died 22 days after the onset of symptoms. The serum HVH complement-fixation titer rose from 1:8 to 1:128 on day 20 of illness.

Autopsy showed bilateral uncal herniation, herniation of the cerebellar tonsils with medullary compression and typical inclusions of HVH in glial cell nuclei in areas of tissue destruction and hemorrhagic necrosis. Extensive hemorrhagic necrosis of the retina was seen, maximal in the inner layers. The retinal pigment epithelium showed focal necrosis, as did the choroid. Retinal vessels showed fibrinoid necrosis of their walls and luminal obstruction and fibrin thrombi were present in the choriocapillaris. The optic nerves were extensively damaged, with near-total demyelination of the anterior portions. Electron microscopy showed viral particles consistent with HVH in the brain, left optic nerve and both retinas.

This case of HVH infection was extremely unusual in first appearing with encephalitis and retinitis. The changes in disc vessels were consistent with direct infection of endothelium by HVH and subsequent thrombosis and hemorrhagic necrosis. The lack of polymorphonuclear cells in the optic nerve head vasculitis excluded the possibility of an Arthus type reaction causing the tissue damage.

▶ [Previous reports of encephalitis and necrotizing retinitis caused by *herpes simplex* type I have been in neonates (see 1965–66 YEAR BOOK, p. 233; and 1970 YEAR BOOK, p. 69), but the present case was in a man age 44. The authors stated that recently, HVH type I was isolated from the cerebrospinal fluid during life (Hartford et al.: Neurology 25:198, 1975).— Ed.] ◀

**Embryologic Pigment Epithelial Dystrophies** are reviewed by J. François[5] (Univ. of Ghent). Pigment epithelial dystrophies have been observed in embryopathies due to chemical factors such as antibiotics and thalidomide, to ionizing radiation and due particularly to infectious factors. An embryopathic pigmentary retinopathy has been observed with chloramphenicol and both retinal dysplasia and pigmentary retinopathy have been associated with maternal thalidomide use. Irradiation undoubtedly causes embryopathies, which are characterized by microcephaly, psychomo-

(5) Ophthalmologica 172:417–433, 1976.

tor retardation and such ocular abnormalities as microphthalmos, congenital cataract and bilateral pigmentary
retinal dystrophy or pigment epitheliopathy.

Pigment epithelial dystrophies have been seen in congenital syphilis and in viral embryopathies. Congenital syphilis
may be accompanied by a bilateral chorioretinitis of either
the "salt-and-pepper" type or the "retinitis pigmentosa"
type. Most embryopathic pigment epitheliopathies are due
to maternal viral infections. Mumps, measles, varicella and
cytomegalovirus have been implicated, but no human viral
infection can be implicated with more certainty than rubella. Ocular malformation in rubella, seen in at least 50–75%
of cases, include congenital cataracts, microphthalmos, congenital glaucoma and, in 45–55% of cases, pigment epitheliopathy. The epitheliopathy is the most common ocular
manifestation of rubella embryopathy. It may be unilateral,
and when bilateral it may be restricted to one or two sectors
of both eyes. Visual functions are unaffected in most cases.
The rubella epitheliopathy is stationary.

A syndrome of macular dystrophy and congenital deaf-
mutism was described by Amalric in 1960. Pigment displacement is seen in the macular area. Visual function is
good and the electroretinogram is normal. Examination of
1,065 deaf-mutes revealed 7 cases of true retinitis pigmentosa and 76 cases of pigmentary macular dystrophy of Amalric's type (7%). Of these 76 cases, 14% were hereditary. Of 38
cases of known etiology, 23 were due to a maternal infection
during pregnancy and 15 to an infection in early childhood.
Macular dystrophy can certainly constitute an abortive
manifestation of a viral or rubella embryopathy.

▶ [In his usual thorough fashion, François has compiled a list of noxious
agents, many of them viral, which can damage the pigment epithelium of
the retina. Perhaps we should add Amalric's syndrome of macular dystrophy associated with deafness to Fishman's list in the Introduction to this
chapter. As it is an active metabolic tissue, perhaps it is not surprising that
the pigment epithelium is affected by many diverse agents either primarily
or secondarily. – Ed.] ◀

**Stargardt's Disease and Fundus Flavimaculatus,**
according to P. François, P. Turut, B. Puech and J.-C.
Hache[6] (Lille, France), are two diseases which, since their

(6)  Arch. Ophtalmol. (Paris) 35:817–846, November, 1975.

first cases, have been associated and have overlapped to such a point that in certain cases they are indistinguishable. At present, there is tendency to differentiate the juvenile macular degenerative forms and to increase the number of entities closely related to the Stargardt disease. Criteria for differentiation used are ophthalmoscopic, photofluorographic, genetic and electrophysiologic.

The patient seeks consultation most frequently because of decreased visual acuity which generally starts in infancy. This decreased bilateral visual acuity is progressive, often more marked on one side, and affects distant vision more than close vision. The age of presumed onset of the first visual involvement was most frequently between 7 and 15 years of age among the 62 personal cases studied.

Although the clinical picture is typical, Stargardt's disease seems to be polymorphic in the age of its appearance, in its ophthalmoscopic features and in the forms observed within the same family. Thus, ways were sought to isolate other juvenile macular degenerative diseases. Only cone dystrophy in the Krill and Deutman concept seemed capable of being individualized from the Stargardt disease or from fundus flavimaculatus.

By study of the 62 cases and review of the literature, the authors showed that ophthalmoscopic, photofluorographic and functional aspects of Stargardt's disease and fundus flavimaculatus are identical, as is also the hereditary transmission, which is generally of the recessive autosomal type and less commonly of the dominant type. The flavimacular lesions found in the perimacular region or at the periphery can coexist in the same family and correspond to a variable expression of the same gene.

It is concluded that the two conditions represent one and the same disease with three forms: pure Stargardt's disease, Stargardt's disease with a perimacular flavimacular crown and Stargardt's disease with peripheral fundus flavimaculatus.

At present, there is no treatment for the Stargardt disease. No therapy can stop its inexorable development even if diagnosis is made early. However, it is useful to make a diagnosis to permit orientation of the patient, to help his behavior by use of optic appliances and to give him genetic counseling.

► [This article, replete with fluorescein angiograms and a beautiful color plate of the various forms of Stargardt's disease and fundus flavimaculatus, culminates years of study and writing on macular and retinal degenerations by François. He and most other investigators of these changes agree that these two conditions are variations of the same disease process. My former brilliant resident at the old Illinois Eye and Ear Infirmary, the late Alex Krill, also wrote prolifically on this subject and considered a primary cone dystrophy to be a separate clinical entity. The rather confusing variations of these hereditary macular dystrophies are clearly discussed and differentiated by Fishman (see the 1975 YEAR BOOK, pp. 225–236).—Ed.] ◄

**Familial Syndrome of Progressive Cone Dystrophy, Degenerative Liver Disease, Endocrine Dysfunction and Hearing Defect: I. Ophthalmologic Findings.** The etiology of progressive retinal cone dystrophy remains obscure, though it is probably heterogeneous. Egill Hansen, Ingegerd Frøyshov Larsen and Kåre Berg[7] (Univ. of Oslo) describe one type of cone dystrophy which may be an ocular manifestation of a systemic disease. Six females and 1 male aged 6–41 were studied for 1–8 years. Three patients were sisters and cousins of 3 others; these patients, all females, belong to a highly inbred kindred. The seventh patient had had an older brother who had died at age 6 months.

One patient had bilateral amaurosis. The least affected patient, aged 13, had fairly good central cone vision but a rod response only outside the central area. Photophobia was present in all patients and decreasing or absent color vision. Typical findings included attenuated retinal vessels, disc pallor and a general atrophic appearance of the fundus without pigmentation. Increasing impairment of vision during pregnancy was observed in 2 patients. Corneal indentation pulse amplitudes were significantly reduced from normal in all patients. Fluorescein angiography, done in 2 patients, was normal. Two patients had had repeated abortions and 2 were probably infertile. The boy was hypogonadic. Defective ACTH reserve was documented in 2 patients. Growth hormone secretion was defective in 2 others and thyroid dysfunction was noted in 2 patients. Three patients had diabe-

---

(7)   Acta Ophthalmol. (Kbh.) 54:129–144, April, 1976.

tes and another had abnormal glucose tolerance. Liver biopsy specimens taken in 4 patients because of slightly elevated transaminase values, showed degenerative changes in all.

This cone dystrophy appears to be part of a disease affecting several organs; its familial occurrence suggests that it is inherited.

**Flecked Retina Secondary to Oxalate Crystals from Methoxyflurane Anesthesia: Clinical and Experimental Studies.** D. M. Albert, J. D. Bullock, M. Lahav and R. Caine[8] (Yale Univ.) recently encountered a patient with an ophthalmoscopic appearance of flecked retina syndrome, possibly accounted for by crystalline calcium oxalate deposits in the retinal pigment epithelium, and a history of prolonged general anesthesia with methoxyflurane, an agent that is degraded in the liver to oxalate and fluoride ions. A second patient with similar appearances who also had had prolonged methoxyflurane anesthesia was later seen. The first patient subsequently developed systemic oxalosis which aggravated preexisting hypertensive renal disease. Barbiturate premedication may have been an aggravating factor; barbiturates are known to accelerate biotransformation of methoxyflurane in experimental animals.

Experimental retinal oxalosis in rabbits was studied. Groups of rabbits received daily subcutaneous injections of 1 – 4 ml dibutyl oxalate, with equal volumes of 0.5M calcium chloride solution given subcutaneously at a distant site. Seven of the 9 treated animals that survived 3 days or longer exhibited a "flecked retina" appearance of the fundus before death; the findings were more extensive in animals living up to 20 days. The earliest change consisted of depigmented areas of the retina, apparently related to a retinal pigment epithelial disturbance. White flecks were seen throughout the posterior pole up to the equator by the 4th day. Intracellular needle-like crystals were present in numerous retinal pigment epithelial cells. Intravitreal injections of sodium oxalate caused necrosis and disorganization of the neural retina and retinal pigment epithelium; also, a line of birefringent crystals was seen along Bruch's membrane.

(8) Trans. Am. Acad. Ophthalmol. Otolaryngol. 79:817–826, Nov.–Dec., 1975.

The presence of multiple calcium oxalate crystals within retinal pigment epithelial cells appears to be a unique feature of this tissue. Of the types of flecked retina syndrome originally described, the stationary form of fundus albipunctatus shows the greatest clinical similarity to oxalate retinopathy. Oxalate retinopathy is a possible cause of the ophthalmoscopic changes of "flecked retina," and should be considered in affected patients.

**Chloroquine Retinopathy in Patients with Rheumatoid Arthritis.** Chloroquine is a useful antirheumatic drug, but disagreement persists as to whether it is a safe alternative in the treatment of rheumatic illness because of its potential retinotoxic effects. A. Elman, R. Gullberg, E. Nilsson, I. Rendahl and L. Wachtmeister[9] (Karolinska Hosp., Stockholm) have used chloroquine to treat patients with active rheumatoid arthritis for many years, excluding pregnant women and patients with renal insufficiency, severe hypertension, dense cataract, diabetes or defective hearing. Doses of 0.25 gm daily are used for 10 months annually. Data were reviewed on 270 patients with seropositive rheumatoid arthritis, who had received totals of from 5 to 1,330 gm chloroquine in up to 15 years. Slight macular changes were not considered to indicate toxic retinopathy, but the "bull's-eye" type of retinal change was regarded as being caused by chloroquine.

The frequency of maculopathy increased from 25% in the lowest-dosage group to about 50% in the highest-dosage group (over 600 gm). The frequency of maculopathy with reduced visual acuity rose from 2% in the low-dosage group to 17% in the high-dosage group. In 15 of 20 patients with reduced acuity, the central visual acuity of the worst eye was 0.6 or greater. The only patient with bull's-eye change had an acuity of 0.2. The correlation of maculopathy frequency with total chloroquine dose was significant apart from age, but age was also an important factor in the development of the macular changes. Electroretinographic study of 99 patients given over 300 gm chloroquine indicated no signs of manifest chloroquine retinopathy. The patient with bull's-eye change had a normal electroretinogram despite marked fundic changes.

(9) Scand. J. Rheumatol. 5:161–166, 1976.

The risk of toxic retinal damage from chloroquine seems small or absent, even with long-term treatment, provided the dose is no greater than 0.25 gm daily for 10 months a year, and that the patient is under age 50 and has no other illness that might affect the retina. If the total annual dose is 70–75 gm, regular ophthalmologic checks should not be essential, but regular checks are advisable for patients over age 50–60 years and should include examination of color sense and visual fields. Pseudoisochromatic plates should be used.

▶ [This aminoquinoline is used in the long-term treatment of rheumatoid arthritis and lupus erythematosus. Although corneal deposits are reversible, they are not correlated with deposits of chloroquine in pigmented tissues such as the retinal pigment epithelium. Corneal deposits are reversible only in earliest stages and may be progressive after withdrawal of the drug. There is some correlation of corneal deposits with changes in the skin, eyelids and hair (Fraunfelder, 1976). In view of the rather high incidence of maculopathy after large doses for long periods, the low-risk dose is important and was determined in this series to be 250 mg a day for 10 months annually (total dose, 75 gm). The earliest to late ocular changes are as follows (see 1969 YEAR BOOK, p. 263; Percival: Trans. Ophthalmol. Soc. U.K. 87:1967): relative central scotoma to red, absolute central scotoma to red and red-green defect on Ishihara color plate, fine pigment mottling of the macula as examined with the Goldmann contact lens with absent foveal reflex, reduction of visual acuity, abnormal electrooculogram defined as a fall of over 15 units to a level below 185% light rise (normal ERG), and "bull's eye macula" (nonspecific and late). – Ed.] ◀

**Aging and Degeneration in the Macular Region: Clinicopathologic Study.** Senile macular degeneration has a wide spectrum of clinical appearances. Currently, interest is centered on recognizing the predisciform state and on using photocoagulation to prevent complications of subretinal neovascularization. S. H. Sarks[1] (Lidcombe Hosp., Sydney) reviewed the clinical and pathologic findings in 378 eyes with various macular appearances, ranging from normal to the late manifestations of senile macular degeneration. The eyes were collected during 1966–75 from 216 patients, 119 men and 17 women, aged 43–97 years.

The histologic classification of the eyes was based on the development of basal linear deposit under the retinal pigment epithelium (Fig 43). Groups I and II represented normal aging; groups III and IV, the progressive development

(1) Br. J. Ophthalmol. 60:324–341, May, 1976.

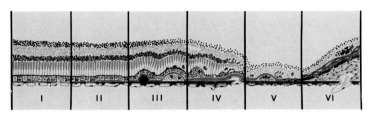

**Fig 43.** – Diagram illustrating histologic classification of 378 eyes according to development of basal linear deposit under retinal pigment epithelium. (Courtesy of Sarks, S. H.: Br. J. Ophthalmol. 60:324–341, May, 1976.)

**Fig 44.** – Electron micrograph of eye. Section taken from area of basal linear deposit. The material was recovered from a paraffin block. This technique results in loss of fine detail but shows a thick layer of amorphous material *(BLD)* lying on Bruch's membrane *(BM)*. The material in intercapillary pillars extends to level of outer surface of choriocapillaris *(CC)* and consists of irregularly banded collagen, vesicles and tubelike structures; reduced from ×6820. (Courtesy of Sarks, S. H.: Br. J. Ophthalmol. 60:324–341, May, 1976.)

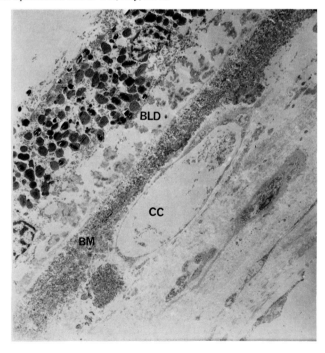

of senile macular degeneration and groups V and VI, the end result. In group I, thickening and hyalinization of Bruch's membrane were noted as early as the 5th decade. Group II showed patchy basal linear deposit in relation to thickened or basophilic segments of Bruch's membrane. In group III, the basal deposit formed a thin, continuous layer associated with moderate degeneration of the retinal pigment epithelium. Vision was reduced in most of these eyes. In group IV, the deposit was thicker and most eyes showed coarse pigmentary changes. In group V, circumscribed areas of depigmentation were noted and thin fibrovascular sheets were present beneath the pigment epithelium in about 40% of eyes. Group VI represented disciform degeneration, an alternative end result to geographic atrophy.

The basal linear deposit consisted of banded fibers embedded in granular material lying between the plasma infoldings and the basement membrane of the retinal pigment epithelium (Fig 44). This deposit seems to be a manifestation of gradual failure of the pigment epithelium and is the most suitable criterion by which to study the natural history of senile macular degeneration.

► [This extensive histologic examination of the maculas of older eyes has enabled the author to formulate a logical sequence of changes in aging and development of senile macular degeneration. According to this, the pigment epithelium does become fatigued by its enormous work over many years and progressively shows pigment dispersion and later atrophy, and deposits an amorphous material with later hyalinization on Bruch's membrane. Bruch's membrane gradually thickens with hyalinization, calcification and formation of drusen. Photoreceptors are gradually lost. Ruptures of Bruch's membrane and subretinal neovascularization from the choriocapillaris with hemorrhage and a fibrovascular scar produce the clinical "disciform degeneration", perhaps influenced by the variable amounts of atrophy of the choriocapillaris. This sequence does not support what many of us tell our patients with senile macular degeneration, that it is caused by "poor circulation," and explains why treatment directed toward improving the circulation is fruitless. — Ed.] ◄

**B-Scan Ultrasonography in the Diagnosis of Atypical Retinoblastomas.** Jerry A. Shields, Brian C. Leonard, Joseph B. Michelson and Lov K. Sarin[2] (Philadelphia) reviewed the B-scan ultrasonographic findings in 14 retinoblastoma patients seen in 1973 – 75. Four patients presented with atypical signs and symptoms which caused diagnostic

(2)   Can. J. Ophthalmol. 11:42 – 51, January, 1976.

confusion initially. The tumor was unilateral in 12 patients and bilateral in 2. Of the 13 enucleated eyes 12 exhibited acoustically dense focal areas compatible with calcification in the tumor, and in each case areas of calcification were found in the tumor on gross and histologic examination that correlated with the dense areas seen on ultrasound study. Ten patients presented with leukocoria and were diagnosed clinically. The sonographic findings in 1 patient are shown in Figure 45 and the gross pathologic findings in Figure 46.

A simple contact B-scan ultrasonoscope permits the rapid screening of children of all ages without anesthesia. It was helpful in the diagnosis of all the present cases of retinoblastoma. An intraocular mass containing focal densities, suggesting calcification, is observed. Routine x-rays did not show calcification in 3 of the 4 patients who presented with atypical features. Echoes from areas of calcification within the tumor tend to persist at low sensitivities, a phenomenon rarely noted in vitreous hemorrhage. Intraocular calcifica-

**Fig 45.** – The B-scan ultrasonographic findings in patient with retinoblastoma and heterochromia iridis. **A,** at 80 decibels a bilobed intraocular mass was seen. **B,** at 40 decibels dense focal areas suggestive of calcification were shown. (Courtesy of Shields, J. A., et al.: Can. J. Ophthalmol. 11:42 – 51, January, 1976.)

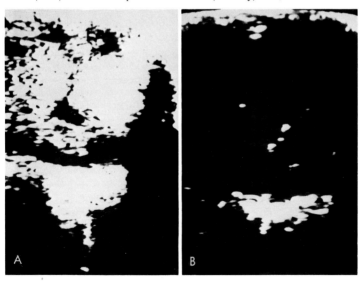

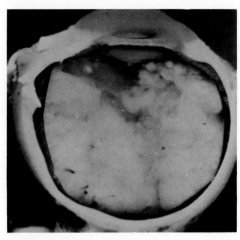

**Fig 46.** – Bilobed fluffy white tumor with areas suggestive of calcification replaces vitreous cavity. (Courtesy of Shields, J. A., et al.: Can. J. Ophthalmol. 11:42–51, January, 1976.)

tion may, however, also occur in other conditions and the finding is not pathognomonic of retinoblastoma. Ultrasonography provides a means of determining and comparing the sizes of the two eyes, thus helping differentiate retinoblastoma, which usually occurs in normal-sized eyes, from such conditions as persistent hyperplastic primary vitreous and congenital glaucoma in which the size of the eye is often abnormal.

The use of contact B-scan ultrasonography is recommended for all children who have eyes with opaque media or suspicious fundus lesions.

**Blindness Caused by Photoreceptor Degeneration as a Remote Effect of Cancer.** Ralph A. Sawyer, John B. Selhorst, Lorenz E. Zimmerman and William F. Hoyt[3] documented blindness caused by retinal degeneration of obscure pathogenesis in 3 patients with cancer.

Woman, 65, noticed sudden hoarseness and episodic dimming of vision in both eyes. Recovery of vision was abrupt but often incomplete. Color vision discrimination was moderately impaired in each eye, and acuity was 20/25 bilaterally. Bilateral modified ring scoto-

(3) Am. J. Ophthalmol. 81:606–613, May, 1976.

mas at 15 degrees were detected. Acuity decreased to hand motions 3 months later, and large central scotomas were present bilaterally. An infiltrate was seen in the left upper lobe of the lung, but repeat bronchoscopies showed no abnormalities. Acuity declined to light perception next month, when tomograms demonstrated a mass beneath the aortic arch, and thoracotomy revealed a poorly differentiated squamous cell carcinoma. An electroretinogram showed no photopic response and a 10% scotopic response bilaterally. Prednisone therapy for 10 days did not improve visual function or alter the periarteriolar sheathing that was present. The patient underwent radiotherapy but died 11 months after presentation.

Autopsy showed pneumonia, chronic bronchitis and metastases of lung carcinoma in the liver. A microscopic focus of tumor cells was present in the basis pontis, but examination of the visual pathways showed normal findings. The eyes exhibited advanced disintegration of inner and outer segments of rods and cones, widespread degeneration of the outer nuclear layers and scattered melanophages in the outer retinal layers. Minimal lymphocytic infiltration was seen around retinal arterioles in several areas.

These 3 older patients with cancer had early ophthalmologic symptoms and signs of retinal origin. The rods and cones appeared to be the anatomical site responsible for the visual loss in these patients. Examination of the visual pathways in 2 showed no significant alterations. Oat cell carcinomas may produce a number of pharmacologically active, hormone-like substances. One or more of these or other tumor products may have been responsible for the damage to photoreceptor cells in these patients.

**Nonocular Cancer in Retinoblastoma Survivors.** Recently, patients with second tumors in the field of low-dose irradiation of retinoblastoma have been seen, and a significant number of patients have appeared with second tumors clearly distant from the irradiation site. David H. Abramson, Robert M. Ellsworth and Lorenz E. Zimmerman[4] reviewed all case reports of second malignancies occurring in survivors of retinoblastoma therapy seen during 1922–72 at the Columbia-Presbyterian Medical Center (CPMC), and cases on file at the Armed Forces Institute of Pathology (AFIP) through 1972. The respective numbers of charts reviewed were 1,093 and 1,209.

Eighty patients had 84 nonocular neoplasms. All but 2 of

(4)   Trans. Am. Acad. Ophthalmol. Otolaryngol. 81:454–457, May–June, 1976.

the 80 patients had bilateral retinoblastomas. The incidence of second tumors in survivors of bilateral retinoblastoma was 10% in the CPMC series and 12.6% in the AFIP series. Fifty-seven patients manifested tumors in the field of irradiation after an average latent period of 11.4 years. Osteogenic sarcoma was by far the most common tumor. Fifteen patients had tumors outside the radiation field after radiotherapy. The average latent period was 11.1 years. Osteogenic sarcoma was also most common in this group. Three patients had second tumors, even though radiotherapy was not given. The average latent period was 10.3 years. In 5 cases, clear clinicopathologic differentiation between late metastasis of retinoblastoma and a second primary neoplasm could not be made. Two patients had two second tumors each. Of the 80 study patients, 85% have died as a result of the second tumors. No patient has survived an osteogenic sarcoma at any location.

The incidence of multiple malignancies in patients successfully treated for retinoblastoma appears to be higher than for any other primary malignancy, whether or not they receive radiotherapy.

► [As pointed out by the authors, only 25% of retinoblastomas are bilateral, but 97% of those who developed second tumors had bilateral retinoblastomas, suggesting that their germinal mutation harbored this cancer diathesis. Although the always fatal osteosarcoma of the orbit must be related to previous irradiation of the retinoblastoma, this does not explain late primary osteosarcoma of the femur, or many types of other malignancies appearing elsewhere in the body, even in 3 cases without any previous irradiation. — Ed.] ◄

**Natural History of Senile Retinoschisis.** Norman E. Byer[5] (Univ. of California, Los Angeles) studied 193 eyes of 108 patients (42 men and 66 women) in whom retinoschisis was observed without any surgical intervention for 2–11 years. Ages at outset ranged from 19 to 83 years. The lower temporal quadrant was maximally involved in about 69% of the eyes and the upper temporal quadrant in about 31%. At the end of the study, 71.5% of the eyes showed lesions extending four disc diameters or more behind the ora, which could be considered postequatorial. Initially, 6 eyes of 5 patients had holes; all these patients were more than 40 years of age when first seen.

(5) Trans. Am. Acad. Ophthalmol. Otolaryngol. 81:458–471, May–June, 1976.

New retinal holes appeared in 9 eyes of 8 patients during follow-up. Four eyes of 4 patients showed definite posterior extension, but, in all cases, this was slow and produced no symptoms. Definite lateral extension was observed in 7 eyes of 6 patients, all of whom were more than 40 years of age. One eye showed a definite increase in height of the inner layer. Twenty-seven eyes of 22 patients showed new areas of retinoschisis during the study. Seven eyes of 4 patients showed definite regression of retinoschisis. No frank, progressive, symptomatic retinal detachment was observed. One small localized detachment did not progress during follow-up. However, 1 patient had an outer layer hole which caused no symptoms, but the condition has not progressed during a follow-up period of over 1 year.

The calculated risk of a retinal detachment developing from double layer holes in retinoschisis is about 1.4%, and, in all patients with retinoschisis, the risk is 0.04%. The risk appears to be analogous to that in cases of asymptomatic retinal breaks. Indications for surgical and prophylactic intervention in senile retinoschisis include (1) secondary retinal detachment due to breaks in both layers; (2) secondary retinal detachment due to outer layer breaks if it progresses beyond the boundaries of the retinoschisis; (3) posterior extension of the retinoschisis to within 25 degrees of the macula; and (4) retinoschisis with outer layer breaks, if the other eye has suffered a retinal detachment caused by retinoschisis.

**Primary Retinal Detachments without Apparent Breaks.** From 3 to 14% of primary retinal detachments have no apparent retinal breaks. Roger D. Griffith, Edward A. Ryan and George F. Hilton[6] (Univ. of California, San Francisco) observed 462 eyes with primary retinal detachments in a prospective study done during 1968–73. Of these, 415 eyes were operated on and followed for at least 6 months.

Forty-one of the 415 eyes had no apparent breaks preoperatively or at operation. These eyes more often had detachments present for more than 1 month, and the incidences of aphakia, four-quadrant detachment, macular detachment

---

(6)   Am. J. Ophthalmol. 81:420–427, April, 1976.

and massive preretinal retraction were greater than in the eyes with retinal breaks. A three-step operation was used (Fig 47). Cryotherapy was followed by drainage of subretinal fluid, and a buckle was then placed just anterior to the equator. If massive preretinal retraction was present, a high buckle with an overlap of 20–25 mm was used.

Surgical cure, defined as anatomic reattachment for at least 6 months, was achieved in 92% of eyes. The cure rate was 85% for eyes without apparent breaks and 93% for those with breaks. Eight of 25 eyes with massive preretinal retraction had reattachment; with exclusion of these eyes, the cure rate was 91% for the group without breaks and 96% for eyes with breaks. Reoperation was required more often for eyes without apparent breaks, being required for cure in 8 of them. Of all reattached eyes, 55% achieved visual acuities of

**Fig 47.**—Three-step operation for primary retinal detachment. **A,** two rows of cryotherapy were applied to all detached periphery. **B,** length of the 4-mm silicone band was cut to equal the circumference of the undrained globe, and subretinal fluid was drained. **C,** ends of the band were overlapped 10–12 mm and tied, and the band was secured to the globe with mattress sutures in each quadrant. (Courtesy of Griffith, R. D., et al.: Am. J. Ophthalmol. 81:420–427, April, 1976.)

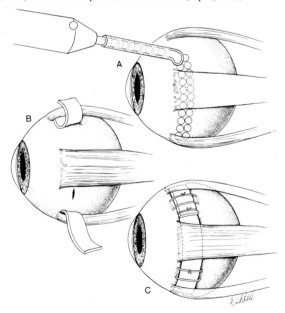

20/50 or better 6 months postoperatively; 15% had acuities of 20/400 or worse. Acuities were considerably worse in the group without breaks.

Operative complications were comparable in the two groups of eyes. Postoperative massive preretinal retraction in eyes without such retraction preoperatively was found in 4.5% of eyes with apparent breaks and in 12.2% of those without apparent breaks.

In diagnosis of retinal detachment without apparent breaks, the differential diagnosis should include secondary detachments (pseudodetachment, such as choroidal detachment). Secondary detachments are usually associated with some other disease, frequently show shifting subretinal fluid and may have bullae just behind the lens. The most likely place for inapparent retinal breaks is near the ora serrata. The chief prognostic factor in the preoperative examination is presence or absence of preretinal fibrosis.

**Angle-Closure Glaucoma Following Scleral Buckling Operations.** Rudolfo N. Perez, Charles D. Phelps and Thomas C. Burton[7] (Univ. of Iowa) reviewed 1,558 consecutive patients having scleral buckling operations for retinal detachment in 1969–75. Twenty-two patients had acute angle-closure glaucoma postoperatively, for an incidence of 1.4%; 9 cases occurred in the last 6 months of the survey, for an incidence of 7.2% in this period. Predisposing factors were, with one exception, not identified. Glaucoma occurred in 3.4% of eyes with episcleral implants and in only 0.6% of eyes with intrascleral implants, a significant difference.

Angle-closure glaucoma was recognized in 16 patients in the 1st postoperative week, usually on the 1st or 2d day. A hazy cornea most often suggested the diagnosis when intraocular pressures ranged from 24 to 50 mm Hg. The midperiphery of the iris usually fell away from the cornea rather than being bowed forward with a bombé appearance. Four of 8 patients failed to respond to conventional treatment and required surgery. Fourteen patients were treated intensively with steroids and acetazolamide or with cycloplegics; only 2 of them required surgery to lower the pressure. The glaucoma resolved slowly; in 8 patients, part or all of the

(7) Trans. Am. Acad. Ophthalmol. Otolaryngol. 81:247–252, Mar.–Apr., 1976.

angle remained permanently closed by peripheral anterior synechiae. Only 1 patient continues to have an intraocular pressure over 20 mm Hg; 2 others are on topical antiglaucoma medication. In 5 eyes the retina has redetached.

This condition is probably due to congestion and swelling of the ciliary body from temporary interference by the scleral buckle with venous drainage. The complication was significantly more frequent with episcleral than with intrascleral implants. Episcleral procedures tend to result in scleral indentations of greater circumference and width that may cause the silicone to be oriented over a greater number of vortex veins and be placed more posteriorly. Episcleral sutures near vortex veins may result in distortion and compression of the veins against the posterior edges of the silicone.

# Neuro-ophthalmology

The evaluation of patients with optic nerve disease is a vexing problem for ophthalmologists. The vast array of diseases, tumors and toxic substances which may affect the optic nerve may dissuade the average physician from his own evaluation of the problem. Patients are referred to neurologists, neurosurgeons or neuro-ophthalmologists for what are assumed to be more sophisticated studies. Despite such studies, no specific etiology for 40% of patients with some type of optic neuropathy is shown. Nevertheless, the reasonable evaluation of a patient with optic nerve disease is not necessarily complicated if the clinician uses some schema of organization. It is useful to evaluate patients with optic neuropathy by considering specific features of the clinical history and examination.

One of the most important aspects of the history is the mode of onset. It is important to determine whether the visual loss occurred acutely or insidiously. The answer to this question is not always obvious. Many persons notice visual loss in one eye while inadvertently covering the better eye. If the patient is an unreliable historian, it is important to document progression of visual loss during repeated clinical examinations. Examples of acute optic neuropathies are those with a vascular origin such as temporal arteritis, migraine and ischemic optic neuropathy. Inflammatory diseases such as collagen vascular disease, postviral demyelination and multiple sclerosis occur acutely. Leber's hereditary optic atrophy frequently has a relatively acute course of visual loss. Traumatic disorders also occur acutely.

Examples of disorders causing progressive insidious loss include compressing lesions such as tumors and aneurysms, toxic optic neuropathies including those associated with alcohol, tobacco, drugs and nutritional deficiencies. The dominant and recessive forms of hereditary optic atrophy may progress slowly. Syphilis may cause acute or chronic visual changes. Optic atrophy is associated with the tapetoretinal diseases, such as retinitis pigmentosa and Leber's congenital amaurosis, and visual loss may occur slowly. Visual loss from functional cause may occur acutely or chronically.

Specific optic neuropathies have varying patterns of symmetry. Disorders which usually affect one eye are vascular disturbances, compressing lesions, trauma, inflammation and functional disturbances. Hereditary optic atrophy and toxic optic atrophy are the most common examples of bilateral visual loss. Obviously there are cases in which trauma or inflammation may cause bilateral visual changes.

The patient should be specifically questioned with regard to coexisting vascular disease such as hypertension, diabetes, peripheral vascular insufficiency or migraine. Obviously, associated neurologic symptoms such as headaches, paresthesias, ataxias, urinary problems and diplopia indicate a more diffuse neurologic disorder. The patient should be questioned specifically with regard to his tobacco and alcohol habits. It is important to know what drugs have been ingested within the several months prior to the onset of the problem. Are there toxic agents at the place of employment? The patient should be specifically asked about the quality of his diet. Patients may have participated in some type of fad diet. Family history is extremely important and if there are family members with possibly related disorders, they should be queried with regard to sex and age of onset.

In persons with optic nerve disease the most informative features of the ophthalmologic examination are visual acuity, visual fields, color vision testing, pupillary reactions, photostress test and ophthalmoscopic observation. If functional origins are suspected then optokinetic targets may elicit eye movements in patients who claim to have light perception or hand motion vision.

Visual acuity may be normal in the presence of certain optic neuropathies. Retinitis pigmentosa, glaucoma, optic neuritis, compression of the optic nerve and interruption of the vascular supply are examples of processes which may affect the optic nerve and cause field defects without affecting the visual acuity, at least in the initial stages of the disorder.

Visual field examination is extremely important. Certain patterns of visual field indicate specific categories of disease. Demyelinating lesions and compressing lesions typically show central scotomas with minimal peripheral depression. Vascular processes affecting the optic nerve typically cause altitudinal, arcuate or sector defects. Hereditary optic atrophies and toxic optic neuropathies are associated with centrocecal scotomas. One of the most common results of visual field testing is constricted visual fields without a central defect. Functional visual field loss is one of the most common conditions causing this type of visual field and if this is suspected, it is important to perform visual fields at varying test distances. Diseases which may result in this type of visual field include glaucoma, tapetoretinal disease, chronic disk edema, quinine intoxication, bilateral occipital lobe infarctions and functional visual loss. Ninety-five percent of visual field defects attributable to optic nerve pathology may be found in the central 30 degrees of vision.

Color vision may be tested in a number of ways. The easiest is to use books commonly available for the evaluation of hereditary forms of color blindness. The preservation of normal color vision implies that a significant number of macular fibers are functioning. Preservation of normal color vision is not compatible with compression of the optic nerve nor with optic neuritis, both of which are examples of diffuse optic nerve disease.

A Marcus Gunn pupil is one of the most sensitive indicators of unilateral or asymmetric optic nerve dysfunction. Absence of a Marcus Gunn pupil in a patient with unilateral visual loss virtually rules out any possibility of organic optic nerve disease. Obviously visual loss in this situation may be attributed to disease elsewhere in the eye, but in most cases, the pathology will be visible to the examiner.

The photostress test[1] is very useful in differentiating visual loss due to mild optic nerve disease from visual loss due to minimal abnormality of the retina or the retinal pigment epithelium. To perform the photostress test a bright flashlight is directed into the patient's eye at a short distance for a period of approximately 60 seconds. The patient is then asked to read the 20/20 or 20/25 line on the vision chart, assuming that his visual function is at this level. The time that elapses before the patient is able to read the desired line is noted. The process is repeated with the second eye. In patients with optic nerve disease the recovery time after bleaching of the retinal receptors should be the same. In other patients with retinal disease there will be a prolonged recovery time in the affected eye due to disturbance of the normal kinetics of pigment regeneration.

Ophthalmoscopic examination may give specific clues to the origin of optic nerve disease. In patients with Leber's hereditary optic atrophy, certain characteristic vascular changes at the superior and inferior poles of the disk have been described.[2] Patients with vasculitis secondary to a collagen vascular disease may have sheathing of peripheral arterioles indicating a systemic vasculitis. Perivenous sheathing is described in as many as 20% of patients with multiple sclerosis.[3] A dilated fundus examination is imperative since minimal pigmentary disturbances in the far periphery may be the only sign of a patient with atypical retinitis pigmentosa or other tapetoretinal disease. The observation of retinal nerve fiber layer defects in both eyes in a patient with unilateral visual loss strongly suggests an underlying demyelination process.[4]

The information obtained from the historical and clinical examination of a patient with optic nerve disease are the most important factors in determining an etiology for the optic neuropathy. A basic laboratory work-up in patients with these types of problem should probably include a complete blood count, sedimentation rate, fluorescent treponemal antibody absorption test, serum B12 and serum folate levels, when these seem applicable. Skull x-rays including views of the optic foramen are important.

In patients with a history and examination strongly suggestive of a compressing lesion, polytomography of the optic foramen and sella or EMI scanning may show lesions despite the presence of a normal skull x-ray.[5] Bilateral abnormal visual-evoked responses in a patient with unilateral visual loss strongly suggests systemic demyelinating disease.[6] If all of these tests are negative, it is unlikely that cerebral angiography or pneumoencephalography will add any startling information. If laboratory examinations are normal, the patient should be followed. Only if the patient continues to show progressive visual deterioration documented by a reliable examiner and reliable visual fields should more significant invasive types of neuroradiologic procedures be suggested.

If the clinician understands the limits and information which can be gleaned from the historical and clinical examination, then we may do the best service to our patients by doing the proper amount of evaluation while not subjecting them to expensive, uncomfortable and potentially dangerous examinations.

Michael Rosenberg, M.D.,
Rush Medical College and University of Illinois

## REFERENCES

1. Glaser, J.: Neuro-ophthalmologic Examination, in Duane, T. (ed.): *Clinical Ophthalmology* (Vol. 2, New York: Harper and Row, 1976 [p. 2, chap. 2]).
2. Smith, J. L., Hoyt, W. F., and Susac, J. O.: Ocular Fundus in Acute Leber's Optic Neuropathy, Arch. Ophthalmol. 90:349, 1973.
3. Rucker, C.: Sheathing of the Retinal Veins in Multiple Sclerosis, Mayo Clin. Proc. 47:335, 1972.
4. Frisen, L., and Hoyt, W.: Insidious Atrophy of Retinal Nerve Fibers in Multiple Sclerosis. Arch. Ophthalmol. 92:91, 1974.
5. Johnson, J. C., Lubow, M., Banerjee, T., and Yashon, D.: Chromophobe Adenoma and Chiasmal Syndrome without Enlargement of the Bony Sella. Ann. Ophthalmol. 8:1043, 1976.
6. Halliday, A., McDonald, W., and Muchin, J.: Visual-Evoked Response in Diagnosis of Multiple Sclerosis. Br. Med. J. 4:661, 1973.

**Effects of Differential Section of the VIIth Nerve on Patients with Intractable Blepharospasm.** Bartley R. Frueh, Alston Callahan, Richard K. Dortzbach, Robert B. Wilkins, Howard L. Beale, Howard S. Reitman and Francis R. Watson[8] (Univ. of Missouri Med. Center, Columbia, Mo.) made a retrospective study of the records of 100 consecutive patients who had differential section of the 7th nerve per-

(8) Trans. Am. Acad. Ophthalmol. Otolaryngol. 81:595–602, July–Aug., 1976.

formed by 6 physicians who used essentially the same technique.

METHOD. — The branches of the 7th nerve were dissected within the parotid gland and were excited with a nerve stimulator to determine function. Those branches affecting the orbicularis oculi muscles were dissected as far distally as possible, and the largest possible segment of the nerve was removed. When a nerve affected other muscle groups, it was followed to a distal branching. Where possible, only the branches to the orbicularis oculi were removed, but no nerve that innervated the orbicularis oculi muscles was allowed to remain.

Blepharospasm was reduced to an insignificant degree or abolished after the first operation in over half of the patients. The long-term recurrence rate is about 50%. Half of the significant recurrences appeared within the first 6 months after operation. Recurrences followed second operations in about half of 22 patients. All but 1 of 8 patients are well after a third operation, 4 of them at more than 5 years after operation.

Only 2% of the patients showed no improvement after operation, and 13% had only a slight decrease in spasm, but 65% of the patients were pleased with the outcome, and another 15% were moderately pleased. The 75 patients with bilateral disease had an average follow-up of 3.1 years after the first operation, and the 10 with unilateral disease had an average follow-up of 3 years.

Postoperatively, ectropion was present in 44% of the patients, 35% of whom had surgical correction; epiphora was present in 41%, of whom 50% recovered spontaneously. Moderate lagophthalmos, present in 20% of the patients, never cleared spontaneously. Exposure keratitis was present in 41% of the patients; it was always mild and cleared spontaneously in 82% of the cases. Paresis of the upper lip was noted in 34% of the patients; only 30% recovered spontaneously. A transcutaneous parotid fistula formed in 12% of the patients, but all fistulas closed off spontaneously in the 1st postoperative month.

The secondary effects of differential 7th nerve section are not inconsequential, but they are not a significant factor for most patients with respect to their view of the outcome. The long-term success rate is far from ideal; however, two operations, when needed, will leave 75% of the patients without significant spasm.

**Rapid Eye Movements in Myasthenia Gravis: II. Electro-oculographic Analysis.** Ophthalmoplegia is often the initial and major manifestation of myasthenia gravis (MG) but relative preservation of saccadic movements has been described in some patients with MG, leading to characteristic twitchlike or quiver movements of the eyes on changes of gaze. Robert D. Yee, David G. Cogan, David S. Zee (Nat'l Inst. of Health), Robert W. Baloh and Vicente Honrubia[9] (Univ. of California, Los Angeles) believed that the initial phase of saccades, when the highest velocities are normally generated, is spared in these patients even with severely limited gaze, the resultant saccades being small in amplitude but of high velocity.

Eye movements were recorded by electro-oculography in 10 patients with confirmed MG, aged 17–67, and 5 with progressive external ophthalmoplegia (PEO), aged 14–68. Two patients with internuclear ophthalmoplegia (INO) due to multiple sclerosis and 1 with 6th nerve palsy due to meningeal carcinomatosis were also examined.

The range of eye movements in patients with MG ranged from 20 degrees to full range. Glissade-like waveforms were present in both eyes of myasthenic patients. Three patients with MG had hypermetric waveforms during 20-degree movements. All those with PEO had glissade-like waveforms during 20-and 40-degree saccades but the rapid initial phase of the saccade was slower than in myasthenic patients. In all patients except those with INO and cranial nerve palsy, saccadic waveforms were similar in both eyes and were not altered by occlusion of each eye.

Two myasthenic patients clinically had quiver movements during voluntary refixations. Maximum saccadic velocities were abnormally low in patients with PEO but not in those with MG. The duration of glissade-like saccades was prolonged in PEO, INO and cranial nerve palsy. All patients were unable to generate a smooth pursuit movement greater than 15 degrees per second during tracking and no patient could consistently match a target velocity greater

(9)   Arch. Ophthalmol. 94:1465–1472, September, 1976.

than 10 degrees per second. Several patients with MG exhibited fatigue of eye movements during smooth tracking.

Patients with MG can clearly be distinguished from those with other forms of ophthalmoplegia on the basis of maximum saccadic velocity. Testing of voluntary saccades of small and large amplitudes, with particular attention to estimating the velocity of the initial phase of the movement and recognizing quiver eye movements, is helpful in the differential diagnosis of ophthalmoplegia.

► [The authors demonstrated by electro-oculographic analysis that the initial rapid saccades in myasthenia gravis have a higher velocity than in other nerve disorders such as progressive external ophthalmoplegia, internuclear ophthalmoplegia and cranial nerve palsy. If the observer is sharp, quiver eye movements can be noted in myasthenics. – Ed.] ◄

**Opsoclonus: Pattern of Regression in a Child with Neuroblastoma.** Opsoclonus is a rare disorder of ocular motility characterized by grossly chaotic, semiconjugate eye movements of large amplitude and random direction that continue during eye closure or sleep. Peter J. Savino and Joel S. Glaser[1] (Univ. of Miami) observed an infant with opsoclonus and neuroblastoma and documented regression of the eye movement disorder cinematographically after removal of the tumor.

Girl, 1 year, acquired unsteadiness on standing and spontaneous eye movements. Examination showed involuntary limb jerks, ataxia, wildly chaotic, random eye movements and a left-sided abdominal mass. The large retroperitoneal tumor was totally removed and found to be a neuroblastoma. The opsoclonus regressed in the 2 weeks after removal of the tumor and was replaced by flutter-like bursts of saccades accompanied by a head shudder, separated by quiet intervals which became progressively longer. Violent head-thrusting developed 3 weeks postoperatively on viewing targets to the left. The eyes made a leftward saccade to initiate the movement, with the head overshooting the end-point violently; a controversive eye movement ended the thrust. The child could sit up 8 weeks postoperatively but still had head and truncal ataxia. Gaze to the left was achieved smoothly without thrusting at this time and all flutter and opsoclonus had ceased although occasional dysmetric eye movements were detected.

Opsoclonus in children is most often due to encephalitis,

(1) Br. J. Ophthalmol. 59:696–698, December, 1975.

but a significant number of children have neuroblastomas. In adults malignancy with opsoclonus is very rare, most cases being attributable to a viral encephalitic process. Only a few children with neuroblastoma will recover completely even with successful treatment, whereas in the encephalitic group the reverse is the case. In the present case the opsoclonus regressed through phases of ocular flutter and then dysmetria after removal of a neuroblastoma. The ocular motor phenomena are apparently related to cerebellar dysfunction. The head-thrust was indicative of a dysmetric head movement due to cerebellar disease, rather than being caused by an oculomotor abnormality.

▶ [The association of opsoclonus with occult neuroblastomas of the adrenal was first stressed by Solomon and Chutorian (N. Engl. J. Med. 279:475, 1968) and is of obvious clinical importance in promoting earlier removal of the tumor. — Ed.] ◀

## Horner's Syndrome in Childhood. Curtis Sauer and Morris W. Levinsohn[2] (Cleveland) have seen 7 patients,

| DIFFERENTIAL DIAGNOSIS OF HORNER'S SYNDROME IN CHILDHOOD: COMMON ETIOLOGIES | | |
|---|---|---|
| LOCATION | ETIOLOGY | CASE |
| Brain stem, spinal cord, and ciliospinal center | Brain stem glioma | 3 |
| | Spinal cord tumor | 3 |
| | Syringomyelia | |
| | Poliomyelitis | |
| | Traumatic brachial plexus palsy | 6 |
| Sympathetic trunk and superior cervical ganglion | Intrathoracic tumor | |
| | Intrathoracic aneurysm | 1 |
| | Neural crest tumors (neuroblastoma, ganglioneuroma) | 4 |
| | Metastatic tumor, leukemia, lymphoma | 5 |
| | Cervical trauma | |
| | Cervical adenitis | |
| Postganglionic fibers (internal carotid artery plexus) | Internal carotid artery thrombosis | 2 |
| | Internal carotid artery aneurysm | |
| | Internal carotid artery trauma | |
| | Otitis media | |
| | Nasopharyngeal tumor | 7 |

(2) Neurology (Minneap.) 26:216–220, March, 1976.

aged newborn to 10 years, with Horner's syndrome during the past 3 years. Several different causes were found, but in each case the syndrome was associated with serious underlying disease.

Fully-developed Horner's syndrome consists of miosis due to paresis of the pupillary dilator; ptosis, which is often slight and anhidrosis on the affected side with deficient vasoconstriction. Any lesion interrupting the complex sympathetic paths to the head and neck may cause Horner's syndrome. Horner's syndrome due to intrinsic lesions of the brain stem and cord was rare in this series, occurring in only 1 case. Traumatic brachial plexus palsy is a very common cause of Horner's syndrome in childhood. The differential diagnosis is summarized in the table.

Chest, cervical spine and skull x-rays should be obtained routinely and urinary assays for catecholamines are indicated, especially if a cervical or pulmonary mass is present. If other cranial nerve lesions are found, careful radiologic evaluation of the middle cranial fossa is necessary. Cerebral angiography should be considered, especially if earlier studies are unrevealing.

**Tonic Pupil: A Simple Screening Test.** Testing for tonic pupil with Mecholyl is impossible, since the drug is no longer made. Brian R. Younge and Z. John Buski[3] (McGill Univ.) saw 25 patients with a clinical diagnosis of tonic pupil in 1973–75. Pupillary responses to one drop of 0.05, 0.1 and 0.2% pilocarpine were determined after 20 minutes.

The 20 female and 5 male patients had an average age of 41.5 years. Fifteen had unilateral dilated tonic pupil. Twenty-two had abnormally depressed ankle jerks. All 3 patients tested with 0.05% pilocarpine had constriction of 0.5 mm in the involved eye only. One of 5 patients failed to respond to 0.1% pilocarpine, and 1 of 6 failed to respond to 0.2% pilocarpine. Patients with bilateral involvement had the same general pattern of response. Three of 10 controls responded to pilocarpine in normal light and 3 others in subdued light. Pupillary response to dilute pilocarpine were greater in the patients with tonic pupil than in the controls. A concentration of 0.1% is recommended.

(3) Can. J. Ophthalmol. 11:295–299, October, 1976.

## Light Microscopic, Autoradiographic Study of Axoplasmic Transport in Optic Nerve Head during Ocular Hypotony, Increased Intraocular Pressure and Papilledema.

Don S. Minckler, M. O. M. Tso and L. E. Zimmerman[4] (Armed Forces Inst. of Pathology) demonstrated marked alterations of both rapid and slow components of axoplasmic transport in ocular hypotony, hypotony-induced papilledema and increased intraocular pressure in rhesus monkey eyes. Autoradiographs were prepared on eyes of adult monkeys by use of tritiated leucine or tritiated proline administered intravitreously. Increased intraocular pressure and ocular hypotony with papilledema were induced by

Fig 48. – Autoradiographs of optic nerve heads of rhesus monkeys 6 hours after intravitreous injection of ³H-leucine. **A,** control eye with normal intraocular pressure. **B,** experimental eye 6 hours after cyclocryotherapy and onset of increased intraocular pressure (50 mm Hg). There is 2+ accumulation of label (black grains) in emulsion over lamina scleralis, indicating interference with rapid axoplasmic transport at that level. AFIP neg no. 74-19156; 30-day exposure autoradiograph, counterstained with toluidine blue; reduced from ×50. (Courtesy of Minckler, D. S., et al.: Am. J. Ophthalmol. 82:741–757, November, 1976.)

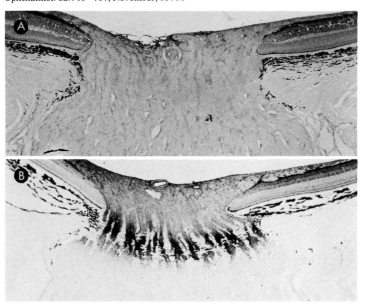

(4) Am. J. Ophthalmol. 82:741–757, November, 1976.

cyclocryotherapy. Hypotony and papilledema were also induced by surgical fistulization of the anterior chamber.

Autoradiographs obtained 6 hours after intravitreous injection of ³H-leucine with normal and elevated intraocular pressure are shown in Figure 48. In ocular hypotony with papilledema, the most abundant accumulations of radionuclide injected 12 days previously were in the swollen axons at the edge of the optic disc at the level of the lamina retinalis (Fig 49). Similar alterations in the rapid and slow components were produced by either cyclocryotherapy or by surgical fistulization.

In other experiments using horseradish peroxidase as a tracer, extravasation of fluid from the central retinal vein to the intercellular spaces of the optic nerve head did not appear to be the major component of disk swelling caused ei-

**Fig 49.** – Autoradiographs prepared 12 days after injection of ³H-leucine. **A,** control eye with normal intraocular pressure. **B,** eye with established papilledema and intraocular pressure of 0 mm Hg after cyclocryotherapy. There is striking retention of label in swollen axons. AFIP neg no. 74-12151; 30-day exposure, toluidine blue; reduced from ×50. (Courtesy of Minckler, D. S., et al.: Am. J. Ophthalmol. 82:741–757, November, 1976.)

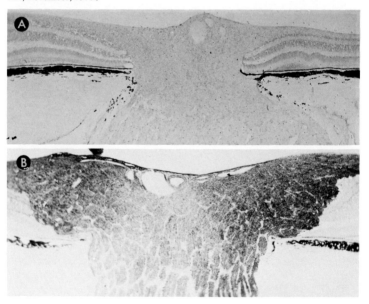

ther by ocular hypotony or by increased intracranial pressure. Instead, there appears to be swelling of the axonal elements.

**A-Scan Ultrasonography in Unilateral Optic Nerve Lesions** is discussed by W. Schroeder[5] (Univ. of Hamburg), based on observations during a 3-year period. An Echo-Ophthalmograph Kretz 7,200 MA with an 8-MHz sound head was used and gauged according to Ossoinig and Blodi. Figure 50 shows the modified Ossoinig technique. The bulbus is in maximal abduction, in which the adjoining bordering surfaces of the bulbus wall, optic nerve, rectus internus

**Fig 50.**—Technique of ultrasonic measurement in distal diagonal section of optic nerve; right eye, viewed from above. (Courtesy of Schroeder, W.: Klin. Monatsbl. Augenheilkd. 169:30–38, July, 1976.)

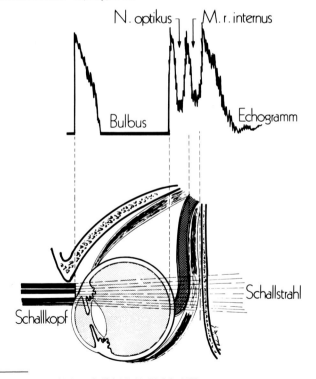

and nasal orbit wall will produce the characteristic ultra-sonogram (echogram) The distance between the 2d and 3d peak marks the sound-course time within the distal optic nerve diagonal section, allowing determination of optic nerve thickness and evaluations based on lateral comparison.

A total of 156 patients was examined, including 74 with papilledema as a major symptom. Broadening of the optic nerve echogram was found in neuritis of the optic nerve, in papilledema due to increased orbital or intracranial pressure, in tumors of the optic nerve and in direct or indirect trauma. A second group included 35 patients with functional disturbance without observable papillary symptoms. A broadening of the optic echogram was seen in 75% with retrobulbar neuritis up to 21 days after the onset of the functional disturbance. Most patients of the third group of 60 had been referred for clarification of a unilateral optic atrophy. A period of months or years had elapsed between the onset of subjective symptoms and echography, which showed alterations only in relatively few cases, aside from instances of tumor.

The present study showed that alterations in the thickness of the distal optic nerve are associated with certain diseases and may be included in an evaluation of clinical symptoms. In acute functional deficit without fundus alterations the broadened optic echogram is an objective indication of a retrobulbar neuritis or hematoma (after trauma). In unilateral papillary edema the echogram furnishes data regarding possible edema of the optic nerve. A broadened echogram is seen in neuritis, tumors and increased orbital or intracranial pressure but only rarely in anterior ischemic neuropathy. Given the presence of a (partial) optic atrophy, the broadened optic ultrasonogram indicates an optic nerve or sheath tumor.

**Nasal Fundus Ectasia.** Dag Riise[6] (Copenhagen) describes a distinctive eye anomaly with a series of characteristic findings that usually consist of an inferonasal crescent, dysversion of the optic disc with inverse vessel emergence, nasal fundus ectasia with scleral thinning, choroidal and

---

(6)　Acta Ophthalmol. (Suppl. 126) (Kbh.):1975.

retinal thinning, myopia, astigmatism and a relative temporal visual field defect. Patients are mostly encountered in hospital outpatient clinics during routine perimetry in connection with other diseases. Some have emerged from examination of close relatives of patients and from patient material in a neurosurgical department.

Study was made of 115 eyes in 66 patients with visual field defects and fundus ectasia. The incidence of the anomaly is about the same in men and women. About one quarter of the eyes had an acuity of 1; most were in the range 0.33 – 1. Myopia was found in 90% of affected eyes and astigmatism of over 1 diopter in 70%. Over half the patients exhibited a distinct inferonasal crescent on ophthalmoscopy. Dysversion was present in 65% of the eyes and inverse vessel emergence in 80%. The fundus ectasia was deeper than 2 diopters in 102 of the 115 eyes; in most cases the depth was 4 to 8 diopters. In most cases the fundus was pale in the region of the ectasia. Degenerative lesions were present in 14 eyes, mainly of elderly patients. Perimetry showed bitemporal relative field defects, which usually were reduced or absent on correction of the eye with glasses corresponding to the floor of the ectasia. Orbital x-rays and electroretinograms, obtained in a few cases, showed normal conditions. Three patients were subjected to exploratory craniotomy for suspected pituitary tumor. Other eye disorders included slight exophthalmos in 6 patients, detached retina in 4 and squint in 3. There was no evidence that general diseases were associated with the anomaly.

The etiology of this disorder is not known. Histologic study shows thinning of the sclera, choroid and retina nasally, down from the optic disc in a location corresponding to the embryonic cleft of the eye, but the disorder cannot be a pure coloboma because there are no duplication or defects. Familial concentration of cases is evident; there is probably a polymeric mode of inheritance similar to that of refraction anomalies. The most important investigation is perimetry with corrective glasses corresponding to the bottom of the fundus ectasia.

▶ [An entire monograph is devoted to these defects in the lower nasal disc and fundus, and rightly so, because 3 cases in the series had exploratory craniotomies for suspected pituitary tumor because of the upper temporal field defects. Photographs of the fundus and visual field defect in this type of case were given in an article by Graham and Wakefield (1974 YEAR BOOK, p. 324). Young, Walsh and Knox (Am. J. Ophthalmol. 82:16, 1976) reported 12 additional cases, which they term "tilted-disc syndrome." — Ed.] ◄

**Optic Pits and Posterior Retinal Detachment.** Robert J. Brockhurst[7] (Retina Found., Boston), states that congenital pits of the optic nerve head are usually unilateral, and they may be associated with other abnormalities such as enlargement of the nerve head, coloboma of the nerve head and atrophy of the pigment epithelium at the temporal edge of the disc. Associated macular changes may include frank serous detachment of the retina, cystic macular degeneration, macular "holes" and pigmentary degeneration. Serous detachments associated with pits have been attributed to a true macular hole, to central serous choroidopathy due to fluid leakage via defects in the retinal pigment epithelium, although fluorescein angiography is negative, and to a mechanical leak of fluid from the subarachnoid space or vitreous through the optic pit into the subretinal space.

Six patients with congenital pits of the optic nerve head and serous retinal detachment were treated by xenon and argon laser photocoagulation. Reattachment of the retina in 5 patients followed induction of a watertight chorioretinal scar by photocoagulation at the disc margin. A tiny hole was observed biomicroscopically in a membrane over the pit in 2 cases. Steroid therapy is ineffective in this condition, and optic nerve sheath decompression reported in the literature is more hazardous than photocoagulation. Repeated treatment was necessary in 4 patients to obliterate all areas of elevated retina at the disc margin. Secondary treatment is probably more effective because there is more pigment in the choroid from former treatment, permitting greater secondary inflammation to occur. Photocoagulation treatment of the pit itself is difficult. Visual acuity improved in all patients, despite fairly strong chorioretinal scarring, and the scotomas were smaller after treatment.

Prophylactic treatment, with use of a ruby laser, should be considered in view of the morbidity of this condition. At present, however, prophylactic treatment cannot be advised

(7)  Trans. Am. Ophthalmol. Soc. 73:264–291, 1975.

because of lack of knowledge of the pathogenesis and natural course of the disorder and of the efficacy of treatment.

▶ [In discussion of this paper, Donald Gass expressed doubts whether photocoagulation actually closed off a pathway from the optic pit to the submacular space with disappearance of the macular edema, or whether this was the natural course of the condition. The long time required for beneficial effect and need for repeated treatments in some cases might suggest the latter. Gass reported 6 cases treated similarly, and 5 of the 6 maculas reattached after a prolonged period. Two of 4 patients without treatment had reattachment of the macula. Vogel and Wessing had no success in photocoagulation of 22 such cases (see the 1975 YEAR BOOK, p. 281).

Also, in concluding the discussion, Brockhurst reported that Dr. Jerry Shields had observed a collie dog with a congenital pit and detachment of the macula. The dog was sacrificed and dye was injected into the subarachnoid space but it did not enter the subretinal space. Intrathecal fluorescein is toxic and therefore this test has not been performed in humans with this condition. – Ed.] ◀

**Hereditary Optic Atrophies.** Only apparent primary atrophies are reviewed by J. François[8] (Ghent, Belgium).

The recessive form of congenital or infantile optic atrophy is rare. It exists at birth or appears generally before age 3 years or occasionally later. Optic atrophy is bilateral and total. Vision is always very poor and sometimes totally absent. Recessive autosomal heredity is demonstrated by the frequency of consanguinity of the parents (more than 50% of the cases) and by the appearance of the disease in a one and the same sibship where at least 2 members are affected. More than 20 illustrative families are known.

The oculo-auriculo-diabetic syndrome is characterized by presence of bilateral optic atrophy of the primary type, diabetes mellitus, diabetes insipidus, neurogenic deafness and other anomalies, such as hydronephrosis. This syndrome is recessive autosomal. Consanguinity of the parents was identified in 15% of the cases. In 1966, 9 sibships with 2–4 affected members were found in the literature. Since then, more than 30 new cases have been reported.

The dominant form of juvenile optic atrophy is much more frequent and more benign than the recessive form. It starts insidiously in early childhood. Nystagmus is never present. Optic atrophy is bilateral and is seldom total. There are no neurologic or general manifestations. Functional symptoms

(8) Ann. Ocul. (Paris) 209:169–179, March, 1976.

include a variable degree of decreased visual acuity and a normal visual field. The curve of adaptation to darkness is not reduced until after age 50. There is an unusual dyschromatopsia of the blue-yellow axis (tritanopia). Generally, the electroretinogram is normal. The dominant form of optic atrophy is stationary or progresses very slowly.

Behr's infantile hereditary-familial optic atrophy starts between ages 1 and 9 years. It is characterized by bilateral primary optic atrophy, nystagmus in half of the cases and strabismus in two thirds of the cases and neurologic signs, especially pyramidal, recalling Friedreich's disease.

Sex-linked optic atrophy is rare. In 1974, Völker-Dieben et al. described a large family in which 8 male members had optic atrophy. It was manifested in early childhood and progressed slowly.

Leber's optic neuritis (atrophy) is generally incomplete and hereditary, starting after an acute optic neuritis. Men are affected more than women (7:1). Central vision diminishes rapidly, but the visual field remains normal. There is a dyschromatopsia of the green-red axis, and the curve of adaptation to darkness is often subnormal. The electroretinogram is normal. Frequently, there is spontaneous but incomplete visual recuperation. Leber's disease is a genetic puzzle. It seems to be of sex-linked, dominant autosomal heredity, but without the classic mode of transmission. Although cytoplasmic heredity best explains transmission, there are nevertheless several objections to the theory.

**Optic Nerve Manifestations of Human Congenital Cytomegalovirus Infection.** Helen Mintz Hittner, Murdina M. Desmond and John R. Montgomery[9] (Baylor Univ.) have encountered 4 children with congenital cytomegalovirus infection and optic nerve abnormalities in the past 3 years. A Latin American boy and a white girl with cytomegalovirus infection on the 1st day of life had unilateral optic nerve hypoplasia. A white boy from whom cytomegalovirus was isolated at age 5 weeks had a unilateral partial coloboma of the optic nerve. A black infant, aged 4 months, with cytomegalovirus infection diagnosed at age 2 days, had a unilateral complete coloboma of the optic nerve associated

(9) Am. J. Ophthalmol. 81:661–665, May, 1976.

with microphthalmia. The association of these lesions with congenital cytomegalovirus infection has not previously been reported.

Cytomegalovirus infection is present in 3–6% of pregnant women. The incidence in infants is 1–3%, the virus being found in the urine and blood. Ocular findings can be a minor part of a rapidly fatal illness or a significant part of the picture in an otherwise healthy infant. Chorioretinitis may occur in as many as 30% of infants with congenital cytomegalovirus infection. Other reported eye findings include perivascular exudates, retinal hemorrhages, conjunctivitis, corneal clouding, cataract, and optic atrophy. All infants with congenital nerve malformations should be evaluated for cytomegalovirus infection. Optic nerve hypoplasia can occur with good visual acuity. The present cases of optic nerve coloboma demonstrate the large spectrum of optic nerve colobomas. Congenital cytomegalovirus infection must be considered in the differential diagnosis of colobomatous microphthalmia.

**Measles Virus-Specific IgG in Optic Neuritis and in Multiple Sclerosis after Optic Neuritis.** A significantly higher level of measles virus-specific IgG has been found in the serums of patients with multiple sclerosis (MS) than in those with other neurologic diseases and specific IgG is present consistently in the cerebrospinal fluid (CSF) of about 60% of the patients with MS. W. M. Hutchinson and Margaret Haire[1] (Queen's Univ., Belfast) compared titers of specific IgG in the serums of patients with a history of optic neuritis (ON) only with those in patients in whom ON was the first symptom of MS.

Among 100 patients seen during 1960–74 with ON of unknown cause, 41 acquired additional features of MS. In 1973–74, 17 patients were admitted in the acute phase of ON. No patient in either series had symptoms or signs of MS at or before the initial attack of ON.

In the first series, the geometric mean titer of measles virus-specific IgG was greater in patients who subsequently had MS than in those with uncomplicated ON or control. The only significant difference was between patients who

(1)   Br. Med. J. 1:64–66, Jan. 10, 1976.

acquired MS and their matched controls. Nine patients with recurrent uncomplicated ON had titers comparable to those of the patients who acquired MS. The MS patients had higher titers than patients with uncomplicated ON after matching for sex and age.

Measles virus-specific IgG was detected in the CSF of 9 of 17 patients in the second series. Titers were slightly higher in those with higher lymphocyte counts. Serum antibody titers tended to be higher in patients with antibody detectable in the CSF; this relationship was statistically significant. Antibody was present in the CSF of 6 of 8 patients with bilateral or recurrent ON and in 3 of 9 with unilateral ON.

Patients with MS known to occur after a definite episode of ON have significantly higher titers of measles virus-specific IgG in their serums than do patients with ON who do not acquire MS. The findings suggest that it would be worthwhile to carry out serial estimates in serums and possibly in CSF from patients with ON and other initial symptoms suggestive of MS to elucidate the relationship of changes in antibody titer to the clinical progression of the disease.

▶ [These studies correlate clinical findings with indirect immunofluorescent tests to detect measles virus-specific IgG antibodies in the spinal fluid and serum. Patients with higher levels would appear to be more likely to be among the 41% who develop multiple sclerosis (MS) after the initial attack of optic neuritis or have recurrent attacks of optic neuritis. An excellent summary by Burde (see the 1974 YEAR BOOK, p. 312) certainly incriminates the measles virus as the etiologic agent of both optic neuritis and MS, especially in individuals with histocompatibility groups HL-A3 and HL-A7 and the genetic lymphocyte determinant LD-7a. In the discussion of their paper, the authors make such statements as, "we feel that all our cases of optic neuritis represented early manifestations of MS." "We think it unlikely that the differences in antibody titers in the present study groups were simply due to differences in the prevalences of histocompatibility types, but it is more probable that the measles antibody titers were related to the extent of demyelination that had occurred in the central nervous system." – Ed.] ◀

**Subclinical Optic Neuropathy in Multiple Sclerosis: How Early VER Components Reflect Axon Loss and Conduction Defects in Optic Pathways.** Recently, Frisen and Hoyt reported the presence of focal and diffuse axon attrition in the retinal nerve fiber layer in multiple sclerosis, even in patients without visual symptoms or signs. Moshe

Feinsod and William F. Hoyt[2] (Univ. of California, San Francisco) examined the electrophysiologic correlates of axon loss and demyelination as recorded in the visual evoked responses (VER) of 25 patients with multiple sclerosis. Four patients had had retrobulbar neuritis, 6 had signs of chronic bilateral optic neuropathy and 15 had no visual

**Fig 51 (top).** — Normal VER recorded from left *(LT)* and right *(RT)* occipital regions.

**Fig 52 (bottom).** — Visual evoked responses to stimulation of left *(OS)* and right eye *(OD)* in patient with brain stem involvement due to multiple sclerosis. Note breakdown of initial negative component into subcomponents *(arrows)*.

(Courtesy of Feinsod, M., and Hoyt, W. F.: J. Neurol. Neurosurg. Psychiatry 38: 1109–1114, November, 1976.)

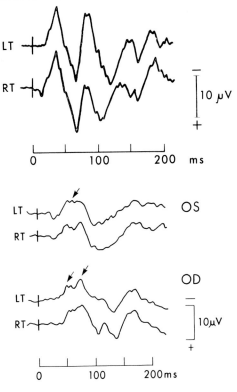

symptoms or signs. The VER was recorded with the pupils dilated in a darkened room, with 100 one-per-second flashes delivered at 20 cm from the pupils by a xenon discharge lamp. The normal VER is shown in Figure 51.

All 25 patients had abnormal latency and shape of the initial negative component of the VER. The patterns seen included prolonged peak latency, multiple subcomponents of the first negative component and delay of the subcomponents after the first (Fig 52) and an extremely low amplitude, bizarre VER with none of the usual single components. The peripapillary nerve fiber layer was abnormal in 17 patients, showing slitlike defects in the arcuate fibers combined with diffuse thinning of the nerve fiber layer, or diffuse thinning of temporal nerve fiber bundles and lesser thinning in the other sectors surrounding the optic disc. The latter pattern included mild temporal pallor of the disc. Only 6 of the 17 patients with nerve fiber layer axon atrophy had corresponding changes in the optic discs. The VER showed clear evidence of optic pathway involvement in 7 patients who met all objective ophthalmologic criteria of normal.

Most of the subclinical electrophysiologic abnormalities observed in patients with multiple sclerosis can be explained by varying degrees of conduction delay in demyelinated axons and depletion of axons in the optic pathways. Tissue culture studies have suggested that delay in conduction and changes in the VER pattern could be caused in part by a humoral factor that impairs synaptic transmission in multiple sclerosis.

**Possible Means of Monitoring Progress of Demyelination in Multiple Sclerosis: Effect of Body Temperature on Visual Perception of Double Light Flashes.** Changes in body temperature can markedly alter the clinical features of multiple sclerosis. For a population of partially demyelinated axons, increasing body temperature mimics the effect of increased demyelination. When a patient with optic neuropathy views a pair of brief light flashes, the interval between them must be considerably greater than normal for the subject to see them as double. R. J. Galvin, D. Regan and J. R. Heron[3] (Stoke-on-Trent, England)

---

(3)   J. Neurol. Neurosurg. Psychiatry 39:861 – 865, September, 1976.

found that the double flash test provides an easily measured index of temperature sensitivity in the partially demyelinated visual pathway.

Patients viewed a small solid-state red lamp giving a pair of brief flashes separated by a variable dark interval, before and after cooling by ingestion of 300 ml of crushed ice and immersion of the hands in iced water. Warming was by immersing the legs in water at 44 C and wrapping the patient in blankets with hot water bottles around the abdomen. Four patients with multiple sclerosis and clinical optic nerve involvement were studied. Three were heated and 3 were cooled.

Heating impaired and cooling improved double flash resolution at demyelinated sites. Visual acuity behaved similarly. The test was extremely sensitive, changing by up to 75 msec in response to simple heating and cooling procedures which produced small variations in acuity. A striking deterioration in double flash resolution was produced in a patient with Uhthoff's syndrome by heating.

This simple double flash test can measure responses to temperature change in patients with optic neuropathy. Apart from its diagnostic value, the test furnishes a simple in vivo model for studying the effects of temperature change and potential symptomatic therapy on conduction in partially demyelinated axons in the visual system. The test might be used to objectively assess the effectiveness of various experimental treatments for multiple sclerosis.

**Dynamic Visual Field Testing Using the Amsler Grid Patterns.** Conventional instruments used for visual field testing require shifting the patient from the examination lane and involve instrumentation of varying expense. Kevin F. S. Chen and Marcel Frenkel[4] (Chicago) developed a rapid, economical, sensitive method of recording visual fields in the examining chair or at the patient's bedside.

The method uses the visual field charts introduced by Amsler. Amsler charts 1, 2 and 3 are sufficient for testing; chart 3 may be used for subjective testing and dynamic field testing with red targets. The patient wears the optical correction and the charts are held 35.6 cm from the eye (Fig 53). A subjective test of field integrity is done by the Amsler

(4) Trans. Am. Acad. Ophthalmol. Otolaryngol. 79:761–771, Nov.–Dec., 1975.

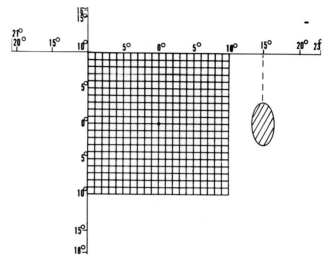

**Fig 53.** – When testing right eye with loose-leaf binder placed inferiorly, temporal field of 23 degrees from fixation can be obtained as well as extent of 20 degrees nasally, 16 degrees regularly and 18 degrees inferiorly. (Courtesy of Chen, K. F. S., and Frenkel, M.: Trans. Am. Acad. Ophthalmol. Otolaryngol. 79:761–771, Nov.– Dec., 1975.)

technique to detect metamorphopsia or minute central or paracentral scotomas. A pinhead test target from the Berens set is used for dynamic testing. The pupils are not dilated for study.

The visual field defects found in dynamic Amsler field testing correlated with 100% accuracy in patients having neurologic defects with the patterns found on conventional testing, including the full spectrum of neuro-ophthalmic lesions. Field defects were found in 139 of 212 glaucomatous eyes by the Amsler technique and in 136 eyes by the Autoplot. The Amsler grid gave false positive readings in 7 eyes and false negative readings in 2. Pickup was inaccurate in 6.5% of the glaucomatous eyes; inaccurate pickup was presumed when a field defect elicited on Amsler testing had different contours or borders from those found on Autoplot or Goldmann testing.

Dynamic visual field testing with the Amsler grid patterns is a sensitive and specific method of determining visual field defects in an economical, time-sparing manner. Full correlation was found between Amsler and conventional test results for neurologic defects. The method is useful at the bedside for chronically ill patients and also is valuable in following the evolution of a scotoma on sequential testing.

**Comparison of Sensitivity of Carotid Compression Tonography with Ophthalmodynamometry in Diagnosis of Internal Carotid Artery Occlusive Disease** is reported by David N. Cohen and Richard Wangelin[5] (Cleveland, Ohio). Carotid compression tonography (CCT) reflects the acute reduction in choroidal blood volume produced by digital occlusion of the ipsilateral common carotid artery, resulting in reduction of intraocular pressure on that side. Normally, the intraocular pressure is independent of flow in the contralateral carotid artery.

**Fig 54.** – Carotid compression tonography technique with cross section of neck at about C4 – C5 level. Common carotid artery well below level of bifurcation is being compressed by fore and middle fingers against cervical vertebrae. (Courtesy of Cohen, D. N., and Wangelin, R.: Trans. Am. Acad. Ophthalmol. Otolaryngol. 81: 882 – 892, Sept. – Oct., 1976.)

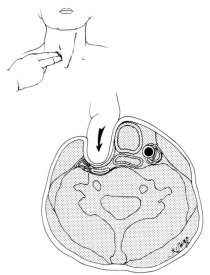

(5)   Trans. Am. Acad. Ophthalmol. Otolaryngol. 81:882 – 892, Sept. – Oct., 1976.

Carotid compression tonography was compared with ophthalmodynamometry (ODMY) in 100 consecutive patients with significant carotid occlusive disease demonstrated by arteriography. All had at least 50% stenosis of the carotid lumen. Ophthalmodynamometry was performed after mydriasis with cyclopentolate hydrochloride and phenylephrine. All CCT recordings were made with an electronic recording tonometer (Fig 54). Compression was exerted at the proximal or lowest part of the common carotid artery and maintained until the pressure no longer fell rapidly,

**Fig 55.** — Carotid compression tonography with occlusion of right internal carotid artery. Upper recording of right eye shows poor ocular pulse. Right carotid compression produces no fall in intraocular pressure; left carotid compression, however, produces marked fall and recovery in intraocular pressure of right eye. (This demonstrates that major portion of blood flow to right eye is being supplied by left carotid system.) Lower recording is normal for comparison. (Courtesy of Cohen, D. N., and Wangelin, R.: Trans. Am. Acad. Ophthalmol. Otolaryngol. 81:882–892, Sept.–Oct., 1976.)

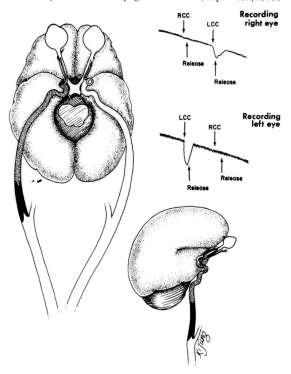

usually for 4–5 seconds but never for more than 8 seconds. Interpretation of the test is illustrated in Figure 55.

A tonographic pattern indicating reduced flow through the carotid system on the appropriate side was recorded in 95 cases. In contrast, a 15% or greater decrease in ophthalmic artery perfusion pressure was found by ODMY on the appropriate side in only 70 patients. Four of the 30 patients with negative correlations had dynamometric pressures that were falsely lateralizing, whereas 26 had completely symmetric pressures. Two patients with complete internal carotid occlusion and normal CCT tests had ODMY pressures indicating a unilateral pressure reduction on the side of disease. The external carotid was supplying the collateral flow in both of these patients. In the 3 other patients in whom the condition was missed by CCT, the ODM readings were also negative.

The CCT test can detect up to 95% of patients with arteriographic evidence of a stenotic lesion in one or both carotid systems capable of interfering with normal blood flow to the brain. The CCT test is easier to perform than ODMY. The CCT test has provided pertinent information when an endarterectomy is contemplated and also for postoperative followup.

▶ [This large documented series of occlusion of the internal carotid artery indicates the much greater diagnostic reliability of carotid compression tonography than ophthalmodynamometry (see also the 1966–67 YEAR BOOK, p. 296; and the 1969 YEAR BOOK, p. 305). Perhaps now the cardiovascular surgeons will have a little more respect for the CCT screening test than they have had for ODMY, which is complicated technically and the results affected by the development of collateral circulation via the external carotids. – Ed.] ◀

**Visually Evoked Response: Use in Neurologic Evaluation of Posttraumatic Subjective Visual Complaints.** The neurologic interpretation of subjective visual symptoms in the absence of abnormal ophthalmic findings is speculative at best. Moshe Feinsod, William F. Hoyt, W. Bruce Wilson and Jean-Paul Spire[6] (Univ. of California) evaluated the visual evoked response (VER) in the validation and clarification of visual complaints in patients with normal neuroophthalmologic findings.

---

(6) Arch. Ophthalmol. 94:237–240, February, 1976.

The VER is recorded with the pupils dilated and in a darkened room, delivering 100 1/second flashes at 20 cm from the pupil by a xenon discharge lamp. The averaged responses to monocular and binocular stimulation are displayed and photographed.

In a girl with short episodes of visual loss and known behavioral problems, the abnormal VER recorded over the injured hemisphere, the site of an epileptic focus, was the cerebral analogue of the hemianopic episodes. In another patient the VER validated his postconcussive complaints; delayed latency of the initial negative wave indicated abnormal conduction along the visual paths. The VER returned to normal as the patient improved. Dimming of vision on hyperextension of the neck in a third patient, probably due to impingement of osteophytes on the vertebral arteries, was validated by changes in the VER. In a fourth patient, the nonorganic nature of posttraumatic visual complaints was identified by recording a normal VER on stimulation of each eye.

The VER is an important means of separating the functional and organic in patients claiming visual disturbance. In complaints associated with late posttraumatic epileptic activity, the VER can show an abnormality even in asymptomatic intervals. In cases of concussion it demonstrates disorganized evoked responses initially and later a return of the normal response. The VER demonstrates an occipital lobe abnormality during and after transient compression of the vertebral artery. A normal response indicates a normally functioning visual system and effectively excludes all but trivial involvement of traumatic origin.

**Eye Signs in Craniopharyngioma.** Craniopharyngiomas are benign tumors of variable size and extent and represent 13% of intracranial neoplasms in childhood and nearly one third of all new growths in the hypophyseal area. Ocular signs often are the presenting feature of these tumors. H. B. Kennedy and R. J. S. Smith[7] (Inst. of Neurological Sciences, Glasgow) reviewed the findings in 45 patients with craniopharyngioma, 22 men and 23 women with a mean age of 25 years, seen over a 20-year period. Over

(7) Br. J. Ophthalmol. 59:689–695, December, 1975.

half the patients presented in the 1st 2 decades of life and over two-thirds presented before age 30 years.

The clinical features are shown in Figure 56. Headache was especially prevalent in children. Half the patients were seen at an eye clinic before being seen by a neurosurgeon. Visual acuity was 6/12 or less in 1 or both eyes in 60% of cases. Half the children and nearly two thirds of adults had diminished vision. Visual field loss was found in half the children and nearly all the young adults. Bitemporal hemianopia was present in 27% of patients at 1st admission. Prechiasmal field defects presented in 9 cases and homonymous hemianopia in 5. A distinct change of field defect type was noted in 10 cases.

Eighteen patients had elevated intracranial pressure initially and 12 of these had papilledema. Over half the patients had optic atrophy when hospitalized. Strabismus was detected in 7 patients. Pituitary and hypothalamic dysfunction was detected in about two thirds of the patients, particularly in older patients. About one third of older adults had a history of mental symptoms. Routine skull films showed abnormalities in all children but in only half the older

**Fig 56.** – Presenting clinical features in 45 cases of craniopharyngioma. (Courtesy of Kennedy, H. B., and Smith, R. J. S.: Br. J. Ophthalmol. 59:689–695, December, 1975.)

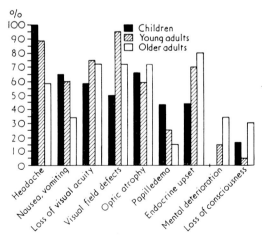

adults. Suprasellar calcification was noted in all children but 1 and in about one third of adults.

**Chromophobe Adenoma and Chiasmatic Syndrome without Enlargement of the Bony Sella.** Visual disturbance is by far the most common clinical manifestation of chromophobe adenoma. In 1 year, John C. Johnson, Martin Lubow, Timir Banerjee and David Yashon[8] (Ohio State Univ.) encountered 4 patients with craniotomy-proved chromophobe adenoma in whom skull films showed no sellar enlargement. All 4 had visual disturbance initially. All had complete development of the sphenoid sinus, apparently predisposing them to predominantly suprasellar, rather than intrasellar, tumor growth. In 2 other patients routine x-rays were initially considered to show normal or questionable findings, and special x-ray studies proved the sellae to be abnormal.

The pneumoencephalogram, especially combined with thin-section tomography, is indispensable in the presurgical work-up of these patients. Computerized axial tomography does not at present provide comparable anatomical detail in the suprasellar area, and nuclide brain scanning and angiography often give equivocal or nonspecific results. Determination of the upper limits of normal sellar size are still somewhat subjective. There is a greater tendency for suprasellar growth of a pituitary mass when the sphenoid sinus is well developed. When the sinus is small and restricted to the area anterior to the pituitary fossa, downward growth of the tumor is favored. Correlation between the presence and degree of visual impairment and the size of the suprasellar mass has not been especially impressive.

A high index of suspicion of a surgically treatable lesion must be maintained in patients with chiasmatic syndrome, despite radiographs showing a normal-sized sella.

**Visual Complications Following Irradiation for Pituitary Adenomas and Craniopharyngiomas.** Deteriorating vision after treatment for pituitary tumors has generally been considered an indication of recurrence, but recurrences have declined significantly with improvements in surgery and radiotherapy. Jay R. Harris and Martin B.

---

(8) Ann. Ophthalmol. 8:1043–1053, September, 1976.

Levene[9] (Harvard Med. School) reviewed the records of 55 patients treated for pituitary adenomas or craniopharyngiomas in 1968–73, 5 of whom were diagnosed as having radiation damage to the optic nerve paths. Initially lateral fields or a coronal five-field plan were used. Most recently patients have been treated by two 90-degree coronal arc-wedged rotations; this technique was used in 25 patients. Fraction size was changed from 250 to 200 rads daily, delivered 4 or 5 days a week. Generally a total dose of 4,500–5,000 rads was given in 4–5 weeks for pituitary adenomas and a dose of 5,500 rads in 5–6 weeks for craniopharyngiomas. All patients were treated with a 2-, 4- or 6-MeV linear accelerator. Two patients were lost to follow-up and 1 patient died. Fifty-five were followed for up to 5½ years after the completion of radiotherapy.

Five patients had visual loss from damage to the optic paths and 1 from an empty sella syndrome. One patient had both radiation damage and recurrence. Optic path damage occurred in 18% of 28 patients given 250 rads or more per fraction per day, a significant association. Four patients with optic nerve damage were treated with the five-field plan; this association was not significant. No areas of increased daily dose ("hot spots") were identified in isodose distributions. The nominal standard dose was not a good discriminant for this complication.

Loss of vision after treatment for pituitary adenomas or craniopharyngiomas can be due to recurrence, empty sella syndrome or radiation damage to the optic pathways. A pneumoencephalogram showing a mass indicates recurrence, whereas air in the sella is characteristic of the empty sella syndrome. In the absence of both these signs, radiation injury to the optic paths should be considered. The daily fraction size should not exceed 200 rads.

**Tilted-Disc Syndrome,** which can be confused with papilledema or visual field defects from chiasmal compression, or both, is characterized by myopic astigmatism, situs inversus of the optic disc, congenital conus, lower nasal thinning of the retinal pigment epithelium and choroid and temporal hemianopia in which the field defects often cross

(9)   Radiology 120:167–171, July, 1976.

the vertical midline. Sue Ellen Young (M. D. Anderson Hosp., Houston), Frank B. Walsh and David L. Knox[1] (Johns Hopkins Hosp.) studied 6 males and 6 females aged 8–61 years, including 2 siblings. Only 2 patients sought help for visual or neurologic symptoms; both were women with headaches. Chiasmatic compression was suspected in 1 of these patients because of bitemporal field depression (Fig 57).

Retinoscopy showed myopia with simple astigmatism at an oblique axis in all patients. Astigmatism originated in the cornea in 2. Most of the visual field defects occurred superotemporally and crossed the vertical meridian with smaller isopters. Three patients had altitudinal defects. The field defects did not progress during 3 years in 2 patients. Fluorescein angiography showed thinning of the retinal pigment epithelium inferonasally, and retinoscopy showed more myopia inferonasally. Study of the eyes of a patient who died of carcinoma showed asymmetric disc tissue elevation, with the retinal pigment epithelium and choroid displaced away from the disc inferiorly. The sclera appeared to be thinner below than above. No apparent cause of the visual field defects was discovered. On several sections there were fewer larger choroid vessels below than above.

Fundic abnormalities comprise the major signs of the tilted-disc syndrome (table). The clinical importance of this syndrome relates to its confusion with papilledema and

**Fig 57.** – Fundus appearance of right eye (**A**) and left eye (**B**). Note situs inversus of optic discs, asymmetric inferonasal conus and better than usual visualization of larger choroid vasculature inferonasally. (Courtesy of Young, S. E., et al.: Am. J. Ophthalmol. 82:16–23, July, 1976.)

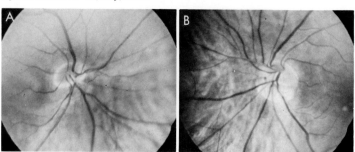

(1)   Am. J. Ophthalmol. 82:16–23, July, 1976.

CHARACTERISTICS OF TILTED-DISC SYNDROME

Fundus:     Tilted appearance (situs inversus)
                of disk (80% bilateral)
            ± conus (congenital)
            Hypopigmentation of inferonasal
                fundus
Refraction: Myopic astigmatism, oblique axis
Visual field: Bitemporal depression, usually
              Lack of true hemianopic defect
              Failure to progress
              Occasional altitudinal defect
X-ray films:  Normal sella turcica

signs of chiasmatic compression. Unnecessary neurodi-
agnostic procedures can be avoided in patients who exhibit
only this benign ocular condition, though its presence does
not exclude the simultaneous occurrence of intracranial
neoplasms or other intracranial disease.

# Medical Ophthalmology and Drug Therapy

INTRODUCTION

Shortly after cortisone and hydroxycortisone were synthesized in 1948 and 1950, they were tried as topical anti-inflammatory agents for ophthalmic use.[1, 2] It was apparent that this class of drugs could be used locally to modify inflammation in ocular disease. However, corticosteroid action was a double-edged sword; it potentiated infection throughout the body including the eye. Other major ocular side effects such as cataract formation and glaucoma were not recognized as complications of systemic and topical corticosteroid therapy until 10–15 years later. Various other ocular complications with topical corticosteroid therapy also have been noted, some of minor consequence, such as ptosis and miosis. Two monographs presented a comprehensive review of ocular corticosteroid therapy.[3, 4] More recent literature has dealt with: (1) penetration and anti-inflammatory efficacy of drug derivatives and their bioavailability; (2) steroid-induced glaucoma and dissociation of this effect from anti-inflammatory action; (3) routine use of topical corticosteroids in the postoperative cataract patient; and (4) new local delivery systems.

## Penetration, Bioavailability, Therapeutic Effectiveness

Over the past 5 years, Leibowitz, Kupferman and their associates developed an experimental model to evaluate ocular penetration of topical steroids into the cornea and anterior chamber. Their work has shown that differences in ocular penetration depend on the specific corticosteroid base, the derivative of that base, corticosteroid concentration, drug vehicle, presence or absence of corneal epithelium and the presence of corneal inflammation.[5-11]

The basic ocular penetration studies performed by Leibowitz and Kupferman involved topical application of a standard dose (0.05 ml) of a radiolabeled ($^{14}$C or $^{3}$H) corticosteroid on a rabbit cornea. Corneal and aqueous humor concentrations were determined from scintillation counting of the sample tissue or fluid. In many instances the radioactive steroid was prepared so that the solution was similar to the commercially available product.

The conclusions reached by Leibowitz and Kupferman confirmed some previous ideas of ocular drug penetration.[12] The epithelium and endothelium are lipophilic coats to a hydrophilic stroma. Therefore, corticosteroid penetration into all layers must be accomplished with biphasic polarity. Removal of epithelium increased stromal penetration of polar, water-soluble solutions, such as the phosphate derivative of corticosteroid preparations. Inflammation permitted some penetration of the epithelial barrier by more soluble polar compounds. The corticosteroid preparation with the best penetration in the cornea with an intact epithelium was 1% prednisolone acetate suspension. The corticosteroid preparation with the best penetration in the cornea with the epithelium removed was 1% prednisolone sodium phosphate solution. Corticosteroid concentrations found in the aqueous humor under the same conditions reflected a pattern similar to the corneal concentrations.

Leibowitz and Kupferman demonstrated that ocular penetration varied according to the corticosteroid base, prednisolone versus dexamethasone, and according to the derivative of the base, acetate, phosphate or alcohol. Important differences in drug penetration due to the vehicle were emphasized by studies of dexamethasone phosphate solution and ointment. Even though increased corneal contact time occurred when dexamethasone phosphate 0.05% ointment was applied, there was no increase in corneal drug concentration when compared with the application of 0.1% dexamethasone phosphate solution. The was true even when the amount of the ointment was doubled to give equal amounts of dexamethasone bases.[12]

Krupin and his co-workers[13] found higher aqueous humor

concentrations of topically applied 0.1% tritiated dexamethasone sodium phosphate in uninflamed rabbit eyes with intact corneal epithelium than were reported by Leibowitz and Kupferman. Some of the difference between their results and those of Leibowitz and Kupferman was attributed to the technique and the sensitivity of their assay. Some of their techniques were challenged by Leibowitz and Kupferman.[14] Sieg and Robinson observed that the corneal concentration of fluorometholone in rabbits could be influenced by the level of anesthesia and head position during application of the drug.[15]

Hull et al., using an isolated rabbit cornea perfusion chamber system, measured corneal permeability of four tritiated 1% corticosteroid preparations (not commercial products).[16] They concluded that prednisolone sodium phosphate, prednisolone acetate and fluorometholone penetrated the cornea equally well. Dexamethasone phosphate showed significantly less corneal penetrability. With removal of the epithelium, the corneal permeability to the phosphate preparations (dexamethasone and prednisolone) increased three- to fourfold, while the corneal permeability to prednisolone acetate and fluorometholone remained unchanged. Leibowitz and Kupferman also noted no significant change in penetration of fluorometholone 0.1% either with removal of epithelium or with corneal inflammation induced by clove oil.[11]

Leibowitz and Kupferman also developed a method for evaluating the anti-inflammatory effectiveness of a corticosteroid preparation.[17-22] This technique involved labeling replicating leukocytes of rabbits with tritiated thymidine and subsequently inducing corneal inflammation with intracorneal inoculation of clove oil. The anti-inflammatory effectiveness of topical corticosteroid preparations was determined by measuring corneal radioactivity. The reduction in migration of labeled leukocytes into the cornea was used as the standard to evaluate anti-inflammatory activity. They reported that 1% prednisone acetate suspension had the greatest anti-inflammatory effect when the epithelium was intact. With removal of the epithelium, the prednisolone acetate preparation was still the most effective agent, although it was not significantly better than the 1% prednisolone phosphate solution or the 0.1% dexamethasone alcohol suspension. The prednisolone phosphate solution was as effective against inflammation as the acetate preparation while at 4 times the tissue concentration. In addition, the anti-inflammatory activity of the prednisolone acetate was similar with or without corneal epithelium even though without epithelium the tissue drug level was almost twice as much. The 0.1% dexamethasone alcohol suspension was equally effective in suppressing inflammation with or without epithelium, although the tissue concentration was doubled without epithelium. The anti-inflammatory activity of 0.1% fluorometholone suspension was equal to 1% prednisolone phosphate solution when the epithelium was intact, and superior to 0.1% dexamethasone phosphate solution. The effect of fluorometholone increased slightly when applied to a cornea without epithelium.

Leibowitz and Kupferman concluded that the 1% prednisolone acetate suspension was the most effective anti-inflammatory agent evaluated by their method. In addition, they documented the fact that a change in the corticosteroid base (prednisolone or dexamethasone) and modification of the derivative of a given base (acetate, phosphate or alcohol) altered the anti-inflammatory capability of an agent. The derivative of a steroid base also affected the anti-inflammatory activity of different concentrations of the corticosteroid base. An increased concentration of the prednisolone acetate preparation (from 0.125% to 1%), produced an increase in corneal concentration and anti-inflammatory effectiveness, while a similar increase in topical concentration of prednisolone phosphate (from 0.125% to 1%) produced a significant increase in corneal concentration, but not in anti-inflammatory activity.

### Steroid-Induced Glaucoma

The second aspect of topical corticosteroid therapy that has attracted much attention is the increase in intraocular pressure which occurs in susceptible individuals. It has been demonstrated that 0.1% dexamethasone phosphate, one of the most potent ocular hypertensive drugs when tested in patients with no ocular disease is the same drug that Leibowitz and Kupferman found to have the poorest corneal penetrability.

Many studies have been done on the dissociation of anti-inflammatory and ocular hypertensive effects of corticosteroids. Some of these studies have been based on dose-response relationships. Armaly showed that a 10-times diluted dexamethasone preparation (0.01%) applied 3 times daily for 4 weeks caused only a mild pressure rise in highly sensitive individuals.[23-25] However, Podos and Becker showed that even 20-times diluted dexamethasone (0.005%) given 4 times a day for 2 to 6 weeks induced significant elevation of intraocular pressure in about half of a group of sensitive individuals.[26, 27] Dose frequency and duration may explain the differences in these results. Dexamethasone 0.001% was much less prone to induce ocular hypertension, but the anti-inflammatory activity of this dose of steroid has not been well studied. However, Lorenzetti et al. showed that dexamethasone in dilutions up to 0.001% effectively prevented heterograft rejection when donor pig cornea was placed in lamellar pockets of rabbit corneas.[28]

New steroid products have been tested in attempts to dissociate the anti-inflammatory and ocular hypertensive effects. Medrysone 1% had very little potential for elevating intraocular pressure but it also was a very weak anti-inflammatory agent clinically. The fact that Lorenzetti et al. showed that medrysone 1% suppressed graft rejection in their model may indicate only that the model is very "steroid sensitive."

It was once thought that the varying ocular hypertensive potential of different corticosteroids was due to differences in ocular penetration. However, this was not true for triamcinolone and tetrahydrotriamcinolone (THTC). Sugar et al. showed that tetrahydrotriamcinolone had significantly less ocular hypertensive effect and anti-inflammatory effect than triamcinolone even though THTC and triamcinolone penetrated the eye equally well.[29, 30] This led some investigators to conclude that there are specialized steroid-sensitive receptors for intraocular pressure in the anterior segment of the eye which have varying sensitivities to different corticosteroid compounds.

Cantrill et al. compared the in vitro potency of various corticosteroids to their ocular hypertensive effects.[31] They pointed out that corticosteroids affect several components of the inflammatory response; among these are vascular permeability, phagocytosis, lymphocyte activation, antibody synthesis and chemotaxis. They selected lymphocyte transformation by phytohemagglutinin as their in vitro model of inflammatory response and measured the ability of various corticosteroids to inhibit this response. The steroids studied for ocular hypertensive effect were dexamethasone phosphate 0.1%, dexamethasone phosphate 0.005%, medrysone 1%, tetrahydrotriamcinolone 0.25%, hydrocortisone 0.5%, prednisolone acetate 1% and fluorometholone 0.1%. Steroids studied for anti-inflammatory potency included dexamethasone phosphate, prednisolone phosphate, fluorometholone, medrysone, tetrahydrotriamcinolone and hydrocortisone phosphate. Dexamethasone and fluorometholone were more than 20 times more potent than hydrocortisone, the reference steroid, in anti-inflammatory effectiveness in vitro. With this in vitro measure of potency, prednisolone acetate, medrysone and tetrahydrotriamcinolone were relatively weak. Medrysone, tetrahydrotriamcinolone and hydrocortisone had modest ocular hypertensive effects in susceptible patients. Dexamethasone 0.1% had the greatest ocular hypertensive effect, 3.5 times that of fluorometholone and 2 times that of prednisolone phosphate. A 1/20 dilution of dexamethasone 0.1% (0.005%) had the same ocular hypertensive effect as fluorometholone 0.1%. Some differences might be explained on the basis of the derivatives, formulation, vehicle or concentration of the drugs tested. For example, Cantrill et al. used fluorometholone, medrysone and prednisolone in a highly viscous vehicle while dexamethasone, hydrocortisone and tetrahydrotriamcinolone were used in buffered aqueous solution. In this study prednisolone acetate was not the most effective anti-inflammatory agent, as Leibowitz and Kupferman reported.

Therefore, studies on the dissociation of anti-inflammatory effects from the ocular hypertensive effects indicate that dexamethasone phosphate is one of the most potent ocular hypertensive steroids, yet it penetrates the cornea poorly after topical administration. However, there is certainly a difference in the mechanism of the two effects: although the anti-inflammatory effect is more immediate and appears to be related to vascular permeability and suppression of leukocyte migration, the ocular hypertensive effect is delayed. This can be related to dose frequency and duration and may be based on a decrease in outflow facility; it may possibly be related to different receptors.

## Routine Postoperative Use of Corticosteroids

A third area of interest is the routine use of corticosteroid therapy after cataract extraction. Knopf in 1970 showed that 0.1% fluorometholone and 2.5% hydrocortisone acetate were equally effective in decreasing postoperative inflammation in cataract patients; however, no untreated control group was included in the study.[32]

Burde and Waltman studied postoperative iritis in a double-blind method using dexamethasone phosphate 0.1% and its diluent as a placebo.[33] These drops were used three times daily for the first 20 postoperative days. No differences were noted in conjunctival reaction, keratopathy, applanation pressures or vitreous reaction. The code was broken in 27 patients in order to place them on dexamethasone because of severe anterior chamber reaction. Thirteen patients were already on the steroid. In addition, a significantly higher incidence of iris prolapse and filtering blebs developed in patients treated with steroids.

Mustakallio et al. conducted a two-center double-blind study of steroids in postoperative uveitis.[34] In one center, Isopto Tears, 0.1% dexamethasone alcohol and 2.5% hydrocortisone acetate were compared on a once-a-day dose. The second center compared dexamethasone phosphate 0.1% and saline on a regimen of 2 drops 3 times daily. Although a significant difference in flare was seen on days 5–7 between steroid and placebo in one center, no other significant difference was found. The conclusion was that topical steroids had minimal effect on postoperative inflammation with a dose 1–3 times daily.

A more recent study by Corboy compared betamethasone phosphate 0.1%, 5 times daily for 2 weeks, with a placebo.[35] Patients with minimal postoperative reactions were excluded. Improvement was judged by conjunctival and corneal reactions; no measure was made of anterior chamber cell and flare. The steroid treated group showed improvement related to conjunctival parameters and overall symptoms. No ocular complications were noted in the steroid group. These data may show the drug's efficacy in postoperative keratoconjunctivitis but they do not provide information on postoperative iritis. Of concern is the relatively heavy dose of steroids for what appears to be a benign process in most instances.

Several studies have shown decreased tensile strength of wounds treated in the early postoperative period with steroid. The Burde and Waltman study revealed an increase in iris prolapse and filtering blebs. Wound problems were not seen in Corboy's study. Rabbit corneal wound healing studies by McDonald et al. also showed inhibition of stromal healing by dexamethasone derivatives.[36] In these experiments, dose response inhibition studies revealed anti-inflammatory effectiveness with dexamethasone alcohol at the 0.001% concentration, dexamethasone phosphate at the 0.01% concentration and dexamethasone acetate at the 0.1% concentration. The anti-inflammatory potency of the acetate derivative differed from studies by Leibowitz and Kupferman. Wound healing and suppression of leukocyte migration apparently were not related. Wound healing effects, however, should be considered in the risk-benefit ratio for routine use of corticosteroids in the cataract patient.

## New Delivery System

Although continuous release systems for topical corticosteroids are not yet commercially available, they appear to have clinical potential. Dohlman et al. used a model of corneal xenograft rejection in rabbits to compare the continuous Ocusert delivery of hydrocortisone acetate versus various doses of topical hydrocortisone acetate drops.[37] Ocuserts with release rates of $0.1 - 9 \mu g$ per hour had anti-inflammatory effects equal to topical preparations in concentrations of $0.0025 - 2.5\%$, 4 times daily. Topical applications of $0.25 - 2.5\%$ or Ocuserts with release rates of $0.1 - 7 \mu g$ per hour had equal inhibitory effect on the onset and development of corneal and uveal inflammation. In other experiments, the corneal and uveal inflammations were allowed to reach maximum, and equal therapeutic effects were achieved with 0.25% drops or a 2 $\mu$g per hour continuous-release system, and with 2.5% drops or a 9 $\mu$g per hour continuous release system. The amount of drug delivered to the eye was about 700–7,000 $\mu$g/24 hours with topical medication compared to between 2.5 and 215 $\mu$g/24 hours with the continuous steroid delivery.

Lerman et al. compared the effectiveness of the continuous delivery of hydrocortisone acetate to drop therapy.[38] Using an experimental model of immune keratitis, induced by bovine serum albumin (BSA), they found the amount of corticosteroid required to suppress inflammation with the Ocusert system was only $\frac{1}{6}$ to $\frac{1}{7}$ of the dose required by topical hydrocortisone ointment, and $\frac{1}{12}$ the dosage when compared with prednisolone.

Keller et al. employed another model of ocular inflammation.[39] Rabbits sensitized to BSA were challenged with BSA without any surgery or abrasion (as in previous models). The continuous delivery systems with hydrocortisone acetate or prednisolone acetate suppressed the immunologic conjunctivitis equally or better than the comparable steroid eye drop.

Allansmith et al. reported the use of sustained release hydrocortisone ocular inserts in humans with ocular atopy induced by pollen extract.[40] With inserts releasing about 10 $\mu$g per hour hydrocortisone, a small but significant suppression of inflammation occurred. A second trial in 8 patients with external ocular disease of immunologic origin showed clinical improvement in 7 of the 8 patients. Retention of the ocular inserts proved to be a problem; 85% were retained in trained volunteers and 50% in untrained patients. In addition, mild discomfort occurred on insertion but the device was generally well tolerated.

Continuous-release steroid devices may be effective in the treatment of ocular inflammation, and they deliver a much smaller total drug dosage than do conventional drops or ointment therapy. These lower doses may obviate apparent dose-related side effects such as steroid-induced glaucoma and cataracts.

## Conclusion

Rational use of various topical corticosteroid preparations calls for studies of differences in ocular penetration, bioavailability and anti-inflammatory effectiveness. The results of any investigation must be evaluated according to the experimental model used. Ultimately all animal models must be evaluated with regard to their applicability to human therapeutics. The new sustained release delivery systems, if proved practical, may eliminate certain side effects by decreasing the total dosage of drug delivered while maintaining prolonged therapeutic levels.

S. Lance Forstot, M.D.
Philip P. Ellis, M.D.
University of Colorado

## REFERENCES

1. McClean, J. M., Gordon, D. M., and Kateen, H.: Clinical Experiences with ACTH and Cortisone in Ocular Diseases, Trans. Am. Acad. Ophthalmol. Otolaryngol. 55:565, 1951.
2. Woods, A. C.: The Present Status of ACTH and Cortisone in Clinical Ophthalmology, The Gifford Memorial Lecture, Am. J. Ophthalmol. 34:945, 1951.
3. Schwartz, B. (ed.): *Corticosteroids and the Eye,* Int. Ophthalmol. Clin., Vol. 6, No. 4 (Boston: Little, Brown and Company, 1966).
4. Kaufman, H. E. (ed.): *Ocular Anti-inflammatory Therapy* (Springfield, Ill.: Charles C Thomas, Publisher, 1970).
5. Cox, W. V., Kupferman, A., and Leibowitz, H. M.: Topically Applied Steroids in Corneal Disease: I. The Role of Inflammation in Stromal Absorption of Dexamethasone, Arch. Ophthalmol. 88:308, 1972.
6. Cox, W. V., Kupferman, A., and Leibowitz, H. M.: Topically Applied Steroids in Corneal Disease: II. The Role of Drug Vehicle in Stomal Absorption of Dexamethasone, Arch. Ophthalmol. 88:549, 1972.
7. Kupferman, A., Pratt, M. V., Suckewer, K., and Leibowitz, H. M.: Topically Applied Steroids in Corneal Disease: III. The Role of Drug Derivative in Stromal Absorption of Dexamethasone, Arch. Ophthalmol. 91:373, 1974.
8. Kupferman, A., and Leibowitz, H. M.: Topically Applied Ste-

roids in Corneal Disease: IV. The Role of Drug Concentration in Stromal Absorption of Prednisolone Acetate, Arch. Ophthalmol. 91:377, 1974.

9. Kupferman, A., and Leibowitz, H. M.: Topically Applied Steroids in Corneal Disease: V. Dexamethasone Alcohol, Arch. Ophthalmol. 92:329, 1974.

10. Kupferman, A., and Leibowitz, H. M.: Topically Applied Steroids in Corneal Disease: VI. Kinetics of Prednisolone Sodium Phosphate, Arch. Ophthalmol. 92:331, 1974.

11. Kupferman, A., and Leibowitz, H. M.: Penetration of Fluorometholone into the Cornea and Aqueous Humor, Arch. Ophthalmol. 93:425, 1975.

12. Leibowitz, H. M., and Kupferman, A.: Bioavailability and Therapeutic Effectiveness of Topically Administered Corticosteroids, Trans. Am. Acad. Ophthalmol. Otolaryngol. 79:OP 78, 1975.

13. Krupin, T., Waltman, S. R., and Becker, B.: Ocular Penetration in Rabbits of Topically Applied Dexamethasone, Arch. Ophthalmol. 92:312, 1974.

14. Leibowitz, H. M., and Kupferman, A.: Ocular Penetration in Rabbits of Topically Applied Dexamethasone, Arch. Ophthalmol. 93:315, 1975.

15. Sieg, J. W., and Robinson, J. R.: Corneal Absorption of Fluorometholone in Rabbits: A Comparative Evaluation of Corneal Drug Transport Characteristics in Anesthetized and Unanesthetized Rabbits, Arch. Ophthalmol. 92:240, 1974.

16. Hull, D. S., Hine, J. E., Edelhauser, H. F., and Hyndiuk, R. A.: Permeability of the Isolated Rabbit Cornea to Corticosteroids, Invest. Ophthalmol. 13:457, 1974.

17. Leibowitz, H. M., Lass, J. H., and Kupferman, A.: Quantitation of Inflammation in the Cornea, Arch. Ophthalmol. 92:427, 1974.

18. Leibowitz, H. M., and Kupferman, A.: Anti-inflammatory Effectiveness in the Cornea of Topically Administered Prednisolone, Invest. Ophthalmol. 13:757, 1974.

19. Kupferman, A., and Leibowitz, H. M.: Anti-inflammatory Effectiveness of Topically Administered Corticosteroids in the Cornea without Epithelium, Invest. Ophthalmol. 14:252, 1975.

20. Leibowitz, H. M., and Kupferman, A.: Pharmacology and Topically Applied Dexamethasone, Trans. Am. Acad. Ophthalmol. Otolaryngol. 78:856, 1974.

21. Kupferman, A., and Leibowitz, H. M.: Therapeutic Effectiveness of Fluorometholone in Inflammatory Keratitis, Arch. Ophthalmol. 93:1011, 1975.

22. Leibowitz, H. M., and Kupferman, A.: Topically Administered Corticosteroids and Treatment of Inflammatory Keratitis, Invest. Ophthalmol. 14:337, 1975.

23. Armaly, M. F.: Dexamethasone Ocular Hypertension in the Clinically Normal Eye: II. The Untreated Eye, Outflow Toxicity and Concentration, Arch. Ophthalmol. 75:776, 1966.

24. Armaly, M. F.: *Steroids and Glaucoma.* In Symposium on Glaucoma, Trans. New Orleans Acad. Ophthalmol. (St. Louis: The C. V. Mosby Company, 1967 [pp. 74–128]).

25. Armaly, M. F.: Factors Affecting the Dose-Response Relationship in Steroid-Induced Ocular Hypertension. In Kaufman, H. E. (ed.): *Ocular Anti-inflammatory Therapy* (Springfield, Ill.: Charles C Thomas, Publisher, 1970 [pp. 88–105]).

26. Podos, S. M., Kolker, A. E., and Becker, B.: Topical Corticosteroids: Dissociation of Effects. In Kaufman, H. E. (ed.): *Ocular Anti-inflammatory Therapy* (Springfield, Ill.: Charles C Thomas, Publisher, 1970 [pp. 106–116]).

27. Podos, S. M., and Becker, B.: Intraocular Pressure Effects of Diluted and New Topical Corticosteroids. In Leopold, I. H. (ed.): *Symposium on Ocular Therapy,* Vol. 5 (St. Louis: The C. V. Mosby Company, 1972 [pp. 90–95]).

28. Lorenzetti, D. W. C., Ellison, E. M., and Kaufman, H. E.: Quantitative Steroid Effect on Graft Rejection, Arch. Ophthalmol. 79:64, 1968.

29. Sugar, J., Burde, R. M., Sugar, A., Waltman, S. R., Kripalani, K. J., Weliky, I., and Becker, B.: Tetrahydrotriamcinolone and Triamcinolone: I. Ocular Penetration, Invest. Ophthalmol. 11:890, 1972.

30. Sugar, J., Sugar, A., and Burde, R. M.: Tetrahydrotriamcinolone and Triamcinolone: II. Effect on Xenograft Reaction in Rabbits, Invest. Ophthalmol. 11:894, 1972.

31. Cantrill, H. L., Palmberg, P. F., Zink, H. A., Waltman, S. R., Podos, S. M., and Becker, B.: Comparison of In Vitro Potency of Corticosteroids with Ability to Raise Intraocular Pressure, Am. J. Ophthalmol. 79:1012, 1975.

32. Knopf, M. M.: A Double-Blind Study of Fluorometholone, Am. J. Ophthalmol. 70:739, 1970.

33. Burde, R. M., and Waltman, S. R.: Topical Corticosteroids after Cataract Surgery, Ann. Ophthalmol. 4:290, 1972.

34. Mustakallio, A., Kaufman, H. E., Johnston, G., Wilson, R. S., Roberts, M. D., and Harter, J. C.: Corticosteroid Efficacy in Postoperative Uveitis, Ann. Ophthalmol. 5:719, 1973.

35. Corboy, J. M.: Corticosteroid Therapy for the Reduction of Postoperative Inflammation after Cataract Extraction, Am. J. Ophthalmol. 82:923, 1976.

36. McDonald, T. O., Borgmann, A. R., Roberts, M. D., and Fox, L. G.: Corneal Wound Healing: I. Inhibition of Stromal Healing by Three Dexamethasone Derivatives, Invest. Ophthalmol. 9: 703, 1970.
37. Dohlman, C. H., Pavan-Langston, D., and Rose, J.: A New Ocular Insert Device for Continuous Constant-Rate Delivery of Medication to the Eye, Ann. Ophthalmol. 4:823, 1972.
38. Lerman, S., Davis, P., and Jackson, W. B.: Prolonged-Release Hydrocortisone Therapy, Can. J. Ophthalmol. 8:114, 1973.
39. Keller, N., Longwell, A. M., and Birss, S. A.: Intermittent vs. Continuous Steroid Administration. Efficacy in Experimental Conjunctivitis, Arch. Ophthalmol. 94:644, 1976.
40. Allansmith, M. R., Lee, J. R., McClellan, B. H., and Dohlman, C. H.: Evaluation of a Sustained Release Hydrocortisone Ocular Insert in Humans, Trans. Am. Acad. Ophthalmol. Otolaryngol. 79:OP 128, 1975.

**Prematurity and the Eye: Ophthalmic 10-Year Follow-up of Children of Low and Normal Birth Weight.** Hans Fledelius[2] (Copenhagen) reports the results of a prospective pediatric study done in 1959–61 on 9,006 consecutive pregnancies. The present material consists of 302 surviving children who weighed under 2,000 gm at birth and 237 full-term control children weighing 3–4 kg at birth. The groups are comparable; the respective follow-up rates were 90 and 74%. Refraction values showed leptokurtosis around a slightly hypermetropic mean value and a skewness toward myopia. The premature group showed little shift toward myopia compared with the mature children, due to a percentage of eyes with early myopia. Ultrasonic oculometry showed a size deficit of the average premature eye of about 0.3 mm in axial length and vitreous length and of 0.18 mm in corneal curvature radius. Exophthalmometric values were lower in the premature children.

Blindness occurred in 1% of the premature children. The rates of attainment of 6/18 or better acuity were 96.2% for premature eyes and 98.2% for mature eyes. Prematures showed a significant shift toward lower scores. Heterotropia was noted in 22.5% of premature and 5.9% of mature children. In both groups, about a third of the children with heterotropia had squint amblyopia; concomitant squint was the

(2) Acta Ophthalmol. (Suppl. 128) (Kbh.):1976.

predominant type. Fusion was entirely lacking in 18.5% of premature and 5.5% of mature cases. Stereopsis was absent in 16.7 and 3.8% of children, respectively. Retrolental fibroplasia was diagnosed in 5 premature children. Ophthalmoscopic signs of "minor" retinal damage were more common in the premature group. Of the 13 children with lens changes 11 were prematures. Ocular malformations were found in 5% of premature and 2% of mature children. Multiple-birth premature children were ophthalmologically like the single-birth prematures. Overall ocular status was not significantly related to such conditions as social status, asphyxia, neonatal jaundice or signs of central nervous system damage in the 1st year of life.

The premature group must definitely be considered one at risk from the ocular point of view. Prophylaxis consists of efforts to reduce the frequency of premature birth, and to have optimal care during the neonatal period especially relative to the use of oxygen. Prematures below a birth weight of 2,000 gm should have ophthalmologic followup for at least the first months of life, and then annually to prevent or correct such abnormalities as amblyopia from strabismus or anisometropia, and myopia and to provide social/educational measures in cases of visual defect.

▶ [This is a monograph of 245 pages, not only containing the author's 10-year follow-up statistics, but also a complete review of the literature. — Ed.] ◀

**Acute Transient Ophthalmomalacia in Giant Cell Arteritis: Report of a Case** is presented by Morten Verdich and Niels Vesti Nielsen[3] (Nykøbing Falster, Denmark). The common manifestations of temporal arteritis leading to severe visual impairment are ischemic optic neuropathy or central retinal artery occlusion. Rarely the disease causes ophthalmomalacia with severe, transient visual impairment due to massive corneal edema. If the nutrition of the optic nerve and retina is unaffected, vision gradually returns.

Woman, 83, was admitted with near-total blindness and a tentative diagnosis of temporal arteritis. Swelling had been noted in the temporal regions a month before, followed by severe pain in the scalp and, over 1 day, progressive visual impairment in both eyes.

(3) Acta Ophthalmol. (Kbh.) 53:875–878, December, 1975.

The patient was under treatment for an ischemic cardiac condition. Hand movements were seen at 2 m on the right and light only on the left. Biomicroscopy showed severe bilateral corneal edema. Intraocular pressures were 6 mm Hg in the right eye and 5 mm Hg in the left. Ophthalmoscopy showed red reflexes only. The blood pressure was 200/100 mm Hg and the pulse was irregular. Tender superficial cutaneous ulcerations were seen on the scalp, with nodular thickening of both superficial temporal arteries. A biopsy specimen from the right artery showed giant cell arteritis. Systemic prednisone was given and hydrocortisone-antibiotic drops were used in both eyes. Vision remitted as the corneas cleared and tension increased in both eyes. At the same time the cranial pain subsided. Acuity was 6/9 on the right and 6/12 on the left with correction, after 2 weeks. Ophthalmoscopy showed a slightly pale left optic disc, a small exudate and narrow retinal arterioles.

This patient fulfilled several criteria for giant cell arteritis. The vascular supply to the anterior part of the left optic nerve was disturbed. The ocular lesion was probably due primarily to a transiently compromised blood supply to the ciliary body caused by giant cell arteritis, which had resulted in occlusion of the long posterior ciliary arteries.

**Leukemic Ophthalmopathy in Children.** Involvement of the central nervous system (CNS) as a complication of acute childhood leukemia is becoming more frequent, presumably because of longer survivals with more effective chemotherapy. Elizabeth W. Ridgway, Norman Jaffe and David S. Walton[4] (Harvard Med. School) studied the clinical manifestations of ocular leukemia in 657 children treated for acute leukemia during 1965–73, 150 of whom were referred for evaluation of eye complaints. The children were treated by sequential single-agent chemotherapy. Prophylactic treatment for CNS disease was not given but established CNS disease was treated by intrathecal methotrexate, sometimes in combination with radiotherapy.

Ocular abnormalities were found in 52 children, most of whom had acute lymphoblastic or undifferentiated leukemia. Concurrent marrow relapse was demonstrated in 30 children. Retinal hemorrhages were found in 37% of the 52 affected patients and in 10 they were seen at initial presentation. Asymptomatic flame-shaped hemorrhages involving

(4)   Cancer 38:1744–1749, October, 1976.

the nerve fiber layer were most frequent. Invasion of the optic nerve, retina, iris or orbit occurred in 56% of the patients. Nine patients had optic nerve infiltration and 6 had orbital infiltration. Nine patients had anterior segment involvement. Retinal infiltration was seen in 6 patients; it was asymptomatic.

Optic nerve infiltration was treated by irradiation, which led to shrinkage of the infiltrates but usually not to improvement in vision. Most patients given topical dexamethasone ointment for anterior segment involvement responded. Retinal infiltrates were treated by local irradiation in 3 patients, with complete clearing resulting. Orbital irradiation led to only partial response of infiltration of the orbit in 1 patient.

Leukemic invasion of the eye should receive appropriate recognition and the posterior pole should be included in the treatment of the CNS when prophylactic radiotherapy is given.

► [A previous study by Allen and Straatsma (see the 1962-63 YEAR BOOK, p. 375) indicated that at the time of death from leukemia the eye was usually involved. Infiltrates of leukemic cells and hemorrhage were seen, most frequently in highly vascular tissues such as the retina. The above study in children showed ocular involvement coincident with or following CNS involvement, that responded poorly to sequential treatment with methotrexate, 6-mercaptopurine, vincristine and prednisone, cyclophosphamide, arabinosyl cytosine, L-asparaginase and daunorubicin. Accordingly, anterior ocular segment involvement was treated with local steroids, and posterior involvement with irradation (1,000 rads in 3–5 days). – Eds.] ◄

**X-Linked Ocular Albinism: Oculocutaneous Macromelanosomal Disorder.** The types of ocular albinism proposed include the Nettleship-Falls classical X-linked type, the Forsuis-Eriksson X-linked type accompanied by an atypical protoanomalous defect and punctate ocular albinism (autosomal). Francis E. O'Donnell, Jr., George W. Hambrick, Jr., W. Richard Green, W. Jackson Iliff and David L. Stone[5] (Johns Hopkins Med. Inst.) report findings in the family of a patient with ocular albinism and severe renal failure and those in 2 unrelated families, indicating that the Nettleship-Falls X-linked type represents a disturbance in the morphogenesis of melanin granules.

(5) Arch. Ophthalmol. 94:1883–1892, November, 1976.

Three unrelated kindreds with the Nettleship-Falls type of X-linked ocular albinism were studied. Biopsy specimens of clinically normal skin were taken from 8 affected males and 9 carrier females. Both eyes of an affected man were examined after death. Specimens of hypopigmented patches in 2 affected male patients and of slate-colored skin in another were also examined.

In this form of ocular albinism, affected men have photophobia, reduced visual acuity, nystagmus and often ocular deviations. The electroretinogram may show a supernormal scotopic response. Ophthalmoscopy showed an apparent macular hypoplasia with absent foveal reflex. At least some pigment can be present. Carrier women are typically asymptomatic but they often have a partial iris translucency. The postmortem study of one proband showed fewer melanosomes than normal and macromelanosomes within the pigment epithelia. Normal skin exhibited giant pigment granules in all affected men and carrier women studied. The hypopigmented areas examined showed only minimal normal pigment granules and no giant melanosomes.

Albinism can be viewed as the consequence of at least two types of disturbed melanogenesis, altered melanin formation and disturbed melanosome formation. In the various types of oculocutaneous albinism, the primary disturbance in melanogenesis at the ultrastructural level appears to be inadequate synthesis of melanin. In contrast, the Nettleship-Falls type of X-linked ocular albinism, like partial albinism in the Chediak-Higashi syndrome, is apparently due to a disturbance in melanosome structure characterized by giant pigment granules.

**Multiple Nevobasocellular Epitheliomatosis Syndrome** is a disease with simultaneous involvement of several systems — skin, orofacial mass, skeleton, endocrine glands, central nervous system and eye and its adnexa. Originally known as Gorlin's syndrome, it was officially named "multiple nevobasocellular epitheliomatosis" by the American Academy of Dermatology in 1963.

H. Hammami, R. Faggioni, E. B. Streiff and B. Daiker[6] (Univ. of Lausanne) report a case.

(6) Ophthalmologica 172:382–399, 1976.

Woman, 50, since age 20 had regularly had either radiotherapy, excisions or cauterizations of many cutaneous lesions on the face, elbow, thorax, abdomen and upper limbs. They were often pigmented lesions of tumoral appearance. Histologically, they were either a simple basocellular epithelioma, a basocellular nevus or an epithelioma with caseation. Since age 16, the patient had had acne on the face and uncomfortable hypertrichosis. At age 32, she underwent removal of a germinal cyst of the left ovary.

Examination confirmed a characteristic facies – a somewhat large nasal base, but without true hypertelorism, and frontal bosses. The face was red and telangiectatic because of marked acne.

From the ophthalmologic viewpoint, in 1969, radiotherapy had been given to palpebral lesions. Also, melanosis of the caruncle of the left eye; vascularized, symmetric, lower and bilateral marginal corneal leukomas; and, in the back of the eye, a pigmented nevus on the edge of the papilla were verified. Visual acuity and field were normal. In 1971, there was decreased vision of the right eye. Radiologic examination of the cranium and carotid arteriography showed ectopic calcification of the dura mater, but ruled out a widespread intracranial process such as meningioma.

Later, the patient was treated for recurrent marginal keratitis which gradually progressed toward the center of the cornea. Radiography of the jaws showed either primary or dental cysts with teeth within.

The endocrine examination confirmed from the adrenal point of view, plasma cortisol, hydroxysteroid and urinary ketosteroids, which gave a clinical impression of atypical Cushing's syndrome of the "thin type" due to adrenal hyperplasia. Study of the parathyroid and thyroid hormones revealed pseudohypoparathyroidism.

Review of 148 cases from the literature revealed that genetic transmission is of the dominant type. The clinical pic-

SYSTEMATIZED PRINCIPAL CHARACTERISTICS OF THE
MULTIPLE NEVOBASOCELLULAR EPITHELIOMATOSIS SYNDROME

| SYSTEM | CHARACTERISTICS |
|---|---|
| Skin | Multiple malignant nevobasocellular lesions. |
| Skeleton | Multiple cysts of the mandibles; costal anomalies (bifid ribs); vertebral anomalies; anomalies of the sella turcica. |
| Central nervous system | Predisposition to medulloblastoma (infantile form); mental retardation; intracranial ectopic calcifications of the falx cerebri and dura mater. |
| Endocrine system | Pseudohypoparathyroidism; ovarian or testicular involvement; Cushing's syndrome. |
| Eye and adnexa | Hypertelorism; basocellular epithelioma of the eyelids; strabismus; congenital or early cataract. |

ture of the patient studied was similar to the Gorlin syndrome in regard to the various systems involved (table). An associated neoplastic pathology provoking cutaneous lesions and tumors secreting hormones or similar substances is suggested.

**Ocular Pathology in the Elfin Face Syndrome (Fanconi-Schlesinger Type of Idiopathic Hypercalcemia of Infancy): Histochemical and Ultrastructural Study of a Case** is reported by O. A. Jensen, Mette Warburg and Annalise Dupont[7]. The Fanconi-Schlesinger type of idiopathic hypercalcemia of infancy (IHI) is characterized by mental retardation and a characteristic facies. The infants are often small for dates and fail to thrive. The serum calcium is elevated for only the first $2-3$ years of life. Pathognomonic cardiovascular anomalies are seen. The ocular pathology was studied in a patient with IHI, admitted to an institution for the retarded at age 13 and examined at age 40. The patient died at age 42 shortly after rupture of a diverticulum of the sigmoid. Autopsy showed supravalvular aortic stenosis, a hypoplastic aorta, pancreatic carcinoma with nodal metastases and perisigmoiditis.

Stains for calcium were strongly positive in corneal epithelial and endothelial cells, corneal keratocytes and the stroma, as well as in conjunctival and scleral epithelial cells. Needle-like deposits were seen in the cells staining for calcium, usually in both the nucleus and cytoplasm, on ultrastructural study. Single crystals were about 50 Å wide and 0.1 $\mu$m or less in length that formed star-shaped aggregates $0.2-0.5$ $\mu$m in diameter. The crystals were morphologically identical with experimentally produced precursors of calcium hydroxyapatite crystals. The electron diffraction pattern was similar to that of calcium hydroxyapatite. Extracellular deposits were found in the corneal stroma that resembled the extracellular conjunctival deposits seen in renal failure and in band keratopathy. Stains for calcium were also positive in the aortic wall, kidneys, the adrenals and spleen.

It may be possible to verify abnormal calcium metabolism in autopsies of patients suspected of having this syndrome.

(7) Ophthalmologica 172:434–444, 1976.

A conjunctival biopsy specimen stained for calcium and ultrastructural study may be diagnostically helpful.

► [This report describes the deposits of calcium hydroxyapatite in the conjunctiva, cornea and sclera in one of the 4 patients reported previously (Dupont et al.: Dan. Med. Bull. 17:33, 1970). A biopsy of the conjunctiva in infants suspected of this disorder can be helpful. — Ed.] ◄

► ↓ The following four articles by "splitters" of somewhat similar clinical syndromes with autosomal recessive inheritance are valuable in that usually a single enzyme deficiency can explain the accumulation and storage of complex sugars, lipids and amino acids in the lysosomes of many diverse tissues. Although replacement of the deficient enzymes is not yet possible, reduction of intake of the storage material can be helpful clinically (see article by Goldsmith and Reed). Detection of an enzyme deficiency can be done conveniently by analysis of tears (see articles by Johnson et al. and Libert et al.), urine, plasma and biopsies of conjunctiva and skin and cultures of fibroblasts to demonstrate the storage material in the lysosomes. — Ed. ◄

### New Mucolipidosis with Psychomotor Retardation, Corneal Clouding and Retinal Degeneration.

Frank W. Newell, Reuben Matalon and Steven Meyer[8] (Univ. of Chicago) report data on a patient with I cell disease, who has survived to age 22 with corneal clouding and extensive retinal degeneration.

Man, 22, had been seen in the 1st year of life with inguinal hernia and slow psychomotor development. A toxic goiter was removed from the mother in the 2nd month of pregnancy. Generalized hypotonia was present with brisk deep reflexes at age 13 months and a left esotropia was noted. Severe corneal clouding was noted at about age 2; it was variable and appeared as a smoky haze of gray-brown color, involving mainly the anterior stroma. Intermittent severe eye pain was noted; the cause was never discovered. Gingival bleeding at age 14 years was corrected by ascorbic acid. Truncal ataxia and muscular hypotonia of the extremities were noted at this time. Vision was estimated at finger counting at 2 feet. The esotropia was less marked than before. The corneal clouding was severe centrally. The optic discs were atrophic and hypoplastic. The scotopic and photopic electroretinogram was extinguished. Conjunctival biopsy specimen at age 21 showed single membrane-limited vacuoles filling numerous epithelial cells, some containing a polymorphous material. Similar inclusion bodies were found in cultured skin fibroblasts ("I-cells"). Lysosomal hydrolases were normal.

Features of the various mucolipidoses are summarized in

(8) Trans. Am. Ophthalmol. Soc. 73:172-186, 1975.

CLINICAL AND DIAGNOSTIC FEATURES OF MUCOLIPIDOSIS

| Name of disorder | Skeletal dysplasia. Course facies | Corneal clouding | Intracellular lesions | | Enzyme deficiency | Fibroblast inclusions | Onset |
|---|---|---|---|---|---|---|---|
| | | | Membranous lamellar bodies | Single membrane limited vacuoles | | | |
| Mucolipidosis I[3] | ±<br>± | ± | + | + | 0 | + | 6 months |
| Mucolipidosis II[11] (Inclusion-cell disease) | +<br>+ | ±<br>1 of 10 cases | + | + | + | + | Birth † |
| Mucolipidosis III[10] pseudo-Hurler polydystrophy | +<br>+ | + | + | + | N.R. | + | 7 years |
| Mucolipidosis IV[12] (Berman) | 0<br>0 | + | + | + | 0 | + | Birth* |
| Present case | 0<br>0 | + | + | + | 0 | + | 9 months |

*Findings described at age 8 months.

†$\beta$-Galactosidase of liver 20–30% normal; $\beta$-N-acetylhexosaminidase 60–90% normal; lysosomal hydrolases 5–20% normal.

N.R., not reported.

the table. Patients with lysosomal storage disease constitute a unique clinical and biochemical resource. The enzymatic deficiency and chemical nature of the storage substance in the present case are not known.

McCulloch points out that variants of the standard patterns of mucolipidosis are now appearing. Maumenee believes that the deposition of abnormal amounts of acid mucopolysaccharide in the pigment epithelium disturbs the essential metabolic functions of the retinal pigment epithelium, and that photoreceptor degeneration may be secondary to interference with pigment epithelial function. Study of the mucolipidoses will give further insight into the function of the retina under normal and pathologic conditions.

**Fabry's Disease: Diagnosis by $\alpha$-Galactosidase Activities in Tears.** Fabry's disease, an inborn error of glycosphingolipid metabolism, is characterized by visceral deposit of trihexosyl ceramide and related glycosphingolipids with terminal $\alpha$-galactosyl moieties, due to defective activity of the lysosomal enzyme ceramide trihexosidase, a specific, X-linked α-galactosyl hydrolase. Human tears are a convenient enzyme source for diagnosis of Tay-Sachs disease, a related glycosphingolipidosis. D. L. Johnson, M. A. Del Monte, E. Cotlier and R. J. Desnick[9] devised a sensitive, rapid assay, using commercially available synthetic substrate, for determination of α-galactosidase activities in tears. Tears were collected from hemizygotes and heterozygotes with Fabry's disease and from age- and sex-matched normal subjects. Tears were collected without use of lacrimating agents, and total α-galactosidase and α-galactosidase A and B activities were determined essentially by the method of Desnick et al., with 4-methylumbelliferyl-α-D-galactopyranoside as substrate and ion-exchange chromatography.

Two components of total α-galactosidase activity were differentiated by thermostability and by chromatography on DEAE-cellulose. The major component, α-galactosidase A, was thermolabile and represented about 90% of total activity, whereas α-galactosidase B was thermostable and eluted at a slightly higher salt concentration. A single, symmetric pH optimum was observed for total α-galactosidase activities from heterozygotes and normal subjects, whereas total activity from hemizygotes, which was about 10% that in controls, had a broad pH profile identical with those for α-galactosidase B activities from all subjects. Apparent $K_m$ values for total activities were 3.2, 4 and over 13 mM for normal subjects, heterozygotes and hemizygotes, respectively. Apparent $K_m$ values for α-galactosidase B were above 13 mM for all subjects. Of the potential inhibitors studied, α-D-melibiose was found competitively to inhibit total α-galactosidase activity.

Tears provide an easily obtainable source of freshly secreted enzyme for diagnosis of hemizygous and heterozygous Fabry's disease. This approach may also be useful for diagnosis and mass screening of patients and carriers for other inborn metabolic errors.

**Fucosidosis: Ultrastructural Study of Conjunctiva and Skin and Enzyme Analysis of Tears.** Fucosidosis is

---

(9) Clin. Chim. Acta 63:81 – 90, Aug. 18, 1975.

an autosomal recessive lysosomal disease characterized by a profound deficiency or absence of $\alpha$-L-fucosidase, resulting in the widespread accumulation of fucose-containing glycosphingolipids, oligosaccharides and polysaccharides and increased excretion of fucosides in the urine. Both severe and mild phenotypes have been described. Severely affected patients have progressive psychomotor retardation and a moderate chondrodystrophy and die at about age $3-5$. J. Libert, F. Van Hoof and M. Tondeur[1] (Free Univ. of Brussels) report results of ultrastructural and tear enzyme studies in 2 patients with the severe form of fucosidosis. One patient is a sister of the first patient in whom $\alpha$-L-fucosidase deficiency was evidenced. Conjunctival and skin biopsy specimens were obtained and tears were collected for enzyme studies.

Clear vacuoles were present in the epithelial cells of the apical conjunctiva and in the endothelial cells of capillaries in both the conjunctiva and skin. The sweat glands of the skin were also heavily involved. Numerous cytoplasmic inclusions distended the fibroblasts, endothelial cells and lymphatic capillaries in the conjunctival stroma. Both clear and dense inclusions were observed. Inclusions were seen in histiocytes and fibroblasts of the superficial dermis and in capillary endothelial cells and perineural cells but not in epidermal cells. Some inclusions were stained by silver and iron staining gave a positive reaction in the periphery of vacuoles of the conjunctival epithelial and stromal cells.

Acid hydrolase activity was not detected in the tears of the patients. A liver biopsy specimen from one patient lacked $\alpha$-fucosidase activity, whereas the other lysosomal enzymes assayed were hyperactive. Leukocytes from both patients lacked $\alpha$-fucosidase activity at any pH from 3.1 to 8.6. The enzyme was present but markedly reduced in plasma from both patients. In the urine of one patient the enzyme was barely detectable between pH 5 and 6.

These patients have the severe phenotype of fucosidosis. The ultrastructural changes resemble those described in Hurler's disease. In contrast to the mucopolysaccharidoses with mucopolysacchariduria, the blood capillary endothelial cells were filled with abnormal inclusions. The fine structure of the stored material is pathognomonic, appearing as both clear vacuoles containing a finely reticular structure and less numerous dark inclusions with a dense, almost homogeneous content. Tear analysis is useful in diagnosing fucosidosis.

**Tyrosine-Induced Eye and Skin Lesions: Treatable Genetic Disease.** Tyrosinemia type II, or Richner-Hanhart syndrome, consists of characteristic eye and skin lesions inherited in an autosomal recessive manner, probable deficiency of enzyme soluble tyrosine aminotransferase and increased levels of tyrosine in the plasma and urine. Permanent neurologic damage, mental retardation and blindness frequently occur. Early diagnosis is important in effectively treating the disorder. Lowell A. Goldsmith and John Reed[2] (Duke Med. Center) have had recent experience with 2 cases of this rare disease.

Girl, the first child of a consanguineous marriage of parents from an inbred rural community, acquired photophobia at age 5 weeks. Examination at 8 months showed long lashes and a diffusely hazy cornea with epithelial ridges radiating out from the central cornea and neovascularization at the corneal periphery. Considerable papillary hypertrophy was present at age 14 months and the corneas were markedly vascularized at this time. Painful erosions appeared on the palms and soles at age 5 months and skin lesions of several types appeared at various times on the palms and soles, some having definite linear configurations. A skin biopsy specimen showed hyperkeratosis and acanthosis. The tyrosine content was increased in the plasma and urine and fell on a low-tyrosine, low-phenylalanine diet. The patient became less irritable and had less photophobia and the skin lesions resolved. After 6½ months of treatment she was growing and actively playing and had normal vision and normal skin. Mental development is presently normal for her age. A liberalized 3,200 AB diet and small amounts of regular food are being given. Blood tyrosine content is maintained at 3–4 times normal levels. The plasma phenylalanine value has been normal on this regimen.

The diagnosis of tyrosinemia II is confirmed by amino acid analysis. Corneal lesions usually appear in the first months of life. Lesions have ranged from delicate dendritic corneal erosions to severe keratitis and ulcers. Skin lesions are limited to the palms and soles and usually are present at the

(2)  J.A.M.A. 236:382–384, July 26, 1976.

same time as the eye lesions. Mental retardation varies widely in severity. No other syndrome of the eyes and palms and soles occurs in the pediatric age group.

Management is with a low-tyrosine, low-phenylalanine milk substitute (Mead-Johnson 3,200 AB). The diet can be liberalized after the skin and eye manifestations are controlled.

**Further Observations on the Diagnosis, Etiology and Treatment of Endophthalmitis.** Richard K. Forster, Ihor G. Zachary, Andrew J. Cottingham, Jr. and Edward W. D. Norton[3] (Univ. of Miami) describe a technique for obtaining cultures in cases of endophthalmitis, and present a study of the relative frequency of etiologic agents in specific types of infectious endophthalmitis.

Fifty-four cases of suspected endophthalmitis were seen during 1969–75. The anterior chamber and vitreous were aspirated for culture in the operating room by a limbal-corneal keratotomy; a 25-gauge needle was used to enter the anterior chamber. The yield of 0.1–0.2 ml fluid was immediately inoculated onto blood agar, thioglycolate liquid, brain-heart infusion and on fungal media. The vitreous was also sampled in aphakic patients. Antibiotics were injected into the vitreous or anterior chamber or both. Gentamicin was injected into the vitreous, cephaloridine into the anterior chamber or vitreous and amphotericin B into the vitreous. Subconjunctival or periocular injections of gentamicin and triamcinolone were given and patients usually received cephaloridine parenterally. Appropriate topical antibiotics and steroids also were used.

Organisms were isolated in 27 cases; in 5 cases, cultures were considered equivocal. Ten of 18 anterior chamber paracenteses in eyes yielding positive results of cultures were culture-positive, as were all 20 vitreous aspirates. All 4 cultures from dehiscent wounds or ruptured blebs also gave positive results. Gram-positive bacteria were identified in 15 cases, gram-negative bacteria in 7 and fungi in 5. Five of 6 traumatic cases yielded gram-positive bacteria. Acuity of 20/400 or better was achieved in 7 of the 27 culture-positive eyes and in 18 of 22 culture-negative eyes. Five of the 14

---

(3)  Trans. Am. Ophthalmol. Soc. 73:221–230, 1975.

eyes that retained some vision yielded *Staphylococcus epidermidis.* Electroretinograms were moderately abnormal in 8 of 12 successfully treated eyes examined 1 – 4 months after treatment. A markedly abnormal record was obtained in 1 instance. Of 12 electroretinograms, 7 primarily showed a decrease in the B-wave with a relatively normal A-wave. Examination of smears contributed little to treatment selection in these cases. *Staphylococcus epidermidis* may be a more common cause of bacterial endophthalmitis than has been thought. Intraocular antibiotics are reasonably safe clinically and add a new dimension to the treatment of endophthalmitis. Allen believes that intraocular antibiotics have not been shown to be better than the same antibiotics delivered by a combination of topical, episcleral and parenteral routes.

► [In this and the following article the current attitudes of early and aggressive attack on endophthalmitis are expressed. These include the use of cultures of aqueous and vitreous with sensitivity tests, intravitreal injections of antibiotics and, in severe cases, vitrectomy with intravitreal injection of antibiotics. – Ed.] ◄

**Vitrectomy in Endophthalmitis: Results of Study Using Vitrectomy, Intraocular Antibiotics or Combination of Both.** Andrew J. Cottingham, Jr. and Richard K. Forster[4] (Univ. of Miami) developed a rabbit endophthalmitis in rabbits by intravitreal inoculation of *Staphylococcus epidermidis* or *S. aureus.* Elimination of organisms was compared using intravitreal administration of 0.1 mg gentamicin alone, vitrectomy alone and a combination of these treatments. Forty-two eyes were used in an *S. epidermidis* study and 54 in the *S. aureus* study.

Six of 11 *S. epidermidis* eyes having vitrectomy alone had negative cultures at 1 week. All 8 eyes treated by the combination were negative a week after treatment. All 9 *S. aureus*-infected eyes having vitrectomy alone had culture growth at 1 week. Four of 12 eyes treated with intravitreal gentamicin 25 – 31 hours after inoculation were negative after 1 week. Ten of 12 eyes treated by both methods were negative at 1 week. Evaluation of eyes treated at 40 – 49 hours gave similar results.

Vitrectomy offers no advantage over intraocular gentami-

(4)   Arch. Ophthalmol. 94:2078 – 2081, December, 1976.

cin in treating endophthalmitis caused by *S. epidermidis* in the rabbit eye. Antibiotics will eradicate *S. aureus* endophthalmitis for a certain time but beyond 24 hours, the addition of vitrectomy to intraocular antibiotics offers a substantial advantage in ridding the eye of infection, both 25–31 and 40–49 hours after infection.

**New Dimensions in Ocular Pharmacology, 1975,** are discussed by Irving H. Leopold[5] (Univ. of California, Irvine). The availability and variety of effective and potentially toxic drugs have increased sharply in this century. New drugs and a wide array of minor modifications are introduced each year. The likelihood of drug interaction increases with the number of drugs used. Topically applied autonomic agents, such as anticholinesterases, cholinergic blocking agents and sympathomimetic agents, can influence enzyme systems and receptors throughout the body and alter many functions and organ systems (Table 1). Systemically administered agents may affect various ocular tissues as well as other organs (Table 2). There is a real possibility that compilations of drug reactions will lead to therapeutic paralysis and a return to therapeutic nihilism, with the risks to patients of inadequate therapy made far greater than the risks of drug interactions. This is most undesirable, since the incidence of clinically important drug interactions is still relatively low.

TABLE 1.—SYSTEMIC EFFECTS OF TOPICALLY APPLIED AUTONOMIC DRUGS

| SYSTEM | EFFECTS | DRUGS |
|---|---|---|
| Cardiovascular | Palpitation, extrasystoles, arrhythmias, hypertension | Adrenergics |
| | Hypotension | Cholinergics |
| | Bradycardia | Anticholinesterases |
| Central nervous | Cortical disturbances, hallucinations-convulsions, cerebellar dysfunctions, ataxia, dysarthria, psychosis, disorientation | Anticholinergics |
| Gastrointestinal tract | Nausea, vomiting, abdominal cramps, salivation, obstruction | Cholinergics, anticholinesterases |
| Respiratory | Bronchiolar spasms | Cholinergics |
| | Pulmonary edema | Anticholinesterases |
| Hematopoietic | Enzyme depression, blood dyscrasia | Anticholinesterases |

(5) Trans. Am. Acad. Ophthalmol. Otolaryngol. 81:19–23, Jan.–Feb., 1976.

TABLE 2. — OCULAR EFFECTS OF SYSTEMICALLY ADMINISTERED DRUGS

| OCULAR STRUCTURE/SYSTEM | EFFECTS | DRUGS |
|---|---|---|
| Conjunctiva | Hyperemia | Reserpine, methyldopa |
| | Allergies | Antibiotics, sulfonamides |
| | Discoloration | Phenothiazine, chlorambucil, phenylbutazone |
| Cornea | Keratitis | Antibiotics, phenylbutazone, barbiturates, chlorambucil, corticosteroids |
| | Deposits | Chloroquine |
| | Pigmentation | Vitamin D |
| Extraocular muscles | Nystagmus, diplopia | Anesthetics—ketamine, sedatives, pentobarbitol, anticonvulsants, propranolol, antibiotics, phenothiazines, carbamazepine, monoamine oxidase inhibitors |
| Intraocular pressure elevations | Open angles | Cholinergic blocking agents, caffeine, corticosteroids |
| | Narrow angles | Cholinergic blocking agents, phenothiazine, tricyclic antidepressants (?) |
| Lens | Opacities— cataract | Corticosteroids, phenothiazine, phenmetrazine, ibuprofen, allopurinol |
| Lid | Edema | Chloral hydrate |
| | Discoloration | Phenothiazines |
| | Ptosis | Guanethidine, propranolol, barbiturates |
| Optic nerve | Atrophy | Diiodohydroxyquin, ethambutol, chloramphenicol |
| | Neuritis | Ethambutol, isoniazid, sulfonamides, digitalis, ibuprofen, imipramine |
| | Papilledema | Corticosteroids, vitamin D, tetracycline, phenylbutazone |
| | Refractive changes | Digitalis, anticholinergics, spironolactone, tetracycline, acetylsalicylic acid (?), fenfluramine, monomine oxidase inhibitors, phenothiazines, carbonic anhydrase inhibitors, antineoplastics, cholinergic blocking agents, sulfonamides, antihistamines |
| Retina | Edema | Chloramphenicol, diiodohydroxyquin, indomethacin |
| | Hemorrhage | Anticoagulants, ethambutol |
| | Vascular damage | Oral contraceptives, oxygen |
| | Degeneration | Phenothiazines, indomethacin, nalidixic acid, ethambutol, sodium chromoglycolate |

Even proved drug interactions are difficult to remember. Not all drug reactions are predictable, but many are preventable without compromising treatment. Pathologic states may modify drug responses. Patient age is also an important factor.

A therapeutic end point should be set for each drug used and a therapeutic objective kept in mind. This is a simple commitment to treat, requiring that drugs be given in doses sufficient to produce an expected effect based on the ophthalmologist's earlier experience with the drug. Failure to improve after an increase in dosage or shortening of the intervals between doses may indicate a need to try another route of administration or another drug. If therapeutic objectives have not been predetermined, lack of efficacy may be difficult to recognize and potentially toxic agents may continue to be administered. A high index of suspicion of drug reactions and interactions and a knowledge of their potential for toxicity must be maintained.

▶ [This address by the guest of honor at the 1975 meeting of the American Academy of Ophthalmology and Otolaryngology contains the usual encyclopedic information and good advice expected from Leopold. Since then, there have been other reports of ocular toxicity from systemic drugs; viz., development of a dry eye after long-term use of practolol (see next article), posterior subcapsular cataracts following use of sodium cyanate (see article by Nicholson et al.) and retinal degeneration in rabbits after administration of vincristine. — Ed.] ◀

**Pathology of Practolol-Induced Ocular Toxicity.** Practolol is a potent $\beta$-adrenergic blocking drug which is widely used to treat angina, cardiac dysrhythmias and hypertension. The incidence of ocular lesions attributable to the drug is second only to that of skin changes. A. H. S. Rahi, C. M. Chapman, A. Garner and P. Wright[6] (London) report on the ocular pathology in 6 patients with lesions attributable to practolol toxicity and the results of antibody-labelling studies. The ocular side effects of prolonged practolol therapy are related to deficient tear secretion and to the formation of an autoantibody having an affinity for the intercellular zones of squamous epithelium. The findings included destruction of lacrimal gland tissue, epidermalization of the conjunctival epithelium and epitheliolysis and stromal ulceration of the cornea leading to perforation in 2 patients. Immunoperoxidase studies showed fixation of specific antibody in the corneal and conjunctival epithelium, but complement fixation was not noted in the one evaluable case.

The conjunctival lesions associated with prolonged practolol therapy include thickening and acanthosis of the epithe-

(6) Br. J. Ophthalmol. 60:312–323, May, 1976.

lium with loss of goblet cells and chronic inflammation leading to stromal fibrosis. The corneal epithelium is less obviously affected, but may show cystic degeneration. Stromal or subepithelial vascularization is seen in corneas showing epitheliopathy and ulceration. The epidermalization of the conjunctival epithelium is probably attributable to an inadequate flow of tears, since dryness of the eyes is a constant finding in patients with ocular lesions. In neither of the autopsies of 2 patients was functional lacrimal gland tissue found. Disappearance of goblet cells probably contributes to the corneal epithelial changes. The cause of the intrinsic epithelial defect is uncertain and the cause of the lacrimal gland damage is also uncertain. Probably an individual idiosyncrasy is involved. The immune response in patients with practolol-induced ocular damage may be secondary to the epithelial disturbance, rather than its cause.

**Cyanate-Induced Cataracts in Patients with Sickle Cell Hemoglobinopathies.** Sodium cyanate reduces the rate of hemolysis and the frequency of painful crises in patients with red blood cell sickling. Don H. Nicholson, Donald R. Harkness, William E. Benson (Univ. of Miami) and Charles M. Peterson[7] (Rockefeller Univ.) report data on 2 patients who had bilateral posterior subcapsular cataracts while receiving oral sodium cyanate for the treatment of sickle cell hemoglobinopathy. A man, aged 24, with S-$\beta$ thalassemia and normal initial ocular findings received 30 mg sodium cyanate per kg daily, orally, for 6 months before tiny axial posterior subcapsular cataracts were noted. These were absent after 6 months of placebo therapy. A second course of cyanate was given in a daily dose of 25 mg/kg and ocular symptoms appeared after 4 months with decreased visual acuity and a discrete posterior subcapsular plaque in each eye. Cyanate therapy was stopped and acuity was normal 3 months later, when the opacities had nearly disappeared. A man, aged 27, with SS hemoglobin received 35 mg sodium cyanate per kg daily and later 20–25 mg/kg daily. Bilateral posterior subcapsular cataracts were seen after 15 months. Cyanate was stopped, but no change in the cataracts occurred in the next 6 months.

(7) Arch. Ophthalmol. 94:927–930, June, 1976.

Cyanate forms an irreversible carbamyl bond with the amino-terminal valine of hemoglobin. The carbamylation reaction with proteins is not specific for hemoglobin, however. The first of the present patients had cataracts consisting of refractile granules, whereas the second patient had cataracts with a ground-glass appearance, showing minimal iridiscence. Reports of spontaneously regressing drug-induced cataracts in man are rare. Cataracts regressed spontaneously after cyanate was withdrawn in the first of the present patients, probably because of the early detection of toxicity and the patient's young age. Most cataractogenic agents exert their effects only after a prolonged latent interval and periodic eye examinations should be continued for several years in all patients in cyanate studies, even though treatment has been terminated.

**Histologic and Electron Microscopic Findings on Rabbit Retina after Application of Vincristine** are described by G. Koniszewski, R. Rix and P. Brunner[8] (Univ. Erlangen-Nürnberg). This substance is obtained from the periwinkle *Vinca rosea* and used in chemotherapy of neoplasms, particularly of the blood. Because a variety of chemical substances are associated with transitory or permanent retinal damage, patients taking vincristine underwent electroretinographic examination and were found to have diffuse and vacillating alteration of potentials.

Six rabbits received a twice weekly dose of 0.04 vincristine per kg (Oncovin) and 6 others a weekly dose of 0.1 mg/kg, injected into the auricular vein; 3 other animals served as controls. Electroretinograms were obtained at regular intervals from all animals.

Determined by dosage and duration of vincristine administration, transient electrophysiologic damage could be demonstrated. Histologic and electron microscopic study revealed cellular destruction in all retinal layers. The outer segments of receptor cells showed diffuse damage, with pigment epithelial cells presenting a higher incidence of reorganization. Follow-up examination 1 year later showed this damage to be partially reversible, particularly when the administered doses had not been extremely high. Pigment

---

(8)  Albrecht von Graefes Arch. Klin. Ophthalmol. 199:147–156, 1976.

epithelial cells no longer showed abnormalities and normal phagocytic activity could be distinguished. Outer segments were largely regenerated; only occasional receptor cells, bipolar ganglion cells and ganglion cells showed nuclear pyknosis and cytoplasmic destruction. This explained the absence of lasting functional disturbances on the electroretinogram and evoked visual potential.

**Ocular Toxoplasmosis in an Adult Receiving Long-Term Corticosteroid Therapy.** Both *Candida* endophthalmitis and cytomegalic inclusion retinitis may be seen in patients whose immune mechanisms are compromised, either by disease or iatrogenically. Don H. Nicholson (Univ. of Miami) and Eugene B. Wolchok[9] (Univ. of Jacksonville) report data indicating that ocular toxoplasmosis should also be considered in this clinical setting.

Woman, 58, had apparent viral pneumonia, followed in 4 months by recurrent fever and hepatosplenomegaly, when splenectomy and liver biopsy showed extensive fibrosis, focal inflammation and necrosis in both organs. Persistent fever and weight loss ensued; systemic steroid therapy was instituted and continued to her death 1½ years later. An apparent paravascular retinal inflammation and granulomatous anterior uveitis developed in the left eye after 9 months of systemic steroid therapy. This progressed to opacification of the vitreous over 2½ months, despite injections of methylprednisolone in the sub-Tenon capsule. Similar uveitis developed in the right eye 6 months after loss of vision in the left eye. Steroids cleared the vitreous and revealed extensive focal, paravascular retinal opacification paralleling both arteries and veins. Methotrexate therapy was not helpful and the patient died suddenly.

Only the right eye was obtained for examination. Multiple focal areas of paravascular retinal necrosis were observed, with scattered intraretinal hemorrhages. Necrosis involved the nerve fiber and ganglion cell layers. Cysts consistent with *Toxoplasma gondii* were present at the margin of each focus of necrosis and free organisms were present at the interface between intact and necrotic inner retina. Encysted organisms were also seen in pigment epithelial cells. The nasal half of the optic nerve was atrophic and contained both cysts and free organisms. Electron microscopy confirmed the presence of *T. gondii.*

Disseminated toxoplasmosis, with a predilection for the

(9) Arch. Ophthalmol. 94:248–254, February, 1976.

CNS, has been reported in association with several diseases and treatments that compromise host immune mechanisms. Electron microscopy was useful for confirming the identity of the infecting organism in the absence of serologic or culture data in the present patient. The efficacy of steroids may depend on the timing of cyst rupture with respect to establishment of the immunosuppressed state. Treatment after cyst rupture but before immunosuppression, when intense inflammation has occurred, will suppress the inflammatory response after immune inactivation of viable organisms has occurred. Treatment when cyst rupture has occurred in a compromised host would be expected to potentiate the infection.

▶ [Gross and microscopic pictures of both retinas in the original article illustrate the destructive nature of actively proliferating toxoplasma, apparently encouraged by long-term steroid therapy. It is unfortunate that this patient being treated for "sarcoid" did not have an autopsy to determine the cause of death, which might have been toxoplasmosis. — Ed.] ◀

# Basic Sciences

INTRODUCTION

It seems particularly appropriate this year to discuss the subject of tissue culture as a research tool because it appears that its use in widely diverse eye research applications is an idea whose time has come.

The value of having cell cultures available does not require belaboring. It would be highly desirable to study some metabolic properties of tissues in culture. Having strains of malignant tumors available to examine the distinctive characteristics of malignancy would be extremely helpful and a tissue culture, where appropriate, would be a highly useful test object to measure the effect of drugs and of toxic substances. However, just as in the case of other research preparations, it is absolutely necessary to know the properties of the cultured cells that one is to use so that the conclusions drawn from experiments will have validity.

Surprisingly, the first use of ocular tissues in culture dates back almost 50 years. Kirby et al. cultured lens epithelium from 52-hour chick embryos in 1929.[1] In 1939 Thygeson, working in Carrel's laboratory, cultivated the epithelium of human conjunctiva and cornea.[2] The organelle culture of whole lens introduced by Merriam and Kinsey in 1950 represented another approach to an in vitro preparation that could be studied by simplified methods.[3]

Just as with any experimental preparation, the use of cultured cells or even organelles requires a certain amount of validation, which cannot be created overnight. Results obtained in a living mouse or in an anesthetized rabbit cannot be translated immediately to the human situation. Even though one may be growing human tissues in culture, a decided advantage in one respect, there are specific types of validation that are peculiar to tissue culture. One of these has to do with the fact that cells placed in culture frequently alter morphologically. Thus, it is not possible to determine from morphology alone that the resultant culture is a pure one of the desired cell type. As in the case of bacterial cultures where a vigorous intruder may overgrow the strain desired by the experimenter, so in tissue culture, contamination by fibroblasts, for example, could conceivably result in a mature culture consisting chiefly of these cells even though the culture was seeded with predominantly epithelial cells. Thus it becomes necessary to validate the cell type in the mature culture as being identical with the type of cell that the experimenter wished to grow.

The correlate of this problem is that because morphology has changed in many instances, one must establish that the aspects of biochemistry that are of particular interest to the experiment have remained unchanged. Then one can consider the tissue preparation as an adequate substrate for experimentation. Achieving these two types of validation sometimes requires considerable ingenuity but the value of such a compact, reproducible, long-lived experimental object makes the effort at validation well worthwhile.

One solution to the wanted-versus-unwanted tissue type was described by Fowle and Ormsby.[4] These workers subcultured corneal epithelium at a time they previously had found would precede fibroblast proliferation. More difficult is the situation of the retinal pigment epithelium grown in tissue culture. If chick embryos are used as a source of pigment epithelium, these cells under proper conditions remain as monolayers in culture and maintain their roughly hexagonal outlines, leaving little doubt that one is dealing with original pigment epithelium.[5] However, if adult tissues are used, the retinal pigment epithelium refuses to maintain its original conformation. It elongates and grows in multilayered cultures. It is incumbent on the experimenters to prove that their experiments are actually being done on retinal pigment epithelium and not on fibroblast overgrowth.[6,7] In my own laboratory, the investigation of individual properties has proved beyond question that the elongated cells are indeed retinal pigment epithelium and that their metabolism in most respects is identical to that of the original tissue.

It is clear that the technique of using tissue culture has come of age when experimenters are growing tissues as explants not merely as an unusual achievement, but for use as a tool in biomedical experimentation. It is worth citing a number of instances in regard to ocular tissues. Buzney et al., who found that mural cells are the cells that grow in tissue cultures of retina capillaries, proposed to use these cultures for studies of the diabetic retinopathy process.[8] Klintworth has reviewed the many instances in which tissue cultures of skin fibroblasts and corneal cells can be analyzed for abnormal substances in inherited polysaccharidosis and can be used to study the basic metabolic defect.[9] Ushida and Itoi studied the effect of dexamethasone on the growth of fibroblasts in tissue culture and demonstrated that there was no significant inhibition by the steroid.[10] These authors suggest that the method of combating inflammation by corticosteroids must work other than by inhibition of fibroblast growth. In unpublished work in my laboratory, Doctor Gonasun and I were able to demonstrate that chloroquine in extremely low concentrations prevents incorporation of radioactive amino acids into mammalian pigment epithelium grown in tissue culture. The excellent work from Kinsey's laboratory on the transport and metabolism in lens grown in isolated culture is classic.

Because virtually every cell structure of the eye has been grown successfully in culture, the application of these techniques to studies that go beyond the morphological are now coming into their own. It is time to recognize that we have with us a new powerful tool that needs only ingenuity and application to deliver much information on the behavior of ocular tissues.

Albert M. Potts, Ph.D, M.D.
University of Louisville

## REFERENCES

1. Kirby, D. B., Estey, K., and Tabor, F.: A Study of the Nutrition of the Crystalline Lens: The Cultivation of Lens Epithelium, Arch. Ophthalmol. 1:358, 1929.
2. Thygeson, P.: Cultivation In Vitro of Human Conjunctival and Corneal Epithelium, Am. J. Ophthalmol. 22:649, 1939.
3. Merriam, F. C., and Kinsey, V. E.: Studies on the Crystalline Lens: I. Technique for In Vitro Culture of Crystalline Lenses

and Observations on Metabolism of the Lens, Arch. Ophthalmol. 43:979, 1950.

4. Fowle, A. M. C., and Ormsby, H. L.: Growth of the Cornea in
Tissue Culture, Am. J. Ophthalmol. 39 (Suppl. 2):242, 1955.
5. Newsome, D., Fletcher, R., Robinson, W., Kenyon, K., and
Chader, G.: Effects of Cyclic AMP and Sephadex Fractions of
Chick Embryo Extract on Cloned Retinal Pigment Epithelium
in Tissue Culture, J. Cell. Biol. 61:369, 1974.
6. Mannagh, J., Arya, D. V., and Irvine, A. R.: Tissue Culture of
Human Retinal Pigment Epithelium, Invest. Ophthalmol. 12:
52, 1973.
7. Gonasun, L. and Potts, A. M.: Unpublished experiments.
8. Buzney, S. M., Frank, R. N., and Robinson, W. C.: Retinal Capillaries: Proliferation of Mural Cells In Vitro, Science 190:985,
1975.
9. Klintworth, G. K.: Tissue Culture in the Inherited Corneal
Dystrophies: Possible Applications and Problems, In Bergsma,
I., Bron, A. J., and Cotlier, E. (eds.): *The Eye and Inborn Errors
of Metabolism,* Vol XII, No. 3, National Foundation of Birth
Defects: Original Article Series (New York: Liss, Inc., 1976).
10. Ushida, Y. and Itoi, M.: Influence of Dexamethasone on Fibroblasts in Tissue Culture, Jpn. J. Ophthalmol. 6:197, 1962.

**Computers in Ophthalmology** are discussed by Aran
Safir[1] (Mt. Sinai School of Medicine, N.Y.). Manipulation
and interpretation of data are easy when they are in numer-
ical form and when agreed-on mathematical manipulations
are performed with the aid of computers. Verbal material
fed into the computer is severely restricted. Ophthalmology
may have a small enough vocabulary on which ophthalmologists could agree so that record keeping would be possible.
Computerization of medical record keeping will probably
depend greatly on an input of information by paramedical
assistants. Practices with several assistants would lend
themselves best to computerized medical record keeping.
Apart from clerical functions, the most natural applications
of the computer in ophthalmology would be in reading instruments and interpreting the results. Tonometers, tonog-
raphers, eye movement measuring devices, objective refractors, keratometers and lens meters or vertometers would be
susceptible to such applications. Even some subjective func-

(1)  Invest. Ophthalmol. 15:163–168, March, 1976.

tions, such as visual acuity measurements and automatic perimetry data, can be converted into objective measurements. The examining functions that require interpretation of image content will be increasingly reserved for the ophthalmologist.

Artificial intelligence, a subdiscipline of computer science, has concerned itself with studying problems of complex decision making. The branching logical tree is one type of decision-making program. The author's group has developed a consultation program in glaucoma that is capable of making diagnostic, prognostic and therapeutic decisions at a high level of expertise. The program is operational and is undergoing clinical testing at several glaucoma research centers. Other consultation systems are also being designed and built. Probably there will soon be computer-guided systems that can do sophisticated work in refraction and perimetry, and consultation systems are planned in such subdisciplines as strabismus, external diseases and neuro-ophthalmology. A complex of overlapping, computer-assisted consultation programs in a variety of ophthalmologic subdisciplines could provide easy access at all times to fellow professionals. Consultation with panels of very specialized colleagues would then be much easier. Perhaps the physician could then resume his former role of patient listener, skilled and unhurried examiner and wise counsellor.

**How Does the External Eye Resist Infection?** Chandler R. Dawson[2] points out that despite constant exposure the conjunctiva and cornea are remarkably resistant to infections from the external environment. Many infectious processes on these surfaces are either self-limited or confer solid resistance to reinfection. The phenomenon of local immunity has been well recognized for many years. Secretory IgA appears to have a major role in protection against viral respiratory tract infection and secretory immunoglobulins in tears are capable of neutralizing viruses. The formation of secretory IgA antibodies is generally thought to be highly localized.

It is usually assumed that cell-mediated immunity is a systemic response to antigenic stimulation but this is not

(2) Invest. Ophthalmol. 15:971–974, December, 1976.

necessarily the case. Work on *Listeria* and chlamydial infections of the guinea pig conjunctiva has indicated that epithelial cells have an active role in the host response to infection. Circulating leukocytes, especially neutrophils, are rapidly mobilized in the conjunctival epithelium in response to specific chemotactic stimuli and polymorphonuclear cells have a crucial role in defense against pyogenic bacteria. Viral replication in cells is inhibited by the interferons and the efficacy of interferon in limiting herpetic eye infection in man has been demonstrated.

Much remains to be learned about immune mechanisms at the conjunctival and corneal surfaces, especially the normal response to organisms at the external surface of the eye. Preliminary attempts have been made to increase resistance to reinfection by local immunization in animal models of herpetic keratitis and trachoma. Immunologic modification of other diseases, such as viral conjunctivitis and the keratitis associated with staphylococcal blepharitis, would be a distinct possibility. The use of "immunopotentiators" such as levamisole is another treatment modality that is being explored in laboratory models and may have application in the treatment of human disease.

**HL-A Linkage Group and Disease Susceptibility** are discussed by Jörg Bertrams and Manfred Spitznas[3] (Essen, West Germany). The indication of HL-A-linked genetic control of immunoresponsiveness makes the HL-A system one of the biologically most important immunogenetic systems in man; the main histocompatibility complex consists of a group of genes on chromosome 6. The antigens are determined by the in vitro microlymphocytotoxicity test. Antigens of the main lymphocyte-defined (LD) locus HL-A-D usually are determined in vitro by the mixed lymphocyte culture (MLC) technique. Some antigens occur often, while others are rare. The HL-A antigen-associated ophthalmic diseases are listed in the table.

Conceivably, HL-A determinants on the cell surface serve as receptors for pathogenic organisms, especially viruses. Another theory is that of "molecular mimicry," according to which the macroorganism is unable to recognize the patho-

(3) Albrecht von Graefes Arch. Klin. Ophthalmol. 200:1–12, 1976.

HL-A ANTIGEN-ASSOCIATED OPHTHALMIC DISEASES

| DISEASE | ASSOCIATED HLA DETERMINANT | REFERENCE |
|---|---|---|
| RETINOBLASTOMA | - BW35, BW12(↓) | BERTRAMS ET AL. 1973B |
| MALIGNANT MELANOMA | - AW32 | BERTRAMS ET AL. 1976C |
| CHORIORETINITIS | NO DEVIATION | " |
| EALES' DISEASE | NO DEVIATION | " |
| CENTRAL SEROUS CHORIORETINOPATHY | NO DEVIATION | " |
| BEHCET'S DISEASE | - B5 | OHNO ET AL 1973, 1975 |
| ACUTE ANTERIOR UVEITIS | - B27 | BREWERTON ET AL. 1973A EHLERS ET AL. 1974 MAPSTONE AND WOODROW 1975 WOODROW ET AL. 1975 BERTRAMS ET AL. 1975 |
| CHRONIC ANTERIOR UVEITIS | NO DEVIATION | EHLERS ET AL. 1975 |

**Fig 58.** — Gene loci of chromosome no. 6 *(upper part of figure)* with particular reference to the HL-A linkage group *(lower part of figure)*. Loci that could be mapped on chromosome no. 6 are the blood group P, the cytoplasmic malic enzyme *(ME1)*, the mitochondrial superoxide enzyme *(SOD2)*, the proteolytic enzyme pepsinogen *(PG5)*, erythrocyte enzymes phosphoglucomutase *(PGM3)* and glyoxalase *(GLO)* and the HL-A loci. The single loci of the HL-A linkage group are the serologically defined loci HL-A-A, HL-A-B and HL-A-C, the lymphocyte-defined (LD) locus HL-A-D and probably a second LD or mixed lymphocyte culture *(MLC)* locus between HL-A-A and HL-A-C *(finely stippled rectangles)*. The locus for the major component of the alternative pathway of complement activation, the Bf-system (Bf-properdin factor B), lies between the HL-A-B and HL-A-D loci, whereas the gene for synthesis of the second complement component *(C2)* is located outside the main HL-A region in close vicinity to HL-A-D *(hatched circles)*. The exact location of the genes responsible for synthesis of the fourth complement component *(C4)* within the HL-A region is still unknown. The same holds true for the position of the B lymphocyte alloantigenic system, called HL-B, probably located outside of the HL-A complex on the side of HL-A-D *(stippled circle)*. The immune response *(IR)* genes most probably lie on the left and right side of the HL-A-D locus *(small black dots)*. (Courtesy of Bertrams, J., and Spitznas, M.: Albrecht von Graefes Arch. Klin. Ophthalmol. 200:1–12, 1976.)

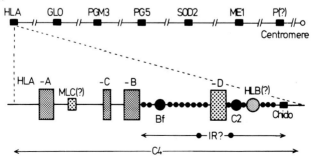

gen and eliminate it by immune reactions. The most attractive hypothesis involves linkage of the known HL-A genes with other poorly identified loci of the HL-A linkage group, which may be more important to disease susceptibility (DS). The deviating HL-A antigens would act merely as markers pointing to the etiopathologically important DS gene or genes.

The interpretation of the DS-genes as immune response (IR) genes is very convincing. Conceivably, IR genes linked with histocompatibility genes predispose to the development of tumors, viral infections and (auto-)immune diseases. This concept is supported by the presence of a genetically controlled alloantigenic system present only on antibody-producing B lymphocytes and macrophages (Fig 58). All HL-A antigen-associated diseases are combined with disturbed immune reactions. Most of the diseases for which an HL-A antigen deviation has been described are associated with one of the typical Europide "HL-A superhaplotypes." This is true of multiple sclerosis, diabetes mellitus and Addison's disease and may apply to all HL-A-B7- and HL-A-B8-associated diseases.

► [This highly technical article is in English. It is bewildering to a clinician how the histocompatibility HL-A genes can be localized on chromosome 6 and how these are closely related to the immune-response genes. The authors state, "The disturbed immune reactions of the HL-A-B7-associated diseases seem to be characterized by a special immune hyporeactivity against different antigens whereas for the HL-A-B8-associated diseases, hyper- and autoimmune reactions seem to be of etiopathogenic importance." See also the comments by Schlaegel on the role of heredity in iridocyclitis (1976 YEAR BOOK, p. 178). – Ed.] ◄

**Plate Thermography Seen by the Ophthalmologist** is discussed by P. Bonnin and M. Passot[4] (Paris). Contact thermography utilizes the fact that certain substances are optically thermosensitive. This is true of liquid crystals whose apparent color is a direct function of their temperature.

A set of Tricoire thermographic plates was used to study the superficial temperature of the forehead, temples, eyeball and mastoids. An interval of $1.5-2$ C was maintained, and plates sensitive beyond 31 C, 33 C and 34.5 C were used in succession. Photographs were taken in daylight on reversi-

(4) Ann. Ocul. (Paris) 209:1 – 10, January, 1976.

ble film with use of an electronic flash, from which heat rays were filtered out.

Plate thermography permitted localization of three types of cutaneous zones. The coldest zones correspond to regions that are deprived of large blood vessels and that rest directly on a relatively neutral plane, such as the frontal bosses. The second type of cutaneous zone overlies a warm organ, allowing the source of heat to be seen: the breast, thyroid and tibial crest. The warmest cutaneous zones are found over the vessels and in the following order of increasing temperature: the cutaneous veins, deep veins, superficial arteries and deep arteries at the point where they emerge.

This method furnishes the following information: basal skin temperature with comparison between the two sides; visualization of arterial courses, of both anatomical and physiologic interest; and evidence of functional anomalies of these same arteries under pathologic conditions.

The great sensitivity of the method confirms that the paramedian frontal warm triangle does not exist by itself; in reality, this warm zone corresponds to the course of the internal frontal artery, a branch of the ophthalmic. The authors have found the internal frontal artery to be more or less warm at least on one side. Among the youngest patients, who are the warmest, the vertical course of the paramedian frontal branch, sometimes its division at half-distance and its anastomoses with the suborbital can be seen very well (Fig 59).

The superficial temporal artery is always easy to see, often too easy, and it is the most radiant vessel of the frontal territory. It is the largest arterial vessel, with its course sinuous with age (Fig 60) and with its two terminal branches, the temporofrontal anterior and the temporoparietal posterior.

Physiologically, the base temperature of the frontal region is low, about 33 C for 81% of the patients studied. Most of the subjects studied, however, were over age 70 years. Also, the prevascular temperature is maximum at the superficial temporal arteries, although this is constantly verified only in the aged patient. The temperature is median over the internal frontal arteries and is lowest at the suborbital artery and external frontal anastomoses. From the

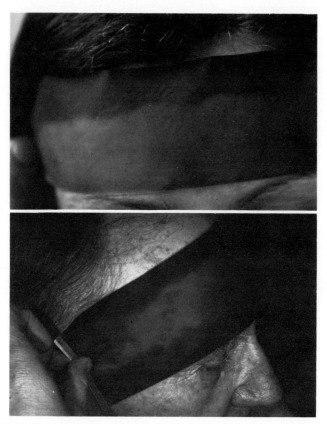

**Fig 59 (top).**—In this young woman, the normal appearance of vascularization is visible on the right side, with the internal frontal artery and its branches, the suborbital artery, the eyebrow anastomosis and the temporofrontal branches of the temporal artery; 33-C plate.

**Fig 60 (bottom).**—Temporal thermogram of a man, aged 65 years, showing the sinuous and very warm course of the temporofrontal branch of the superficial temporal artery; 33-C plate.

(Courtesy of Bonnin, P., and Passot, M.: Ann. Ocul. (Paris) 209:1–10, January, 1976.)

pathologic standpoint, all the necessary vessels have not yet been gathered for statistical analysis.

The Tricoire method of plate thermography is not costly and is totally harmless, reproducible and believable.

**New Method for Determining the Blood Quantity in the Eye in a Unit of Time.** G. Cristini, R. Meduri, G. C. Garbini and A. Giovannini[5] (Univ. of Bologna) describe a new method for semiquantitatively determining blood flow in the eye in a unit of time, using the principles of rheography with an "infinite time constant." Twenty normal subjects aged 30–70 years, were examined.

Electrical impedance variations induced by blood flow through an area between two electrodes connected to a Wheatstone bridge were recorded, using a suction cup electrode device. The vacuum was gradually increased, raising ocular pressure above venous pressure and blocking the venous outflow without a change in arterial inflow, resulting in increased accumulation of blood in the interior of the eye. The resultant impedance variation is shown by a "slow" rising curve maintaining the same pulse morphology, representing the total amount of blood in both continuous and pulsatory volumes. Abolition of the conventional time constant of 2–3 seconds avoided the return to the isoelectric line.

Firm fixation and good respiratory control are essential to obtain error-free records. The calculated arterial minute volume was very close to that obtained by Van Beunigen and Fischer. This method of measuring arterial minute volume offers interesting interpretative, diagnostic and therapeutic prospects. The measurement is technically simple and the stress exerted on the subject is small.

(5)   Albrecht von Graefes Arch. Klin. Ophthalmol. 197:1–11, 1975.

# Surgery

**Distraneurin (Chlormethiazole) as Anesthetic for High-Risk Cases in Ophthalmology.** W. Unger, H. Ortner and A. Benke[6] (Vienna) found Distraneurin to be particularly suited for use in patients with impaired liver function with or without associated cardiac or circulatory diseases. One advantage was the demonstrable diminution of ocular tension.

Chlormethiazole was administered as an 0.8% solution in an isotonic glucose solution (5%); its working substance corresponds to the thiazole fraction of vitamin $B_1$, which possesses hypnotic and anticonvulsive properties. Toxicity is about 20 times less than that of pentobarbital, with only minimal impairment of respiratory and circulatory centers. After it couples with glutamine and acetic acid in the liver, elimination occurs to 95% through the urine during the first 24 hours.

The present study included 50 patients, aged 65–83, undergoing cataract surgery (48 patients) and glaucoma operation. Anesthesia was administered only by infusion, without intubation, with the depth of anesthesia controlled by alteration of the drop rhythm. The use of an airway (Mayo tube) is contraindicated because the choke reflex is present even in deepest chlormethiazole anesthesia and pharyngeal stimuli may cause complications. There is no excitation during induction; 150 ml of the solution usually achieves the necessary anesthesia within 10 minutes and 250–350 ml more is required for a sustained effect. Recovery is calm and without undesirable side effects. One property of this agent is its capacity to reduce intraocular pressure, which is more noticeable with high initial values. It is likely a particularly well-suited anesthetic agent for glaucoma patients, although further study will be necessary.

(6)  Klin. Monatsbl. Augendheilk. 168:341–345, March, 1976.

**New Synthetic Absorbable Suture for Ophthalmic Surgery: Laboratory and Clinical Evaluation** is reported by W. A. Dunlap, W. D. Purnell and S. D. McPherson, Jr.[7] (North Carolina Meml. Hosp., Chapel Hill). Recent advances in microsurgery have called for the development of new suture materials for use in ophthalmic surgery. Glycolic acid and lactic acid have been combined to produce a high-molecular weight glycolactide, polyglactin 910 or Vicyrl, to modify the absorption rate in tissues. It is an ester analogue of a glycine-alanine polyamino acid, and as such is a structural analogue of a simple protein.

The suture was evaluated in 6-0 and 8-0 monofilament sizes in rabbits. The 6-0 suture had a swaged-on G-6 cutting needle and the 8-0 suture had a GS-9 spatula needle. In vivo measurements were made in rabbits with partial-thickness and penetrating corneal wounds and in animals having suture material placed subconjunctivally, within the corneal lamellae and in the anterior chamber. Conjunctival wounds in 12 patients having cataract, glaucoma or muscle surgery were closed with glycolactide suture; the 7-0 size was used in most.

In vitro measurements showed suture diameters to be fairly constant. Suture strength was reduced about 25% after a knot was tied. Little clinical evidence of tissue reaction to the suture material was seen in 28 days in in vivo studies. No corneal wounds leaked after the 2d postoperative day with both sutures and knots in place. The effects of tissue implantation on rupture strength decreased little until the 6th day.

No complications were seen in the 12 patients. The sutures elicited no observable reactions in the eye. In 45 patients in whom the suture was used for corneoscleral wound closure, the glycolactide possessed superior strength and visibility compared with chromic collagen of comparable size. All but 3 of these patients were followed until final disappearance of the glycolactide suture. Disappearance curves indicated that the glycolactide suture more nearly approximated the "ideal" suture than did collagen, disappearing in 6–8 weeks.

---

(7) South. Med. J. 69:588–592, May, 1976.

The marketed braided glycolactide suture of microsurgical caliber approaches silk in handling qualities and is superior to collagen in strength and absorption characteristics.

▶ [It appears that 7-0 Vicryl suture is the most satisfactory absorbable suture to date for cataract surgery. — Ed.] ◀

**Retrievable Suture Idea for Anterior Uveal Problems** is presented by Malcolm A. McCannel[8] (Minneapolis). Mackenson, in 1968, suggested that a monofilament perlon (nylon) suture could be used for an iris suture and remain inert in the anterior chamber. A problem with an iridodialysis with a torn iris border led to the idea that a suture introduced at the limbus under the iris border could be retrieved easily if held vertically by passing the suture up and out through the cornea in a single motion. This suture was reversed in a case of cyclodialysis with hypotonia and a marked cyclodialysis cleft over about half of the eye circumference. In a case of dislocation of an intraocular lens fixation loop, a fine suture was used to hold the repositioned loop in its proper place without need to open the eye widely. A

**Fig 61.** — Iridodialysis repair. (Courtesy of McCannel, M. A.: Ophthalmic Surg. 7:98 – 103, Summer, 1976.)

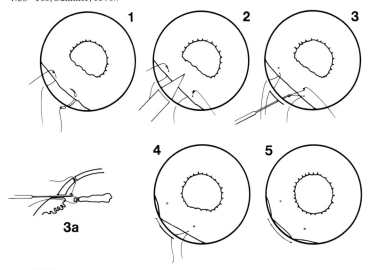

---

flat spatula was useful in carrying the needle point in the short distance available. A sharpened Steven tenotomy hook could also be used.

It has been suggested that by use of a short no. 30 hypodermic needle, with its point slightly barbed, the anterior chamber can be made deep with an injection of acetylcholine as the needle is introduced, and the barb catches the vertical suture so that it can be retrieved and exteriorized without need to open the eye wider than the original stab incision, which rarely requires a closure suture. Use of the fine suture in an iridodialysis repair is illustrated in Figure 61. A 10-0 monofilament suture is used.

**Self-Curing Methylmethacrylate: Is It Safe?** Richard L. Anderson (Univ. of Iowa) and Orkan George Stasior[9] (Albany Med. College) point out that ophthalmic surgeons are performing increasing numbers of reconstructive procedures about the eye and orbit, using self-curing methylmethacrylate. Cardiovascular complications and deaths have recently been associated with the use of this substance in orthopedics and have led some to condemn its use in ophthalmology. Few complications have been noted with this material in neurosurgery or surgical specialties other than orthopedics. Most of the more than 20 deaths attributed to bone cement to date occurred in Great Britain in total hip replacements. The cause of hypotension and cardiac arrest in these patients remains speculative. Skin and mucosal allergies, anorexia and decreased gastric motor activity have also been attributed to methylmethacrylate.

The compound most often used by ophthalmic surgeons is Cranioplastic. Ophthalmic applications include correction of enophthalmos, filling orbital or periorbital bone defects, making socket impressions, use as conformers in the management of socket contraction and formation of exenteration implants. No reports of local tissue necrosis have appeared, but this remains a possibility, and self-curing methylmethacrylate should not be placed posteriorly in the orbits of seeing eyes. No cardiovascular collapse or death has been attributed to the facial uses of freshly mixed methylmethacrylate. There is less free monomer in facial than in orthope-

(9) Ophthalmic Surg. 7:28–30, Winter, 1976.

dic acrylic cement, and in facial procedures the material is not forced into the medullary cavity of a bone. Young, otherwise healthy patients tend to have facial reconstructive procedures, in contrast to elderly patients having hip operations. Extensive procedures and mobilization problems potentiate the danger of cardiovascular problems in hip surgery patients.

At present there is no evidence to condemn the facial use of self-curing methylmethacrylate because of cardiovascular complications, but the search for more inert compounds should continue.

# Miscellaneous

**Aberrant Bacterial Forms from Various Ocular Sites.** A previous study of bacterial conjunctivitis called attention to the possible importance of cell wall-deficient (CWD) bacteria and other aberrant bacterial forms. Yvonne Jacobs and Bruce Golden[1] (Johannesburg, South Africa) surveyed 400 ocular cultures to demonstrate the presence of aberrant bacterial forms at various ocular sites and to compare the incidence in eyes suspected of being bacterially infected with that in apparently uninfected eyes. Specimens were taken from the lower conjunctiva, from the aqueous by paracentesis of the anterior chamber and from open limbal incision sites during cataract extraction operations. Several solid and liquid mediums were used to isolate organisms. Several reversion techniques were used to determine the nature of the parent forms of the CWD bacteria isolated.

There were 224 specimens from patients with no apparent infection at the time of culture and 176 from patients with suspected bacterial infections or with culturally, cytologically or clinically confirmed bacterial infections. Of 386 conjunctival swabs, 50 (12.9%) yielded aberrant bacterial forms. The rate was 12.2% in cultures from patients without apparent bacterial infection. Many of these patients had received prophylactic antibiotics before specimens were taken. Of the patients with suspected infections, 24 (13.9%) had cultures showing aberrant forms. No aberrant forms grew on 4 specimens from limbal incision sites. Three of 7 cultures of aqueous specimens yielded aberrant forms, which grew on a total of 53 (13.2%) of 400 cultures; a total of 59 aberrant forms were isolated. Nearly all these were CWD forms.

Patients may harbor CWD organisms or other aberrant bacterial forms in their eyes. The presence of these orga-

---

(1) Arch. Ophthalmol. 94:933–936, June, 1976.

nisms is another factor to be used in assessing host responses to microbiologic agents.

▶ [As the authors explain, "aberrant bacterial form" is a general term denoting bacteria that are slower growing than normal, cell wall deficient, stain poorly and are pleomorphic, form abnormal colonies and under proper circumstances can be reverted to their normal status. Their response to antibiotics may be different from their parent forms and may be responsible for recurrence of inflammation long after the inciting infection. The technique for the isolation and demonstration of these organisms is described in this article. — Ed.] ◀

▶ ↓ The following three articles contain suggestions for the prevention and management of recurrent anterior chamber hemorrhage after blunt injury to the eye. The oral administration of either of the antifibrinolytic drugs, aminocaproic acid or tranexamic acid, appears to reduce the incidence of this complication significantly. If the "8-ball" hemorrhage persists, with development of secondary glaucoma and beginning blood staining of the cornea, evacuation of the blood and diathermization of any fresh bleeding areas can be done. — Ed. ◀

**Aminocaproic Acid in Treatment of Traumatic Hyphema.** Secondary hemorrhage may occur in 9–38% of patients with traumatic hyphema. This may be more severe than the initial bleeding and result in increased intraocular pressure. Secondary bleeding usually occurs 2–6 days after the initial episode, probably due to lysis and retraction of the clot and fibrin aggregates that occluded the injured vessel.

Earl R. Crouch, Jr., and Marcel Frenkel[2] (Univ. of Illinois) made a prospective study to evaluate the effect of aminocaproic acid, an antifibrinolytic agent, in preventing secondary hemorrhage after traumatic hyphema. The subjects were all patients admitted with traumatic hyphema during 1972–74, with exclusion of those with suspected penetrating ocular injury and those with total hyphemas. Of the 59 patients in the study, 32 received aminocaproic acid orally, 100 mg/kg every 4 hours for 5 days, 27 received a placebo. All patients were managed by elevation of the head of the bed and patching of the involved eye. Moderate ambulation was permitted. Follow-up ranged from 6 months to 2.5 years.

Ten patients had secondary hemorrhage — 9 (33%) of those receiving placebo and 1 (3%) of those receiving aminocaproic acid; the latter patient had sickle cell trait. Two placebo-

(2) Am. J. Ophthalmol. 81:355–360, March, 1976.

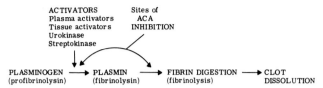

**Fig 62.** – Pharmacologic action of aminocaproic acid by competitive inhibition of conversion of plasminogen into plasmin and a direct antiplasmin effect. (Courtesy of Crouch, E. R., Jr., and Frenkel, M.: Am. J. Ophthalmol. 81:355 – 360, March, 1976.)

treated patients who rebled and 5 (10%) of the 49 patients who did not rebleed also had sickle cell trait. The 2 placebo-treated patients who rebled required clot removal because of increased intraocular pressure and early corneal staining. Among patients without rebleeding, clots persisted for a mean of 2.8 days in the placebo group and 4 days in the aminocaproic-acid treated group, a significant difference. Post-traumatic complications did not differ significantly in the two groups, although 2 placebo-treated patients had non-glaucomatous optic atrophy, and 2 had corneal staining. Final visual acuities were somewhat better in the aminocaproic acid-treated patients, although their initial acuities had been slightly worse.

The action of aminocaproic acid is illustrated in Figure 62. The significant reduction in incidence of rebleeding in patients with traumatic hyphemas treated with aminocaproic acid suggests that the agent may be deterring lysis of the initial clot until the initially ruptured vessels regain their integrity.

**Traumatic Hyphema Treated with the Antifibrinolytic Drug Tranexamic Acid.** Secondary hemorrhage is the most serious complication of traumatic hyphema and usually occurs 2 – 5 days after trauma, suggesting the possibility of a fibrinolytic bleeding which may be avoided by inhibiting the fibrinolysis. Thorkild Bramsen[3] (Univ. of Aarhus) evaluated the use of tranexamic acid, an antifibrinolytic drug which inhibits plasminogen conversion to plasmin, in 72 patients with traumatic hyphema seen consecutively over 1 year. Patients with ocular contusion alone, those with

(3)   Acta Ophthalmol. (Kbh.) 54:250 – 256, April, 1976.

only a hemorrhagic aqueous flare, those admitted with secondary hemorrhage and patients with perforating lesions were excluded.

The 60 men had an average age of 20.8 years and the 12 women, 20.1 years. Patients had complete bed rest for 5 days, were given stenopeic spectacles and received tranexamic acid orally in a dosage of 25 mg/kg 3 times daily for 6 days. Acetazolamide was given if the intraocular pressure rose above 30 mm Hg. Mydriatics and topical steroids were not used. Comparison was made with 135 patients treated individually without tranexamic acid.

Only 1 study patient (1.4%) had secondary bleeding; none had iritis or increased intraocular pressure 12 days after injury. Acuity was 1.0 or greater in 57 cases and 0.1 – 0.3 in only 4 cases; in no case was it below 0.1. Synechias were found at the angle in 2 of the 57 patients over age 10 years; 1 was the patient with secondary hemorrhage. Secondary hemorrhage occurred in 6.7% of controls after 2 – 4 days in all cases. The calculated probability of tranexamic acid therapy having an effect on the occurrence of secondary hemorrhage was 95.8%.

Tranexamic acid therapy seems to improve the prognosis of traumatic hyphema. The only side effect noted was increased peristaltic motion but this has not led to discontinuation of treatment. No ocular pathology was found by Zachariae in a family with hereditary angioneurotic edema, treated with tranexamic acid for 4 years with the same dosage as has been used for hyphema. Patients with hyphema now are being treated solely with tranexamic acid. If this is satisfactory, outpatient treatment will be considered.

**Traumatic Hyphema: Treatment of Secondary Hemorrhage with Cyclodiathermy.** Recurrent anterior chamber hemorrhage, a serious complication of traumatic hyphema, is often associated with a poor visual prognosis. Howard D. Gilbert and Ronald E. Smith[4] (Johns Hopkins Hosp.) report 4 cases in which cyclodiathermy was used to stop recurrent secondary hemorrhage after traumatic hyphema. A relatively simple technique of diathermy is used.

TECHNIQUE. – Under general anesthesia and with use of the op-

(4)   Ophthalmic Surg. 7:31 – 35, Fall, 1976.

erating microscope, and occasionally a gonioscopic lens, the hyphema is lavaged or removed. When fresh bleeding is seen coming from part of the anterior chamber angle, a small conjunctival flap is dissected in this area, and with a 1- to 1.5-mm pin, partially penetrating or penetrating diathermy applications are made to the sclera 2 mm posterior to the limbus, immediately over the suspected source of bleeding. Several applications may be necessary. A broader, horseshoe-shaped row of partially penetrating or surface diathermy spots is then placed to outline and delimit the suspected bleeding area. The open end of the horseshoe is at the limbus, and its most posterior aspect is 3 or 4 mm posterior to the limbus (Fig 63). A setting of 35 on the MIRA RF diathermy unit and an application time of 1 or 2 seconds were used in most applications. The anterior chamber must sometimes be lavaged at this point to insure that bleeding has stopped. The conjunctival flap is closed with plain gut suture, and the eye is dressed with antibiotic ointment and a patch.

Hemorrhage and intraocular pressure were controlled by this method, without major complications, in all 4 cases. The results in this small series are encouraging. Complications included sector iris atrophy in 1 case and an irregular pupil in another; neither was considered to be serious. Indications for this technique include recurrent, fresh anterior chamber bleeding with elevated intraocular pressure resistant to medical therapy, multiple rebleeds requiring prolonged hospitalization and black-ball clotted hyphema with elevated intraocular pressure and bleeding during surgical remov-

**Fig 63.** — Placement of diathermy. Major vessels to area of active bleeding are isolated and treated. (Courtesy of Gilbert, H. D., and Smith, R. E.: Ophthalmic Surg. 7:31–35, Fall, 1976.)

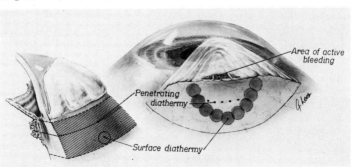

al of the clot. The method is not indicated for prophylaxis in routine traumatic hyphemas, as most of these clear without operative intervention.

**Neutron Therapy** is discussed in an editorial.[5] Neutron therapy, a relatively new form of treatment of malignant tumors, is effective but causes radiation damage to the eye when the eye is unavoidably irradiated. Neutrons are generated in the cyclotron by bombarding a beryllium target with deuterons, generated in turn by the action of an electric field on deuterium gas. Neutrons pass readily through most materials and are best absorbed by hydrogen-containing material such as paraffin wax. They pass easily through blocks of metal. Paraffin wax molds are applied to the patient, but it is not possible to screen the eye completely when it lies in the treatment field.

A cyclotron constructed primarily for clinical purposes has been used at Hammersmith Hospital, London, since 1966 and three cyclotrons have been adapted for clinical use in the United States in the past 2 years.

Neutrons produce ionization in tissues by interacting with atomic nuclei to produce nuclear recoils in the form of protons and alpha particles. Unlike x-rays, neutrons do not require a high oxygen level to be effective. Less cellular recovery occurs between divided neutron doses than with x-rays, and the neutron dose does not have to be increased when it is fractionated. This may have led to overtreatment in early American studies. Penetration of soft tissues is not better than with x-rays, but bone is better penetrated, making neutron therapy advantageous for intracranial tumors. The experience at Hammersmith Hospital showed that the neutron is a particularly effective agent in treatment of tumors. Thus an understanding of its effects and side effects will continue to be necessary. Collaboration by the ophthalmologist will be required whenever tumors of the head are being treated with neutrons.

**Effects of Fast Neutrons on the Eye.** John Roth, Nicholas Brown, Mary Catterall and Anthony Beal[6] (Hammersmith Hosp., London) report the ophthalmic findings in

(5)   Br. J. Ophthalmol. 60:235, April, 1976.
(6)   Ibid., pp. 236–244.

patients with an eye unavoidably irradiated during treatment of advanced head tumors with 7.5-Mev fast neutrons. A total of 93 eyes were examined in patients aged 26 – 82 years. Follow-up from start of treatment ranged from 10 weeks to 31 months. Doses as large as 1,620 rad of 7.5-Mev fast neutrons were given in 12 treatments over 26 – 33 days. The tumor directly obstructed nasolacrimal drainage in 3 patients and caused proptosis in 3. Cranial nerves of ophthalmic importance were involved in 3 patients.

Blurred vision commonly occurred after 14 – 28 days; it tended to remit in most instances after a few months but persisted in patients given 500 rad or more. At levels of 1,500 rad or more, vision deteriorated progressively and was reduced permanently below 6/60 in most cases. Several patients noted eyelid pain or pain or discomfort in the eye, and those given over 1,000 rad had severe, persistent pain. Epiphora occurred in 31 eyes but persisted in only 13.

Clinical signs included cutaneous erythema in 52 cases, eyelid edema in 37, loss of cilia and meibomian gland obstruction. Partial lacrimal punctal obstruction developed in 27 eyes and progressed to become complete in 11. Two patients developed bilateral nasolacrimal duct obstruction. Conjunctival changes included injection in 40 eyes, telangiectasis in 26, chemosis in 17, ulceration in 2, contracture in 6 and keratin plaques in 12. Corneal epithelial keratitis was common. Corneal erosion ensued in 11 eyes and late corneal ulceration in 4 eyes. Corneal sensitivity was reduced in 19 eyes. Iris atrophy was a late sequela in 3 eyes. Radiation cataracts developed in 11 eyes. Three eyes exhibited pigmentary retinopathy. Reduction in intraocular pressure occurred in 9 eyes and persisted in 7 of them. Five eyes lost all useful vision or were damaged beyond hope of recovery. Except for a glaucomatous eye and 1 eye with central retinal artery occlusion, loss of sight occurred only at doses exceeding 1,500 rad.

The clinical effects of fast neutron irradiation of the eye are dose related. The unavoidable damage is similar to that seen with other forms of irradiation. Improved cure rates with neutron therapy are not obtained at the expense of inflicting greater damage to normal structures. The neu-

tron effects of treating extremely extensive tumors are
acceptable.

▶　↓ The following three articles on the practice of medicine are at least
thought provoking. In the first article, the authors "conclude that far too
many physicians perform surgical operations and that work loads of
surgical specialists are modest. The total volume of operations in this
study could have been handled by a substantially smaller cadre of busier
surgical specialists." Lyle, an optometry professor in Ontario, believes
that optometrists have sufficient training to administer diagnostic drugs,
and that this would improve their effectiveness in diagnosis. The Secre-
tary for Continuing Education of the American Academy of Ophthalmology, Spivey, describes the complicated administrative setup and plans designed to keep ophthalmologists well informed on recent advances. – Ed.

**Doctors Who Perform Operations: Study on In-Hos-
pital Surgery in Four Diverse Geographic Areas. –**
*Part 1.* – Rita J. Nickerson, Theodore Colton, Osler L. Peterson, Bernard S. Bloom and Walter W. Hauck, Jr.[7] (Harvard
Med. School) surveyed all in-hospital operations done for the
entire populations of four geographic areas of the United
States, two in the Northeast, one in the Southeast and one
in the Northwest. California Relative Value-weighted operative work served as the basic index of a physician's total
surgical-care productivity. Data were collected for 1970.

General practitioners constituted 27% of physicians who
performed operations, but accounted for less than 9% of total
work. Surgical specialists, about 48% of the physicians in
the study, performed about 90% of total operative work.

*Part 2.* – Nickerson, Colton, Peterson, Bloom and Hauck[8]
found that work loads of surgical specialists varied by certification, specialty, age and practice organization status.
Extreme variation in distributions of physicians of six primary specialty groups, according to their weighted operative work loads, was observed. The median age of the specialists was close to that of all physicians. The mean work
load of Board-certified specialists was about 50% greater
than the mean for those without certification, but this association was less marked for ophthalmologists than for other
specialists.

Even commonplace operations were not frequent events
on the average for the individual specialized surgeon. Few

(7)　N. Engl. J. Med. 295:921 – 926, Oct. 21, 1976.

(8)　Ibid., pp. 982 – 989, Oct. 28, 1976.

individual operations contributed 5% or more of the total weighted work of a specialty. For ophthalmology, lens extraction accounted for two thirds of the total. Over 70% of ophthalmologists performed intracapsular lens extractions and resections of muscle or tendon. Advancement or recession of eye muscles was performed by about 70% of Board-certified and by 50% of noncertified practitioners. Photocoagulation reattachment of the retina was done by 22% of certified surgeons. Nearly half of the noncertified surgeons performed iridectomy.

Far too many physicians of all kinds perform operations. Even among surgical specialists, many have modest work loads, primarily because of their excessive numbers. A substantial reduction in the number of physicians performing operations is possible. The different practice patterns of ophthalmologists on the one hand and general and thoracic surgeons on the other make it evident that manpower planning must be done on a specialty-by-specialty basis. The surgical specialties, however, are interrelated, and planning must involve coordination among all specialties.

**Utilization of Pharmaceuticals in Optometry** is discussed by W. M. Lyle[9] (Univ. of Waterloo School of Optometry, Ont.), an optometrist. The role of optometry within the health disciplines is becoming more clearly defined. The trend toward removal of legislative prohibitions against the use of diagnostic pharmaceutical agents by optometrists is accelerating. At least eight states in the United States and one Canadian province have changed their laws in this direction in the past 5 years and most observers believe that an increased use of diagnostic drugs will and should become an integral part of optometric practice within this decade. British ophthalmic opticians (optometrists) have used such drugs as atropine, pilocarpine and eserine for some decades with no complaints of adverse consequences. A broader use of diagnostic drugs by optometrists would facilitate data collection and extend the data base, increase practitioner efficiency and improve the quality of service. Such optometric procedures as contact lens services are enhanced by use of the full spectrum of diagnostic drugs. Ophthalmoscopy,

(9) Can. J. Public Health 67:217–220, May–June, 1976.

gonioscopy, fundus photography and pupil function tests may be done more efficiently with the use of diagnostic drugs.

Optometrists have adequate basic science education and possess sufficient theoretical and practical experience in the use of diagnostic drugs. At the author's optometry school, more time is devoted to pharmacology than is given to dental students and nearly as much as is given to medical students. Continuing education programs are widely available to provide refresher courses for the active practitioner.

# Subject Index

# Index to Authors